Rapid Fire EM

Jason D. Diyanni, D.O.
Emergency Medicine Physician
Columbus, Ohio

Disclaimer
Please be aware that care has been taken to confirm the accuracy of the information presented and to describe generally accepted practices in emergency medicine. However, the authors, editors, and publisher are not responsible for errors or omissions or for any consequences from application of the information in this book. It makes no warranty, expressed or implied, with respect to the currency, completeness, or accuracy of the contents. Application of this information is a particular clinical situation remains the professional's responsibility of the practitioner: the clinical treatments described and recommended may not be considered absolute and universal recommendations.

The authors, editors, and publisher have exerted every effort to ensure the treatments are in accordance with the current recommendations and practice in emergency medicine at the time of publication. However, in view of ongoing medical specialty and practice changes per the American academy of emergency medicine, and government regulations, the professional's treatment plan should be in concordance with current data, literature, and regulations. Some drugs and medical devices presented in this publication have Food and Drug administration clearance for limited use in restricted research settings. It is the responsibility of the health care provider to ascertain the FDA status of each drug or device planned for use in his or her clinical practice.

To purchase additional copies of this book, contact us at rapidfireem@gmail.com or visit our website at http://www.rapidfireem.com
Follow us on Facebook and Instagram at #rapidfireem

Published in the United States of America

Editors and Contributors

Elizabeth Diyanni, PA-C.
Columbus, Ohio

Rajiv Bahl, M.D., MBA, MS
Orlando, Florida

Matthew Wiepking, M.D.
Los Angeles, California

Shan Gao, M.D.
Burlington, Iowa

Kelley Stanko, M.D.
Biloxi, Mississippi

Asaad Alsufyani, M.D.
Jeddah, Saudi Arabia

Rita Hudec, M.D.
Fort Lauderdale, Florida

Nima Malakooti, M.D.
Columbus, Ohio

Jean-Paul Amegee, M.D.
Toledo, Ohio

Matthew Robinson, D.O.
Columbus, Ohio

Steve Grider, D.O.
Toledo, Ohio

Daniel Kemple, M.D.
Toledo, Ohio

Scott Levitt, M.D.
Albany, Oregon

Kevin Doherty, D.O.
Columbus, Ohio

Michael S.Turner, M.D.
Columbus, Ohio

David Duff, M.D.
Columbus, Ohio

Kimberly Cunagin, D.O.
Columbus, Ohio

Allen Williams, M.D.
Toledo, Ohio

Jacob Smith, D.O.
Roanoke, Virginia

Catherine Osburn
Design editor

Introduction

Rapid Fire EM is a quick-review resource for emergency medicine residents preparing for the American Board of Emergency Medicine (ABEM) certification exam. It is also a relevant tool for practicing emergency medicine attendings, physician assistants (PA), and nurse practitioners (NP), as well as PA, NP, and medical students rotating on their emergency medicine clerkships.

Rapid Fire EM is the most innovative and simplified emergency medicine review resource on the market. It's content has been vetted by emergency medicine attendings to give you a concise and accurate board review of the most commonly asked questions on the ABEM certification board exam. Using a unique question-answer format, **Rapid Fire EM** is proven to help you recall key emergency medicine terms and information found on the ABEM exam, as well as help you apply this knowledge to your current medical practice. In short, **Rapid Fire EM** compiles the most essential emergency medicine facts in their simplest form to save you hundreds of hours and give you the step up you need to pass the ABEM exam, aid in the completion of your EM residency, and make you a shining star on your emergency medicine clerkship.

Let's face it: you don't have all the time in the world to filter through hundreds of pages of text and tedious charts on a yearly basis. You also don't have time to decipher which facts to commit to memory.

THAT'S WHY *RAPID FIRE EM* HAS DONE THE WORK FOR YOU!

Rapid Fire EM is conveniently organized into chapters by organ system and the percentage of questions asked about each system on the ABEM exam. Below is the published ABEM content for the written exam and each subject's percentage of the exam. More information on the certification exam can be found at www.ABEM.com.

Traumatic Disorders: *10%*
Cardiovascular Disorders: *10%*
Signs, Symptoms, and Presentations: *9%*
Thoracic-Respiratory Disorders: *8%*
Abdominal and Gastrointestinal Disorders: *8%*
Resuscitation, Procedures, and Skills: *8%*
Toxicologic Disorders: *5%*
Head, Ear, Eye, Nose, and Throat Disorders: *5%*
Systemic Infectious Disorders: *5%*
Nervous System Disorders: *5%*
Obstetrics and Gynecology: *4%*
Psychobehavioral Disorders: *4%*
Musculoskeletal Disorders (Non-traumatic): *3%*
Renal and Urogenital Disorders: *3%*
Environmental Disorders: *3%*
Endocrine, Metabolic, and Nutritional Disorders: *2%*
Hematologic and Oncologic Disorders: *2%*
Immune System Disorders: *2%*
Cutaneous Disorders: *1%*

Other Content (Administration, EMS, Abuse, Assault, Imaging, Chronic pain, Analgesia): *3%*

Contents

Traumatic Disorders

1) What are the three time windows that traumatic deaths occur after an injury?
   a) Immediate
   b) Within 60 minutes "Golden hour"
   c) Delayed (days to weeks)
2) List the criteria associated with high-risk trauma patients.
   a) < 5 years old, > 55 years old, DM, Hepatic disease, Cardiac disease, Respiratory disease, Obesity, Pregnancy, Immunosuppressed, or Anticoagulant use
3) List the ABCDE steps involved in the primary exam during trauma resuscitation.
   a) Airway
   b) Breathing - Breath sounds and Inspect the chest
   c) Circulation – Pulses, Blood pressure, and Peripheral perfusion
   d) Disability – Brief neurological exam (GCS)
   e) Exposure and environmental control – Undress patient and Control body temperature
4) Describe the first steps in the ATLS protocol during the primary survey exam.
   a) Look, Feel the skin, Check pulses, and Ask the patient's name to assess airway in < 10 seconds
5) List adjuncts to the 1° survey during ATLS.
   a) Chest and Pelvis X-rays, FAST, EKG, Vitals, Blood work, +/-Foley catheter, NG tube placement,
6) What are the most common injuries missed on the 1° survey?
   a) Extremity injuries
7) What is the 2nd most common injury missed during the primary survey?
   a) Spinal injury
8) What is involved in the secondary survey exam during trauma resuscitation?
   a) Head to Toe exam (Injury identification)
9) What part of the body should always be maintained while log rolling a patient during a trauma evaluation?
   a) C-spine

10) At what point during trauma resuscitation should a trauma transfer be initiated if the patient is not at a trauma center?
   a) During or after the 1° survey

11) What two imaging studies are routinely performed on most trauma patients during the 2° exam?
   a) Chest and Pelvis X-ray

12) List the routine labs performed in all trauma patients.
   a) CBC, BMP, Hepatic panel, Lipase, Type and Screen, PT/PTT/INR, Urinalysis, Glucose, Drug panel, ETOH, +/- Cardiac enzymes (Chest trauma), and Pregnancy test (Childbearing age)

13) Why are the trauma rooms set at higher temperatures and hot blankets placed on trauma patients?
   a) To prevent hypothermia

14) What kind of fluid is given to trauma patients to prevent hypothermia?
   a) Warm fluid at 40° C (NS or LR)

15) What procedures can be done to quickly correct breathing issues from trauma?
   a) Needle thoracotomy, Finger thoracotomy, Chest tube, Occlusive dressings, and ETT positioning

16) List the indications for immediate airway management during trauma resuscitation.
   a) GCS < 8, No gag reflex, Unable to speak, Facial trauma, Penetrating neck trauma, Expanding hematoma of the neck, No spontaneous respirations, or Hypoxia

17) What procedure is performed for airway protection during trauma as a last resort?
   a) Cricothyrotomy

18) List the systolic blood pressure level needed to palpate the pulse in each of the following: Carotid, Femoral, and Radial arteries.
   a) Carotid: > 60 mmHg
   b) Femoral: > 70 mmHg
   c) Radial: > 80 mmHg

19) How many liters of blood make up our circulatory system?
   a) 5 L

20) Injuries and fractures to what areas of the body are capable of leading to hypovolemia after trauma?
    a) Pelvic and Femur fractures, Intraabdominal injuries, and Internal Chest injuries
21) How many classes of hemorrhagic shock are there?
    a) 4
22) What class of hemorrhagic shock has a < 15% blood loss (< 750mL), and no vital sign changes?
    a) Class 1
23) What class of hemorrhagic shock has a 15-30% blood loss (750 - 1500mL), HR > 100, anxiety, and ↓Pulse pressure?
    a) Class 2
24) What class of hemorrhagic shock has 30-40% blood loss (1500 - 2000mL), HR > 120, ↓BP, RR 30-40, Capillary refill 3-4 sec, ↓Pulse pressure, and Confusion?
    a) Class 3
25) What class of hemorrhagic shock has a > 40% blood loss (> 2000mL), HR > 140, ↓BP, Capillary refill > 5 sec, RR > 40, Lethargy, and No urine output?
    a) Class 4
26) What is the calculation for the shock index?
    a) HR / Systolic BP
27) What is the shock index normal range?
    a) 0.5 – 0.7
28) What does a shock index > 0.7 indicate?
    a) An increased risk of developing hypotension and need for massive transfusion
29) What type of blood is used as a universal donor in trauma resuscitation?
    a) O negative (males can receive O positive as well)
30) How many mL of crystalloids are required to replace 1 mL of blood during fluid resuscitation in the setting of acute blood loss?
    a) 3-4 mL crystalloids = 1 mL blood
31) What is the best volume expander for fluid resuscitation in the setting of acute blood loss?
    a) Blood products

32) What is the most common side effect of administering the massive transfusion protocol?
   a) Hypothermia

33) What is the ratio of PRBC, FFP, and platelet blood products given during "massive blood transfusion protocol"?
   a) 1:1:1

34) Which vasopressor medications can be given to decrease the likelihood of medication-induced tachycardia in the setting of shock with tachycardia?
   a) Vasopressin or Phenylephrine

35) What antifibrinolytic medication can be given to prevent further bleeding with hemorrhagic hypovolemic shock?
   a) Tranexamic acid (1 g)

36) What are the three components that make up the "trauma death triad" and should be prevented during resuscitation?
   a) Hypothermia
   b) Coagulopathy
   c) Acidosis

37) What medications/products can be given to reverse anticoagulation from Warfarin, in patients with hemorrhagic shock?
   a) Prothrombin complex concentrate (PCC), Fresh frozen plasma (FFP), or Vitamin K

38) What products can be given to reverse anticoagulation from oral anticoagulants (i.e. Rivaroxaban, Apixaban, Fondaparinux) in patients with hemorrhagic shock?
   a) Prothrombin complex concentrate (PCC), Fresh frozen plasma (FFP), or Cryoprecipitate

39) What lab test should be performed on all female trauma patients of childbearing age?
   a) Pregnancy test

40) What is recommended for the evaluation of pregnant patients > 20 weeks, involved in trauma, having < 3 contractions per hour (asymptomatic)?
   a) Maternal-fetal monitoring x 4-6 hours

41) How many hours are recommended for maternal-fetal monitoring after trauma in a pregnant patient with > 3 contractions per hour (symptomatic)?
    a) 24 hours
42) List the criteria for discharge of a pregnant patient > 20 weeks post-trauma.
    a) No Contractions, No Vaginal bleeding, No Uterine tenderness, Reassuring fetal heart tracing, and Intact membranes
43) What lab test measures the amount of fetal Hb transferred from a fetus to the mother's bloodstream and should be tested in a pregnant trauma patient with vaginal bleeding and abdominal pain?
    a) Kleihauer-Betke test
44) What position should all pregnant females > 20 weeks be placed in to prevent hypotension during trauma resuscitation?
    a) Left lateral decubitus
45) What type of trauma is the leading cause of maternal death?
    a) Blunt
46) What is the most common cause of fetal death in trauma victims?
    a) Maternal death
47) What should be considered when placing a chest tube in a pregnant patient due to the displacement of the intestines, organs, and diaphragm?
    a) Placing higher (3rd or 4th intercostal spaces)
48) What signs on a fetal ultrasound suggest fetal demise?
    a) No Movement, No Fetal Heartbeat, or Extended extremities
49) What obstetric complications can occur from trauma?
    a) Uterine rupture, Preterm labor, Fetal demise, Amniotic fluid emboli, or Placental abruption
50) Can a placental abruption be 100% ruled out on ultrasound after maternal trauma?
    a) No
51) Can a placental abruption be present after maternal trauma without signs of vaginal bleeding on a physical exam?
    a) Yes (concealed abruption)
52) Is it recommended to update the Tdap vaccine during maternal trauma?

a) Yes

53) Is Rhogam recommended to be given during maternal trauma if Rh negative?
   a) Yes

54) During the evaluation of maternal trauma, what is the first sign of fetal distress?
   a) Tachycardia followed by decelerations

55) What type of trauma is the most common in pediatrics?
   a) Blunt

56) What anatomic area is the most commonly injured in pediatric patients and is the leading cause of death in pediatric trauma?
   a) Head

57) Due to the larger head to body ratio in pediatrics what should be done during resuscitation to align the patient's airway?
   a) Place a support under the shoulders

58) What type of skull fracture is the most common in pediatric head trauma?
   a) Linear

59) What is the most common skull bone fractured in pediatric head trauma?
   a) Parietal bone

60) What type of brain bleed is most commonly associated with non-accidental trauma?
   a) Subdural hematoma

61) What evidence-based criteria is used to determine whether imaging is required in pediatric head injuries?
   a) PECARN (Pediatric Emergency Care Applied Research Network)

62) List the PECARN criteria recommending a head CT for a closed head injury in children > 2 years old.
   a) AMS
   b) GCS < 15
   c) Signs of basilar skull fracture

63) List the PECARN criteria recommending observation or head CT for a closed head injury in children > 2 years old.
   a) LOC

b) Vomiting
c) Severe headache
d) Severe mechanism: Fall > 5 feet, MVA, Bike/Ped vs vehicle, or Struck by a high impact object

64) List the PECARN criteria recommending a head CT for a closed head injury in children < 2 years old.
a) AMS
b) GCS < 15
c) Palpable skull fracture

65) List the PECARN criteria recommending observation or head CT for a closed head injury in children < 2 years old.
a) LOC > 5 seconds
b) Not acting normal
c) Parietal, Occipital, or Temporal hematoma
d) Severe mechanism: Fall > 3 feet, MVA, Bike/Ped vs vehicle, or Struck by a high impact object

66) Why are skull bone fractures following trauma more common in the pediatric population?
a) The skull bones are thinner

67) What is the most common level of the cervical spine injured in pediatric spine trauma?
a) C1-C2

68) What type of lung injury is more common in pediatric chest traumas due to the increased flexibility of the chest wall?
a) Lung contusions

69) Does hypotension typically occur in head injuries?
a) No (look for other causes)

70) List the findings that make up the Cushing reflex associated with increased intracranial pressure.
a) Hypertension, Bradycardia, and Irregular breathing

71) What injury is the leading cause of death after trauma?
a) Head

72) List the criteria for the Canadian head CT rule.
a) GCS < 15 at 2 hours
b) Suspected open or depressed skull fracture
c) Retrograde amnesia
d) > 2 episodes of vomiting

e) Basal skull fracture

f) Age > 65 years old

g) Dangerous mechanism of injury

73) List the criteria for the New Orleans head CT rule.

a) Headache

b) Vomiting

c) Age > 60 years old

d) Persistent anterograde amnesia

e) Intoxicated

f) Seizure

74) What GCS levels help define mild, moderate and severe traumatic brain injuries and the risk of an intracranial injury?

a) Mild: GCS 14-15

b) Moderate: GCS 9-13

c) Severe: GCS < 9

75) What is the mortality rate for traumatic brain injuries based on a GCS < 9?

a) Estimate of 40%

76) Can hemorrhagic shock occur with scalp lacerations?

a) Yes

77) How do you calculate cerebral perfusion pressure (CPP)?

a) CPP = MAP - ICP

78) What is a normal level of CPP?

a) Between 60 and 80 mmHg

79) Is it recommended to obtain cervical imaging along with brain imaging in the setting of geriatric, unconscious, or nonverbal pediatric patients, or in major traumas?

a) Yes

80) What type of brain bleed occurs after trauma on the opposite side from the site of direct impact?

a) Contrecoup bleed

81) What type of brain bleed is the most common form seen with traumatic brain injuries?

a) Traumatic subarachnoid hemorrhage

82) What type of brain hematoma presents after head trauma with immediate LOC followed by a lucid interval and a dilated pupil on the same side?

a)   Epidural hematoma

83) What type of skull fracture is associated with injury of the middle meningeal artery leading to an epidural hematoma?
a)   Temporal skull fracture

84) What is the CT brain finding with an epidural hematoma?
a)   Biconcave (lens-shaped)-does not cross suture lines

85) What type of brain bleed presents with altered mental status, crescent-shaped bleed on brain CT that crosses suture lines, and is more common in elderly and alcoholics?
a)   Subdural hematoma

86) What type of brain herniation from hematomas or masses causes bilateral temporal lobe herniation, fixed pupils, decerebrate posturing, brainstem compression, and coma?
a)   Central herniation

87) What type of brain herniation from hematomas or masses causes herniation through the foramen magnum leading to acute hydrocephalus, vomiting, and headache followed by respiratory depression and flaccid paralysis?
a)   Tonsillar herniation

88) What type of brain herniation and leads to unilateral fixed dilated pupil, vision field loss, and contralateral motor paralysis?
a)   Uncal (transtentorial) herniation

89) What is the most common type of brain herniation?
a)   Uncal herniation

90) Are antiepileptic medications recommended for seizures associated with traumatic brain bleeds?
a)   Yes

91) Is prophylactic antiepileptic medication recommended in those with high-risk head injuries post-trauma?
a)   Yes

92) What type of ECG findings can be seen with brain bleeds and increased ICP?
a)   Deep T waves

93) What are the physical exam findings of brain death in a patient with a GCS < 3?
a)   Nonreactive pupils, Absent Brainstem reflexes, and No spontaneous respirations

94) What is the treatment for an open skull fracture?
   a) Neurosurgery consult and Antibiotics
95) What is the management of a depressed skull fracture?
   a) Neurosurgery consult for possible surgery
96) What is the management for a linear skull fracture?
   a) Conservative therapy
97) What physical exam findings can be seen with basilar skull fractures?
   a) Mastoid ecchymosis (Battle's sign)
   b) Periorbital ecchymosis (Raccoon eyes)
   c) Otorrhea or Rhinorrhea of CSF
   d) CN deficit (V, VI, or VII)
   e) Hemotympanum
98) What is the most common location of a basilar skull fracture?
   a) Petrous part of the Temporal bone
99) What is the treatment for a basilar skull fracture?
   a) Neurosurgery consult, and +/- Antibiotics
100) Describe the "double ring" or "halo" sign seen on absorbent paper indicating the presence of CSF drainage following a head inury.
   a) Central clearing of blood with an outer clear ring of CSF
101) What type of brain injury can occur after trauma or asphyxiation that shows up on CT or MRI as indistinct grey-white margins and is typically seen in comatose patients?
   a) Diffuse axonal injury
102) What type of brain injury presents after head trauma, with or without LOC, causes dizziness, intermittent blurry vision, headache, GCS 14 or 15, vomiting, and nausea?
   a) Concussion
103) What potential high-risk injury is important to prevent after a concussion and can lead to irreversible brain damage, brain edema, and death?
   a) Second impact syndrome
104) What is the management for concussions?
   a) No exercising until cleared and Brain rest

105) What condition can follow a closed head injury, with symptoms of nausea, blurry vision, insomnia, irritability, trouble concentrating, dizziness, and headaches?
   a) Post-concussion syndrome
106) What is the treatment of post-concussion syndrome?
   a) Brain rest until symptoms resolve (no exercising, reading, watching TV, or using phones or tablets)
107) Is a CT brain required for the diagnosis of a concussion?
   a) No
108) When is a CT brain recommended in the workup of a concussion?
   a) LOC or Amnesia + Headache, Vomiting, Seizure, Neurological deficits, Age > 65, GCS < 15, or Intoxication
109) What brain condition can develop due to multiple repeat concussions?
   a) Chronic Traumatic Encephalopathy (CTE)
110) What type of seizure can occur within minutes after a head trauma and is not associated with a severe head injury?
   a) Impact seizure
111) What maneuver is always necessary during the intubation of a trauma patient?
   a) C-spine stabilization
112) List the NEXUS criteria for cervical spine imaging.
   a) AMS
   b) Intoxication
   c) Distracting injury
   d) Midline tenderness
   e) Neuro deficits
113) List the Canadian Cervical spinal rule for a CT.
   a) > 65 years old
   b) High-risk mechanism: High-speed MVA, Fall > 5 stairs, Bike accident, or Fall > 3 feet
   c) Paresthesia present
   d) Unable to rotate neck 45° right and left
   e) Non-ambulatory after injury
   f) Midline tenderness

114) What are the four anatomic spine lines that should be evaluated on a lateral cervical X-ray after trauma?
   a) Anterior longitudinal ligament line
   b) Posterior longitudinal ligament line
   c) Spinolaminar line
   d) Spinous process line
115) What three cervical X-ray views are performed in neck trauma and are 99% - 100% sensitive for fractures?
   a) Lateral, AP, and Odontoid views
116) Should all head trauma patients be placed in a C-collar during trauma resuscitation?
   a) Yes (Suspected to have a C spine injury until proven otherwise)
117) What imaging studies following a negative cervical CT should be done before clearing the C-collar in trauma patients with ongoing neck pain to rule out ligament injury?
   a) Flexion/Extension cervical X-rays or Cervical MRI
118) What location of the adult cervical spine is the most common site of injury?
   a) C5/C6
119) List stable cervical fractures.
   a) Anterior subluxation
   b) Clay shoveler's
   c) Posterior arch C1 fracture
   d) Unilateral facet dislocation
   e) Wedge fracture
   f) Laminar fracture
   g) Posterior or anterior arch of atlas fracture
120) List unstable cervical fractures.
   a) Jefferson fracture
   b) Bilateral facet dislocation
   c) Type 2 and 3 Odontoid fractures
   d) Hangman's fracture
   e) Teardrop fracture
   f) Occipitoatlantal dissociation
121) What type of spine fracture is stable and from anterior compression of the vertebral body after a forced flexion injury?

a) Wedge fracture

122) What cervical fracture is defined by an avulsion fracture of the spinous process after sudden spinal flexion?

a) Clay shoveler's fracture

123) What type of unstable spinal injury results from severe flexion and disrupted anterior and posterior lines on X-ray and is associated with spinal cord injury?

a) Bilateral facet dislocation

124) What unstable cervical fracture is defined by bilateral fractures of the pars interarticularis of C2 causing displacement of C2 on C3?

a) Hangman's fracture

125) What unstable cervical fracture is defined by a burst fracture of the atlas (C1) and shows a widened predental and periodontoid spaces?

a) Jefferson fracture

126) What type of spinal fracture is a fracture of the anteroinferior aspect of the vertebral body due to flexion or extension injuries, and causes a complete ligamentous disruption and instability?

a) Teardrop fracture

127) What type of odontoid fracture is defined by an avulsion of the tip?

a) Type 1

128) What type of odontoid fracture is defined by a fracture through the base of the neck of the dens below the transverse ligament?

a) Type 2

129) What type of odontoid fracture is defined by a fracture through the body of C2?

a) Type 3

130) What types of odontoid fractures are considered unstable?

a) Type 2 and Type 3

131) What length of the predental space on cervical X-ray is considered pathologic for a fracture in adults after trauma?

a) 3 mm

132) What length of the predental space on cervical X-ray is considered pathologic for a fracture in children after trauma?

a) 5 mm

133) What length is considered normal for the prevertebral cervical spaces at C2 and C6 in adults and children?
   a) C2: < 6 mm
   b) C6: < 22 mm (< 14 mm pediatrics)
134) What part of the spinal cord conducts vibration and proprioception?
   a) Posterior columns
135) Which spinal tract caries the upper motor neurons?
   a) Lateral corticospinal tract
136) Which spinal tract caries the lower motor neurons?
   a) Anterior horn cells
137) Which spinal tract conducts pain and temperature?
   a) Anterior spinothalamic tract
138) What spinal cord syndrome due to a flexion injury causes a complete loss of pain and temperature sensation, and motor function below the injury, with preserved vibration and proprioception?
   a) Anterior cord syndrome
139) What other medical condition can lead to anterior cord syndrome?
   a) Anterior spinal artery thrombosis
140) What unilateral spinal cord injury from a penetrating injury causes ipsilateral weakness and loss of position/vibration sense, with contralateral loss of pain and temperature sensation?
   a) Brown-Sequard Syndrome
141) Which spinal cord syndrome from a hyperextension injury causes loss of motor and sensory deficits more in the upper extremities > lower extremities?
   a) Central Cord Syndrome
142) What is the prognosis for recovery with a central cord syndrome?
   a) > 50 %
143) What spinal cord syndrome caused by tumors, trauma or transverse myelitis, has a complete loss of all sensory and motor pathways below a certain level?
   a) Transverse Cord Syndrome

144) Which spinal cord syndrome from a traumatic extension injury, B12 deficit, or syphilis has a loss of position and vibration sensation only?
   a) Posterior Cord Syndrome
145) What spinal cord injury mimics a complete cord lesion and is transient less than 24 hours with an absent bulbocavernosus reflex?
   a) Spinal shock
146) Which type of shock causes unopposed parasympathetic outflow, hypotension, and bradycardia and is due to a cervical or high thoracic cord injury?
   a) Neurogenic shock
147) What specific anogenital reflexes if intact denote an incomplete spinal cord lesion?
   a) Cremaster reflex, Contraction of the anal musculature, and Bulbocavernosus reflex
148) What spinal cord injury seen in pediatric cervical injuries has no radiographic abnormalities on CT and X-rays but causes neurological deficits?
   a) Spinal Cord Injury Without Radiographic Abnormalities (SCIWORA)
149) What is the recommended imaging study for diagnosing SCIWORA?
   a) MRI
150) Which type of unstable spinal fracture is associated with a flexion, distraction seat belt injury in an MVA and causes a horizontal fracture through L1 or L2?
   a) Chance fracture
151) Which type of spinal fracture is from axial loading with flexion and is stable if it involves less than 50% of vertebral height?
   a) Compression fracture
152) Which type of spinal fracture is caused by axial loading and failure of the anterior and middle spinal column?
   a) Burst fracture
153) What anatomic part of the oral airway is the most common cause of traumatic airway obstruction?
   a) Tongue

154) In what traumatic conditions is nasotracheal intubation contraindicated?

    a) Maxillofacial trauma, Basilar skull fracture, and Apnea

155) List the concerning findings seen in penetrating neck trauma to suggest airway protection with intubation.

    a) Expanding hematoma, Stridor, Muffled voice, Dyspnea, Drooling, Hemoptysis, or Subcutaneous emphysema

156) What muscle divides the anterior and posterior triangles of the neck?

    a) Sternocleidomastoid muscle

157) When pertaining to penetrating neck injuries how many zones is the neck divided into?

    a) 3

158) What are the anatomical borders for zone 1 specified for penetrating neck trauma?

    a) Clavicle-Cricothyroid

159) List the structures located in zone 1.

    a) Carotid arteries, Thoracic vessels, Superior mediastinum, Lungs, Esophagus, Trachea, Thoracic duct, and Spinal cord

160) What is the treatment and workup for penetrating trauma to zone 1 of the neck?

    a) CT Angiography, Esophagography, Esophagoscopy, and Bronchoscopy

161) What are the anatomical borders for zone 2 specified for penetrating neck trauma?

    a) Cricothyroid-Mandible angle

162) List the structures located in zone 2.

    a) Mid-carotid, Vertebral arteries, Jugular veins, Esophagus, Larynx, Trachea, and Spinal cord

163) What is the treatment and workup for penetrating trauma to zone 2 of the neck?

    a) Surgical exploration +/- CT Angiogram, Esophagography, Esophagoscopy, and Bronchoscopy

164) What are the anatomical borders for zone 3 specified for penetrating neck trauma?

    a) Mandible angle-Base of skull

165) List the structures located in zone 3.
   a) Proximal carotid, Vertebral arteries, Pharynx, and Spinal cord
166) What is the workup for penetrating trauma to zone 3 of the neck?
   a) CT Angiography
167) Penetrating trauma of what neck structure warrants further exploration and workup?
   a) Platysma
168) What zone is the most common injury in penetrating neck injuries?
   a) Zone 2
169) What is the most common structure injured in penetrating neck trauma leading to death?
   a) Vascular injuries (internal jugular most common)
170) What is the most common cause of death in penetrating neck injuries?
   a) Exsanguination
171) Should you ever probe a neck wound in the ED after penetrating trauma?
   a) No
172) Should you remove a penetrating foreign body?
   a) No
173) How do you stop an active hemorrhage after a penetrating neck injury?
   a) Direct pressure
174) List the "hard signs" associated with a significant vascular injury from a penetrating neck injury.
   a) Hypotension, Arterial bleed/Pulsating, Thrill, Focal deficits, Bubbling wound, Expanding hematoma, Hemoptysis, or Hematemesis
175) List the "soft signs" associated with a significant injury from a penetrating neck injury.
   a) Stridor, Hoarseness, Subcutaneous air, Vocal cord paralysis, or Facial nerve injury
176) What type of arterial injuries can occur with blunt neck trauma?
   a) Pseudoaneuysm or Dissection

177) What type of injury following blunt neck trauma should be evaluated in a patient with neck pain, stroke-like symptoms, and Horner's syndrome?
   a) Carotid artery dissection
178) What is the most common cause of death from strangulation?
   a) Cerebral anoxia (from vessel occlusion)
179) What complications can follow strangulation and can lead to delayed mortality?
   a) Laryngeal or Pulmonary edema
180) What procedure should be avoided in a suspected laryngeal injury following trauma?
   a) Cricothyrotomy
181) What mechanisms of blunt trauma to the neck have a high risk of injury to the spinal cord?
   a) Hyperextension or Hyperflexion injuries
182) What cardiothoracic injury should be evaluated with a sucking chest wound, hypotension, and respiratory distress?
   a) Tension pneumothorax
183) What location can be used for needle decompression of a tension pneumothorax?
   a) 2nd intercostals space midclavicular line or 5th intercostal space midaxillary line (per 10th edition of ATLS)
184) What is the definitive ED treatment for a tension pneumothorax after needle decompression?
   a) Chest tube (20-40 French)
185) How do you treat a sucking chest wound?
   a) Petroleum gauze with three sides taped
186) What type of lung injury after chest trauma should be suspected with decreased breath sounds, hypoxia, SOB, and an increased consolidation on chest X-ray?
   a) Hemothorax
187) What is the ED treatment for a hemothorax?
   a) Chest tube (20-40 French)
188) What amount of blood return from a chest tube on placement meets the criteria for massive hemothorax and the need for thoracotomy?

a) > 1,500 mL

189) What amount of continuous blood return from a chest tube during treatment meets the criteria for massive hemothorax and the need for thoracotomy?

a) > 200 mL/hr for more than 4-6 hours

190) Can blood from a hemothorax be used for autotransfusion?

a) Yes

191) What trauma injury is an absolute indication for an ED thoracotomy?

a) Traumatic arrest from penetrating chest trauma with signs of life prehospital or on arrival to the ED

192) What is the criteria used to consider performing an ED thoracotomy in blunt chest trauma?

a) Traumatic arrest from blunt chest trauma with loss of vital signs in ED only

193) Where is the incision made for a thoracotomy?

a) 5th intercostal space left side

194) After performing a thoracotomy and opening the chest wall, what is the next step?

a) Open the pericardium

195) What is the definition of a flail chest injury?

a) Multiple rib fractures move paradoxically to the motion of the breathing

196) Fractures to what two ribs should raise suspicion of major coinciding injuries due to large forces required to fracture them?

a) 1st and 2nd ribs

197) What shoulder bone fracture requires large forces to fracture it and may also be associated with occult chest injury?

a) Scapular fracture

198) Fractures to what ribs should raise suspicion of possible coinciding hepatic or spleen injuries?

a) 9th-12th ribs

199) What percentages of rib fractures do not show up on plain chest X-ray films?

a) Up to 50%

200) What is the management for most rib fractures?

a) Incentive spirometry, Pain control, or Nerve block

201) What type of infection can develop over the next few weeks following a rib fracture?
   a) Pneumonia
202) What type of lung injury occurs as a result of chest wall trauma and damage to the lung capillaries leading to lung edema, chest pain, SOB, hemoptysis, and hypoxia?
   a) Pulmonary contusion
203) What ribs are commonly associated with a pulmonary contusion when fractured?
   a) Ribs 4-6
204) What are the lung findings on chest X-ray with a pulmonary lung contusion that present within 6 hours after chest trauma?
   a) Patchy consolidations
205) What bone fracture can be seen in MVA's from a steering wheel injury and is associated with myocardial contusions?
   a) Sternum fracture
206) Can a myocardial contusion from trauma cause ECG changes and elevated cardiac enzymes?
   a) Yes
207) What imaging can be done to diagnose a myocardial contusion?
   a) Cardiac MRI or Echocardiogram
208) What is the treatment of a myocardial contusion?
   a) Supportive
209) What is the term used to explain a sudden cardiac arrest resulting from a blunt chest wall injury directly to the heart?
   a) Commotio Cordis
210) What cardiac emergency can develop after penetrating chest trauma causing hypotension, muffled heart sounds, distended jugular veins, and is diagnosed with the cardiac US?
   a) Cardiac tamponade
211) What cardiac complications from a penetrating chest wound should be suspected in a patient present in PEA?
   a) Cardiac tamponade
212) What type of thoracic injury can occur due to rapid deceleration from an MVA trauma and presents with chest pain, dyspnea, Hamman's crunch, and subcutaneous emphysema?
   a) Tracheobronchial tear

213) What location do most tracheobronchial tears occur in the thoracic cavity?
   a) Within 2 cm of the carina
214) What thoracic organ injury can concomitantly occur with tracheobronchial injuries?
   a) Esophageal injuries
215) What is the treatment of a tracheobronchial injury?
   a) Selective intubation of uninvolved lung and Surgery
216) What type of vascular injury can occur after trauma and presents with chest pain, dyspnea, and a harsh systolic murmur with a widened mediastinum on the chest X-ray?
   a) Traumatic ruptured aorta
217) What is the most common location of the tear in a traumatic ruptured aorta?
   a) Ligamentum arteriosum
218) List the findings of an aortic tear that may be present on a chest X-ray.
   a) Indistinct aortic knob, Apical cap, Tracheal deviation, and Depressed left mainstem bronchus
219) In the ED how do we prevent further injury from shearing forces in a thoracic aortic tear?
   a) Control: Blood pressure and Heart rate
220) What imaging studies can definitively diagnose a thoracic aortic tear?
   a) Angiography, Chest CT with IV contrast, or TEE
221) What diagnostic workup is suggested when you see a patient with a seat belt sign on the chest or abdomen after an MVA and is associated with organ and bowel injuries?
   a) CT with IV contrast imaging
222) What type of abdominal organ injury commonly occurs with a hyperflexion injury from a seat belt in an MVA or injury from bike handlebars?
   a) Pancreatic injury
223) What imaging is recommended as first-line in the ED for detecting thoracic, cardiac, and abdominal injuries and free fluid in trauma patients?

    a)   Focused Assessment with Sonography for Trauma (FAST)

224)   What type of injuries is the FAST exam less sensitive in diagnosing in trauma victims?

    a)   Hollow viscus injury, Solid organ injury, and Retroperitoneal injury

225)   Does an unstable patient with a positive FAST exam and abdominal free fluid, go to CT or the operating room first?

    a)   Operating room (OR)

226)   Does a stable patient with a positive FAST and abdominal free fluid, go to CT or the OR first?

    a)   CT scan first then surgery planning

227)   List the other indications that suggest a laparotomy after abdominal trauma.

    a)   GSW, Free air under the diaphragm on chest X-ray, Hypotension, Positive FAST, Peritonitis, Gross blood per NG tube, Bright red blood per rectum, Impalement, or GI evisceration

228)   What type of traumatic injuries can lead to a diaphragmatic hernia or rupture?

    a)   Penetrating or Blunt

229)   What is the most common location of a diaphragmatic hernia or rupture after penetrating trauma?

    a)   Left posterior lateral (due to right-handed assailants)

230)   What is the most common location of diaphragmatic hernia or rupture after blunt trauma?

    a)   Left anterior

231)   Why are right-sided diaphragmatic hernias or ruptures more commonly missed?

    a)   Due to the liver

232)   How are diaphragmatic hernias diagnosed?

    a)   Chest X-ray, CT chest or Abdomen, Ultrasound, or Laparotomy (incidental)

233)   What are the X-ray findings seen with a diaphragm rupture?

    a)   Elevated hemidiaphragm, Stomach bubble in the chest cavity, or NG tube in the chest cavity

234)   What is the treatment of a diaphragmatic hernia or rupture?

a) Surgical repair

235) What is the most common area injured in blunt trauma that leads to hypotension?
a) Pelvic fracture

236) What intervention during trauma resuscitation should be performed for a suspected open book pelvic fracture with hypotension?
a) Pelvic binder

237) Due to the movement of the diaphragm what anatomical locations on the body should thoracoabdominal injuries be suspected with trauma?
a) 4th rib to the navel anteriorly and 6th rib to the ischial rim posteriorly

238) What imaging study is done to rule out a urethral injury with blood at the meatus during trauma?
a) Retrograde urethrogram

239) What procedure is contraindicated during trauma if there is blood at the meatus of the penis, a high riding prostate, scrotal bruising, or perineal bruising present on an exam?
a) Foley placement

240) What imaging study is done to work up gross hematuria after trauma?
a) IV contrast CT abdomen pelvis or Cystourethrogram

241) List the types of injuries associated with anterior and posterior urethral injuries.
a) Pelvic fracture, Straddle injury, Fractured penis, and Foreign bodies

242) What type of urethral injury, anterior or posterior, causes extravasation into the pelvic cavity?
a) Posterior

243) What imaging study can be used at beside during the primary survey to rule out bladder rupture?
a) Ultrasound during FAST

244) What is the preferred imaging done for diagnosing a bladder rupture?
a) Retrograde cystogram

245) What is the treatment for an intraperitoneal bladder rupture?
   a) Surgery (Urology)
246) What is the treatment for an extraperitoneal bladder rupture?
   a) Supportive therapy with urology consult
247) Which type of bladder rupture is the most common?
   a) Extraperitoneal
248) What is the secondary route of obtaining a urine sample, or placing a bladder catheter when a foley catheter cannot be placed in the presence of urethral strictures, trauma, or retention?
   a) Suprapubic catheter
249) What type of technique is used to place a suprapubic catheter?
   a) Seldinger technique
250) Is a suprapubic aspiration urine sample sterile and can it be used for a urinalysis?
   a) Yes
251) What image study is preferred in the workup of renal trauma?
   a) IVP or CT with IV contrast
252) Can renal injuries also present without hematuria?
   a) Yes
253) What imaging study is preferred to work up renal vascular injuries and pathology?
   a) CT Angiogram of the abdomen and pelvis
254) What is the time window for revascularization of the kidneys with a vascular injury?
   a) Within 12 hour
255) What type of trauma is more associated with ureteral injuries?
   a) Penetrating trauma
256) What imaging study is used to evaluate ureteral injury with blunt or penetrating trauma?
   a) IVP or CT Urogram
257) List the findings that suggest a positive test on a diagnostic peritoneal lavage. (procedure is not recommended by ATLS)
   a) > 100,000 RBCs/mL in lavage fluid
   b) 10,000 RBCs/mL with penetrating trauma
   c) Bile, feces, or urine return with lavage
   d) Aspiration of 10 mL of frank blood

258) What physical exam finding is described as flank discoloration and is associated with hemorrhagic pancreatitis or retroperitoneal hematomas?
   a) Grey Turner's sign
259) What physical exam finding is described as periumbilical ecchymosis and can be with hemorrhagic pancreatitis or an intraabdominal organ injury?
   a) Cullen's sign
260) What is the most common source of bleeding, arterial or venous, in retroperitoneal hemorrhage?
   a) Venous
261) What procedure is used for the treatment of an arterial retroperitoneal hemorrhage?
   a) Angiography and embolization
262) What is the treatment for a retroperitoneal hemorrhage or hematoma?
   a) Surgery
263) What specific symptom after trauma is due to referred pain from a splenic rupture, injury, or subdiaphragmatic injury?
   a) Left shoulder pain
264) What solid abdominal organ is the most commonly injured in blunt trauma?
   a) Spleen
265) What vaccines should be given in a patient with a splenectomy?
   a) Pneumococcal and HIB vaccines
266) What types of bacteria are asplenic patients at risk for?
   a) Encapsulated bacteria (S. Pneumoniae, H. Influenza, and N. Meningitidis)
267) What is the treatment for low-grade spleen laceration?
   a) Non-operative management
268) What are the surgical treatment options for a high-grade spleen laceration?
   a) Splenectomy verse Embolization
269) What solid abdominal organ is the most commonly injured in penetrating trauma?
   a) Liver

270) What are the treatment options for low-grade (1-3) liver hematomas and lacerations?
   a) Non-operative management verse Embolization

271) What is the best imaging study to evaluate solid organ injury following trauma?
   a) CT abdomen and pelvis with IV contrast

272) Is oral contrast required when evaluating for abdominal injury in trauma patients?
   a) No

273) What type of CT study has the highest accuracy for diagnosing all three of the following: solid organ, visceral (colon and rectum), and GU injuries in penetrating trauma?
   a) Triple contrast CT (IV, Oral, and Per rectum)

274) Is CT imaging always required in stable abdominal trauma patients with penetrating trauma that does not violate the fascia or blunt abdominal trauma?
   a) No (may do serial abdominal exams)

275) What type of small intestine injury is commonly seen in trauma to the abdomen from bike handlebars?
   a) Duodenal hematoma

276) What organs are in the retroperitoneal space and injury from trauma can cause a delayed diagnosis?
   a) Duodenum, Ascending and Descending colon, and Pancreas

277) Is an elevated amylase level specific for pancreatic injury after trauma?
   a) No

278) How do hollow viscus injuries from abdominal trauma typically present on an abdominal exam?
   a) Distended and +/- peritoneal signs

279) What section of the colon is the most commonly injured with abdominal trauma?
   a) Transverse

280) Where do most visceral injuries occur with blunt trauma?
   a) At fixation points

281) What type of imaging is used to evaluate testicular lacerations or hematomas after trauma?
   a) Ultrasound
282) What is the most common cause of injury in the geriatric population?
   a) Falls
283) What medications typically mask shock in the elderly?
   a) Beta-blockers or Calcium channel blockers
284) What type of extremity injury is common in an adult pedestrian verse auto accident?
   a) Tibial plateau fracture
285) Name the four types of blast injury classification.
   a) Primary, Secondary, Tertiary, Quaternary, and Quinary
286) Which of the four blast injuries is the most common type?
   a) Secondary
287) What type of blast injury causes gas filled structure injuries to gas filled structures such as the lung, eye, ears, and bowel due to the pressure from the blast wave?
   a) Primary
288) What type of blast injury is the most common and causes injuries due to flying debris?
   a) Secondary
289) What type of blast injury is injury to the person after being thrown from the blast?
   a) Tertiary
290) What type of blast injury is due to burns or crush injuries?
   a) Quaternary
291) What type of blast injury is due to chemical, biological, or radiological substances?
   a) Quinary
292) List the types of injuries that can be seen with primary blast injury.
   a) TM ruptures, pulmonary (contusion, hemothorax, pneumothorax, hemorrhage), Bowel rupture or injury, or Concussions
293) What is the most common type of primary blast injury?
   a) TM rupture

294) What is the law of distance pressure seen with blast injuries?
  a) Pressure received from a bomb = to the cubed root of the distance from the bomb blast
295) List the level 1-trauma facility requirements.
  a) Trauma surgery availability within 15 minutes
  b) Neuroradiology 24 hours a day
  c) Dialysis 24 hours a day
  d) Surgery subspecialties 24 hours a day
  e) Trauma research program
  f) Injury prevention program
296) What college credentials trauma centers?
  a) American College of Surgeons
297) What management should be performed with suspected extremity artery injuries after direct pressure fails?
  a) Tourniquet
298) Is the trajectory of a bullet from a GSW usually strait?
  a) No
299) What are the most common anatomical sites with a GSW that have and increased risk of developing lead poisoning?
  a) Intra-articular, Disk space, and Bursa locations (due to solubility of lead in the synovial fluid)
300) What are the most common causes leading to death from abdominal GSW's?
  a) Hemorrhage or Organ failure
301) Give the four phases of disaster management.
  a) Preparation, Mitigation, Response, and Recovery
302) What is the most common adult triage algorithm followed in mass casualty events?
  a) START
303) What are the questions asked with START triage that helps designate a triage category and treatment?
  a) Able to walk, Spontaneous breathing, Respiratory rate, Capillary refill and pulse deficits, and Mental status
304) What are the four mass casualty triage categories used in START?
  a) Green, Yellow, Red, and Black

305) What mass casualty triage category are patients with minor injuries, and the walking wounded?
   a) Green (minor)
306) What mass casualty triage category are patients with serious and potentially life threatening injuries that require treatment within 6 hours who's transport may be delayed?
   a) Yellow (delayed)
307) What mass casualty triage category are patients who have immediate life-threatening injuries and require immediate intervention for airway, breathing, and circulation issues?
   a) Red (immediate)
308) What mass casualty triage category are patients who have injuries greater than the resources available, and are unlikely to survive given the severity of the injuries?
   a) Black (expectant)
309) What mass casualty triage level would a patient be who has either of the following: respiratory rate > 30, absent radial pulse, prolonged capillary refill > 2 seconds, mental status changes, or not able to follow commands?
   a) Red (immediate)
310) List the "hard signs" associated with a vascular injury.
   a) Massive external bleeding
   b) Rapidly expanding hematoma
   c) Palpable thrill/audible bruit
   d) Signs of Occlusion (pallor, pain, paralysis, pulselessness, paresthesias)

Cardiovascular

311) Give a differential for chest pain in the emergency department.

    a) Aortic dissection, Biliary Colic, Cardiac tamponade, Cardiac valve disruption, Cardiomyopathy, Cholecystitis, Clavicle fracture or dislocation, Coronary artery aneurysm, Costochondritis, Diaphragm rupture or herniation, Esophageal perforation, GERD, Hepatitis, Hemoperitoneum Lung cancer, Myocardial ischemia, Myocarditis, Myocardial wall aneurysm, Pancreatitis, Pericarditis, Pneumoperitoneum, Pneumothorax, Pneumonia, Pulmonary contusion, Pulmonary effusion, Pulmonary emboli, Pulmonary hemorrhage, and Rib fracture or dislocation

312) Give a list of the typical workup for a patient with chest pain.

    a) ECG, CBC, BMP, Troponin, Chest X-ray, Cardiac monitoring, +/- BNP (heart failure), D-Dimer (PE), and LFT (gallbladder), or Lipase (pancreas)

313) What two components make up cardiac output?

    a) HR x SV = CO

314) What is the number one cause of death of adults in America?

    a) Ischemic heart disease

315) What type of heart block is seen with prolonged PR interval > 200 ms?

    a) 1st-degree heart block

316) What type of heart block is characterized by progressive PR interval lengthening with QRS drop?

    a) 2nd-degree Mobitz type 1

317) List common causes that lead to a 1st degree and 2nd degree Mobitz type 1.

    a) Acute MI, Uncontrolled parasympathetic, Drugs (beta-blockers, calcium channel blockers), Myocarditis, Endocarditis, Hypothermia, Lyme disease, or Electrolyte imbalance

318) What type of heart block is characterized by randomly dropped QRS complexes without a change in the PR interval?

    a) 2nd-degree Mobitz type 2

319) What type of heart block is characterized by no relationship between the P waves and the QRS complexes?
   a) 3rd-degree

320) What type of MI are 2nd-degree Mobitz type 2 and 3rd-degree heart blocks associated with?
   a) Anterior MI

321) What is the treatment for a 2nd-degree Mobitz type 2 and a 3rd-degree heart block?
   a) Pacemaker

322) What is the treatment recommendation for asymptomatic 1st-degree and 2nd-degree Mobitz type 1 heart blocks?
   a) Observation and Treat underlying condition

323) What medication should be avoided when treating bradycardia with a 2nd-degree Mobitz type 2 heart block?
   a) Atropine

324) What tick-borne disease should be suspected in a young patient with a high-grade heart block?
   a) Lyme disease

325) Where is the pacer spike on the ECG in a patient with an atrial pacer?
   a) Over the P wave

326) Where is the pacer spike on the ECG in a patient with a ventricular pacer?
   a) Beginning of the QRS

327) Which type of bundle branch block is defined by an RSR pattern in V1-V2, wide complex QRS, and wide S wave in Leads 1, V5 or V6?
   a) Right bundle branch block (RBBB)

328) Which type of bundle branch block is defined by a wide QRS, large R wave in lead 1, slurring of the QRS, and large QS V1?
   a) Left bundle branch block (LBBB)

329) What are some medical causes of LBBB?
   a) MI, Chronic hypertension, Chronic CHF, Valvular disease, or Fibrosis of the conduction system

330) What criteria can be used to diagnose ST-segment elevation MI (STEMI) in LBBB and RBBB?
   a) Sgarbossa criteria

331) List the Sgarbossa criteria for STEMI.
   a) Concordant ST elevation ≥ 1 mm in leads with a positive QRS
   b) Concordant ST depression ≥ 1 mm in V1 - V3
   c) Discordant ST elevation ≥ 5 mm in leads with a negative QRS with an ST/S ratios < - 0.25
332) What is the length of a wide QRS?
   a) > 0.12 sec
333) What is the normal range of the PR interval?
   a) 120-200 milliseconds
334) What is the normal length ranges for QTC in male and females?
   a) Male: 430-450, Female: 450-470
335) What plant does Digoxin come from?
   a) Foxglove plant
336) What ECG changes are seen with Digoxin toxicity?
   a) Alternating positive and negative QRS segments
337) What ECG changes are seen in a patient taking digoxin?
   a) Down sloping slurred ST depression, flattened, inverted or biphasic T waves, and or a shortened QT interval
338) What is the classic name for the ST down sloping seen with digoxin?
   a) Salvador Dali mustache
339) What heart rate defines general sinus tachycardia?
   a) > 100 bpm
340) What heart rate defines a tachyarrhythmia in the ACLS tachycardia with a pulse algorithm?
   a) >150 bpm
341) List the different cardiac rhythm types that are classified under supraventricular tachycardia (SVT).
   a) Sinus tachycardia, Atrial fibrillation, Atrial flutter, Multifocal atrial tachycardia, Atrioventricular Reentry Tachycardia (AVRT), Atrioventricular nodal reentrant tachycardia (AVNRT), Wolf Parkinson white (WPW), Atrial tachycardia, and Premature atrial contractions (PAC)
342) Define orthodromic and antidromic conduction in AVRT.
   a) Orthodromic: anterograde conduction through the AV node

    b) Antidromic: anterograde conduction through the accessory pathway

343) List the classic ECG findings with narrow complex SVT.
    a) Regular narrow QRS with a rate of 150-220 bpm and absent P waves

344) What is the treatment for stable SVT with a heart rate of 150-220 bpm?
    a) Vagal maneuver or Adenosine

345) At what cervical level do you perform carotid massage?
    a) C6

346) What is the first and second Adenosine dose amounts given to treat SVT?
    a) 1st dose: 6 mg
    b) 2nd dose: 12 mg

347) What a common side effect of Adenosine?
    a) Bronchospasm

348) What amount of energy is delivered during ACLS with monophasic and biphasic defibrillation?
    a) Monophasic: 360 J
    b) Biphasic: 200 J

349) Why is biphasic defibrillation used in cardiac resuscitation?
    a) It decreases the number of shocks and increases the likelihood of a 1st-time success rate

350) What is the treatment for unstable SVT with hypotension, altered mental status, signs of shock, chest pain, or heart failure?
    a) Synchronized Cardioversion (50-200 J biphasic)

351) What are the second and third-line medications for SVT?
    a) Beta-blocker or a Calcium channel blocker

352) What type of arrhythmia is irregularly irregular, without defined p waves?
    a) Atrial Fibrillation (A. fib)

353) What ECG rhythm has regular narrow complex QRS's with multiple P waves preceding it in a sawtooth pattern at rates 200-350?
    a) Atrial flutter (A. flutter)

354) List causes of A. fib or A. flutter.

a) MI, Thyrotoxicosis, CHF, PE, Alcohol, Caffeine, Infections, Cocaine, or Amphetamines

355) What type of cardioversion is used for unstable A. fib or A. flutter?

a) Synchronized

356) What treatment can be used for rapid correction of stable new-onset A.fib < 48 hours?

a) Cardioversion (electrical vs chemical- i.e. Flecainide)

357) What risk stratification score is used to determine the risk of stroke and need for long term anticoagulation for a patient with new-onset A. fib or flutter?

a) CHA_2D_2-VASc score

358) What is the treatment for a symptomatic stable atrial flutter or atrial fibrillation with RVR?

a) Beta-blockers, Calcium channel blockers, or Digoxin

359) What medications used to slow the heart rate in a stable patient with A. fib have the least effect on the blood pressure?

a) Digoxin or Amiodarone

360) What arrhythmia is defined as an irregularly irregular narrow complex tachycardia rhythm with at least three distinct P wave morphologies with variable PR intervals?

a) Multifocal atrial tachycardia (MAT)

361) What is the preferred treatment for MAT?

a) Magnesium sulfate

362) What arrhythmia is defined by a short PR interval, a slurred upstroke and widened QRS and reentrant tachycardia through a bypass tract of the heart?

a) Wolf-Parkinson-White Syndrome (WPW)

363) What is the accessory pathway called in WPW?

a) Bundle of Kent

364) What is the pathognomonic wave called that is seen with WPW?

a) Delta wave

365) Define the ECG findings in type A and type B WPW.

a) Type A: Positive delta wave in precordial leads with R/S > in V1

b) Type B: Negative delta wave in leads V1 and V2 (pseudo-infarction pattern)

366) What is the treatment for WPW based on?
   a) Width of the QRS

367) What is the treatment for stable narrow complex orthodromic WPW?
   a) Adenosine

368) What is the treatment for stable wide-complex WPW?
   a) Procainamide or Amiodarone

369) What is the treatment of WPW with atrial fibrillation and tachycardia?
   a) Procainamide or Cardioversion

370) What is the treatment for unstable WPW?
   a) Synchronized Cardioversion

371) What antiarrhythmic medication is contraindicated in myasthenia gravis patients?
   a) Procainamide

372) What specific medications are contraindicated in the treatment of WPW due to an increased risk of sudden death from blocking the AV node?
   a) Digoxin and Calcium channel blockers

373) What arrhythmia is defined as a regular wide complex rhythm with rates between 100-150 bpm?
   a) Ventricular tachycardia (V. Tach)

374) How do you tell is a rhythm is SVT with aberrancy from V. Tach?
   a) If any one of the following is a yes then it is V. Tach:
      i) Absent RS complex
      ii) R to S interval > 100 msec
      iii) AV dissociation
      iv) V. Tach morphology in V1 – V2
      v) LBBB morphology with a dominant S wave in V1 - V2
      vi) RBBB morphology with a dominant R wave in V1 - V2

375) What helps distinguish SVT with aberrancy from V. Tach on ECG?
   a) P wave preceding aberrant beat

376) What are the medication treatment options for wide complex tachycardia?
   a) Procainamide, Amiodarone, or Sotalol
377) What is the IV Procainamide dose given for wide complex QRS tachycardia?
   a) Bolus 20-50 mg/min until corrected and infusion 1-4 mg/min
378) What is the bolus and infusion dose of Amiodarone IV given for wide complex QRS tachycardia?
   a) Bolus 150mg and infusion 1mg/min
379) What is the treatment for unstable ventricular tachycardia?
   a) Synchronized cardioversion
380) What arrhythmia from electrolyte abnormalities has a wide complex V. Tach with alternating heights and can be seen in alcoholics?
   a) Torsades de pointes
381) What is the cause of Torsades de pointes?
   a) Prolonged QT interval
382) What is the treatment of Torsades de pointes (polymorphic ventricular tachycardia)?
   a) Magnesium sulfate
383) If the administration of magnesium sulfate fails to convert or control Torsades de pointes what other mechanical treatment can be performed?
   a) Overdrive pacing
384) What is the treatment for unstable Torsades de pointes?
   a) Cardioversion
385) What antiarrhythmic should not be used to treat Torsades de pointes?
   a) Procainamide
386) What electrolyte abnormalities are associated with Torsades de pointes and a prolonged QT?
   a) Hypokalemia, Hyperkalemia, Hypomagnesemia, Hypocalcemia, and Hyperphosphatemia
387) List common medications classes that can lead to a prolonged QT and Torsades de pointes.

a) Tricyclic antidepressants, Antipsychotics, Phenothiazines, Macrolides, Fluoroquinolones, Methadone, Procainamide, and Quinidine

388) What are the names of the two congenital QT prolongation syndromes?

a) Jervell-Lange-Nielsen syndrome and Romano-Ward syndrome

389) What heart rate is the definition of bradycardia?

a) ≤ 50 bpm

390) What is the first-line treatment of symptomatic bradycardia?

a) Atropine

391) What is the dose, frequency, and max of Atropine used in bradycardia?

a) 1st dose 0.5mg,

b) Repeated every 3-5min

c) Max of 3mg

392) List the causes of bradycardia.

a) Sick sinus syndrome, Hypothyroidism, Hypothermia, Hypoglycemia, Increased vagal tone, Drugs, Parasympathetic drugs, Cerebral Vascular Accident (CVA), Sinoatrial (SA) node dysfunction, and AV blocking medications

393) What type of infections can lead to relative bradycardia?

a) Typhoid, Rocky Mountain Spotted Fever (RMSF), Pneumocystis pneumonia (PCP), and Legionella

394) What are the treatments for symptomatic bradycardia if atropine fails?

a) Transcutaneous pacing, Dopamine, or Epinephrine

395) What is the dose for dopamine in the treatment of bradycardia?

a) 2-10 mcg/kg/min

396) What is the dose for Epinephrine in the treatment of bradycardia?

a) 2-10 mcg/min

397) What are 5 H's of the reversible causes of cardiac arrest?

a) Hypovolemia, Hypoxia, Hydrogen ion, Hypo-/Hyperkalemia, or Hypothermia

398) What are the 5 T's of reversible causes of cardiac arrest?

a) Tension pneumothorax

b) Tamponade

c) Toxins

d) Thrombosis pulmonary

e) Thrombosis coronary

399) What are the three drugs used for the treatment of hypotension in return of spontaneous circulation (ROSC)?

a) Epinephrine, Dopamine, or Norepinephrine

400) What ECG rhythms are reassuring after ROSC?

a) Bradycardia

b) Accelerated idioventricular rhythm

c) 3rd AV block with inferior MI

d) 2nd-degree Mobitz type 1 AV block (Wenckebach)

e) PVC's

f) PAC's

g) Non-sustained V. Tach

401) What is the target PEtCO2 with CPR and ventilation?

a) 35-40 mmHg

402) What arrhythmia is defined as a disorganized non-perfusing rhythm that is associated with heart disease, MI, or toxic ingestion?

a) V. Fib

403) What arrhythmia is defined as a wide complex QRS without a preceding P wave and can be unifocal or multifocal, single or in runs, and is associated with electrolyte abnormalities, CHF, or MIs?

a) Premature ventricular contractions (PVC)

404) What is the treatment for chronic PVCs that are asymptomatic?

a) Supportive

405) What are common causes of PVCs?

a) Electrolyte abnormality, ETOH, Caffeine, Stimulants, CAD, MI, or HTN

406) Which medications are used for frequent PVC's seen with acute ischemia?

a) Amiodarone or Lidocaine

407) What narrow complex of rhythm has rates between 40-60 bpm and inverted p waves?

a) Junctional rhythm

408) What is the treatment of a symptomatic junctional rhythm with a rate of 40?

a) Atropine

409) What are the two cardiac rhythms that require defibrillation (non-synchronized shock) with CPR during ACLS?

a) Ventricular fibrillation and Pulseless Ventricular Tachycardia

410) Which two cardiac rhythms during ACLS due not require shocks with CPR?

a) Pulseless Electrical Activity (PEA) and Asystole

411) What bedside imaging-resource can be used in the ED to evaluate cardiac activity during ACLS?

a) Cardiac ultrasound

412) What medications are recommended during ACLS for V. Fib, PEA, Asystole and Pulseless V. Tach?

a) Epinephrine and Amiodarone

413) What mediation is administered first after two minutes of CPR during ACLS?

a) Epinephrine

414) What is the dose of Epinephrine used in ACLS in a pulseless arrest?

a) 1 mg

415) How often is Epinephrine given during ACLS in a pulseless arrest?

a) Every 3-5 min

416) What is the dose for the 1st and 2nd rounds of Amiodarone given during ACLS with CPR?

a) 1st dose 300 mg

b) 2nd dose 150 mg

417) How often are pulse checks during pulseless arrest in ALCS?

a) Every 2 min

418) Is the pulse supposed to be checked immediately after defibrillation is administered during a pulseless arrest with ACLS?

a) No resume CPR then recheck after 2 min

419) What specific intervention can be attempted in refractory ventricular fibrillation, and has limited data on effectiveness?

a) Dual sequential defibrillation (DSD)

420) What is the target temperature for post-arrest cooling?
   a) 34°-36° C
421) List the unfavorable resuscitation features that determine the risk-benefit ratio of early catheterization post-arrest.
   a) Lactate > 7, PH < 7.2, Unwitnessed arrest, No bystander CPR, > 30 min to ROSC, Ongoing CPR, Age > 85, ESRD, or Non-VF initial rhythm
422) What is the treatment for the disease of the sinoatrial node and sick sinus syndrome?
   a) Pacemaker
423) What ECG abnormalities are seen with sick sinus syndrome?
   a) Tachycardia-bradycardia syndrome, and Fast and Slow alternating rates.
424) What cardiac emergency presents with hypotension, JVD and muffled heart sounds?
   a) Cardiac tamponade
425) What is the triad called for the symptoms seen with cardiac tamponade?
   a) Beck's triad
426) What is the sign called when the neck veins dilate and distend with inspiration with a cardiac tamponade?
   a) Kussmaul's sign
427) What chest X-ray finding can suggest a large pericardial effusion?
   a) Enlarged heart/cardiomegaly or "Water bottle heart"
428) What ECG finding can be seen with large pericardial effusion?
   a) Electrical alternans (beat to beat change in QRS heights)
429) What is the diagnostic study of choice for cardiac tamponade?
   a) Echocardiogram
430) How much fluid may be present at baseline in the pericardium?
   a) 50 ml or less
431) What finding on a cardiac echocardiogram suggests tamponade physiology with a significant restriction?
   a) RV collapse in diastole
432) What is the treatment for cardiac tamponade?
   a) Pericardiocentesis

433) How much fluid do you need to remove to see a hemodynamic improvement during a pericardiocentesis when treating cardiac tamponade?
   a) 20-50 mL

434) List the indications for immediate pericardiocentesis with a cardiac tamponade.
   a) Cardiac arrest, Vascular collapse, or Cyanosis/Hypoxia

435) What is the most common clinical scenario for an emergency pericardiocentesis?
   a) PEA in cardiac arrest

436) List criteria for the diagnosis of Kawasaki disease.
   a) Conjunctivitis
   b) Rash adenopathy
   c) Strawberry tongue
   d) Fever
   e) Hand or Feet Edema/Desquamation

437) What is the treatment of Kawasaki disease?
   a) IVIG and Aspirin

438) What is the most common cause of pediatric acquired heart disease?
   a) Kawasaki disease

439) What vascular emergency presents with sudden onset tearing chest pain radiating to the back, with a BP of 220/110, asymmetric blood pressure readings and pulses in the upper extremities, and a widened mediastinum on chest X-ray?
   a) Aortic dissection

440) What part of the vessel wall is weakened due to high pressures in an aortic dissection creating a false lumen?
   a) Media

441) Define LaPlace's law determining wall tension leading to an aortic dissection?
   a) Wall tension = Pressure x Radius

442) What collagen vascular disease is associated with a high risk of aortic dissection?
   a) Marfan's

443) List the risk factors for aortic dissection.

a) Hypertension, Trauma, Age > 50, Marfan's, Ehlers danlos, Bicuspid aortic valve, Methamphetamine or Cocaine abuse, Syphilis, Aortic coarctation, and Male

444) What is the number one major risk factor for aortic dissection?
   a) Hypertension

445) Define the Stanford classification for a type A aortic dissection.
   a) Type A: Ascending aortic dissection

446) What is the definitive treatment for a type A aortic dissection?
   a) Surgical

447) Define the Stanford classification for a type B aortic dissection.
   a) Type B: Descending aorta

448) What is the definitive treatment for a type B aortic dissection?
   a) Medical management

449) Give the three types of the DeBakey classification for aortic dissection.
   a) Type 1: Ascending and Descending (Whole aorta)
   b) Type 2: Ascending
   c) Type 3: Descending

450) List the chest X-ray findings seen with an aortic dissection.
   a) Displaced aortic knob, Widened mediastinum, Left apical cap, Left hemothorax, Left pleural effusion, Depressed left mainstem bronchus, Loss of aortic pulmonary window, Change of aortic configuration

451) Does a normal chest X-ray exclude an aortic dissection?
   a) No

452) What EKG findings can be seen with an aortic dissection that involves the coronary arteries?
   a) ST elevations

453) What are the imaging modalities that can be used to diagnose an aortic dissection or thoracic aortic aneurysm?
   a) MRI or CT chest angiogram, TEE, or Aortogram

454) What imaging modality is used most in the ED for diagnosing an aortic dissection?
   a) CT chest angiogram

455) What bedside imaging modality can be performed in the ED for an unstable patient with suspected aortic dissection?

a) Cardiac US

456) What is the preferred class of medications to be given to lower the BP and control tachycardia with an aortic dissection?
   a) Beta-blockers (Esmolol IV infusion)

457) What is the target systolic blood pressure for stabilizing the shearing forces in a patient with an aortic dissection?
   a) 100-120 mmHg

458) What is the target heart rate for stabilizing a patient with an aortic dissection?
   a) < 60 bpm

459) What medications should not be given before a beta-blocker when controlling the blood pressure in an aortic dissection due to reflex tachycardia?
   a) Nitroprusside or Nitroglycerin

460) What complication from an aortic dissection, should be suspected in a patient with chest pain, hypertension, syncope and hemiplegia, visual changes and altered mental status?
   a) CVA from a spreading aortic dissection

461) What vascular emergency should always be suspected with hypertension and pain above and below the diaphragm?
   a) Aortic dissection

462) What diameter in centimeters is an elective repair for a thoracic aortic aneurysm recommended?
   a) > 5.5 cm for non-Marfan patients

463) Give the contraindications for using beta-blockers.
   a) CHF, AV blocks, or History of Bronchospasm

464) Which ECG leads reflect the inferior wall?
   a) II, III, and aVF

465) Which ECG leads reflect the septum?
   a) V1 and V2

466) Which ECG leads reflect the anterior wall?
   a) V3 and V4

467) Which ECG leads reflect the lateral wall?
   a) V5, V6, I, and aVL

468) Which ECG leads reflect the anterolateral wall?
   a) V3, V4, V5, V6, I, and aVL

469) Which artery supplies the septum, inferior wall, right side of the heart, and the AV node?
   a) Right coronary artery (RCA)
470) Which two coronary arteries supply the sinus node?
   a) RCA and Circumflex
471) Which artery supplies the posterior wall of the heart?
   a) Posterior descending artery
472) Which artery supplies the anterolateral heart?
   a) Left anterior descending artery (LAD)
473) Which artery supplies the left lateral heart?
   a) Circumflex artery
474) What are the three diagnoses that makeup acute coronary syndrome (ACS)?
   a) Stable angina, Unstable angina, and Acute MI
475) List ACS risk factors.
   a) Diabetes, Hypercholesterolemia, Hypertension, Smoker, Family history, Drug abuse, Male, HIV, Age, and Lupus
476) What patient populations commonly present with atypical ACS symptoms?
   a) Diabetics, Elderly, and Women
477) What associated symptoms with chest pain increase the suspicion of ACS?
   a) Radiation of pain to neck, jaw, or arm, Substernal or Left side pressure aching or squeezing pain, Diaphoresis, Shortness of breath, or Nausea
478) What cardiac marker is the first to rise within 1-2 hours after an acute myocardial infarction (AMI), although it is not often used due to poor sensitivity?
   a) Myoglobin
479) What is the time frame for troponin to start to show elevations in the blood?
   a) 3-6 hours
480) How many days following an MI does the troponin level trend down to normal levels?
   a) 7-10 days

481) What cardiac enzyme can also be elevated with pathologies such as AMI, renal failure, muscle exertion, and rhabdomyolysis?
   a) CK-MB

482) What medication has been shown to decrease mortality in ACS and should always be unless there is an allergy?
   a) Aspirin

483) What is the dosing of Aspirin given in ACS?
   a) 162 – 325 mg

484) What medication can be given during ACS to vasodilate the coronary arteries or lower the blood pressure?
   a) Nitroglycerin

485) Does response to Nitroglycerin or a GI cocktail rule in or rule out ACS as a diagnosis?
   a) No, they are not sensitive

486) List the contraindications of giving Nitroglycerin during ACS.
   a) Hypotension (Systolic BP < 90 mmHg)
   b) Bradycardia (< 50 per min)
   c) Tachycardia
   d) Posterior MI
   e) Inferior MI
   f) Concurrent use of PDE- 5 inhibitors (Sildenafil, Vardenafil, etc.)

487) Why can too much oxygen be harmful in ACS if the patient is not hypoxic?
   a) It can extends infarct and can cause vasoconstriction

488) What symptom has the highest positive predictive value for ACS?
   a) Right-sided chest pain

489) What type of ECG findings with reciprocal changes indicates ischemia?
   a) T wave inversion, ST-segment elevation or depression, Q waves > 1mm, Biphasic T waves, New LBBB, or New directional change in the QRS

490) What are the ECG findings associated with a transmural infarct from an AMI?
   a) ST elevation, Q waves, and T wave inversions

491) What are the ECG findings seen with a subendocardial infarct from an AMI?

a) ST depression and T wave inversion

492) What findings on ECG indicate reperfusion during an AMI?

a) Improved T wave inversion, Normalized ST segments, or Accelerated idioventricular rhythm

493) What rhythm is a wide complex rhythm with variable rates 40-100 bpm, and is associated with acute MIs and reperfusion?

a) Accelerated idioventricular rhythm

494) What is the recommended treatment for an accelerated idioventricular rhythm?

a) Observation (can resolve spontaneously with minutes)

495) T wave inversion within what time frame after an acute MI indicates reperfusion?

a) Within 4 hours

496) What rhythms are associated with a worse prognosis in an acute MI?

a) Atrial fib, V. Fib, and Sustained V. Tach

497) What is the most common physiological cause of ACS that leads to heart tissue damage and is defined as an imbalance in the oxygen supply and demand?

a) Atherosclerosis

498) List the non-atherosclerotic causes of ACS.

a) Vasculitis, Congenital anomalies, Infectious Emboli, Drugs (Cocaine, Meth), DIC, Metabolic disease, Trauma, and Dissection

499) What is the physiologic mechanism of cocaine or methamphetamine-induced ACS that leads to ECG changes?

a) Vasospasm

500) Do most drug-induced ACS patients require stenting and a catheterization?

a) No (less than 5% with MI)

501) What type of ACS has constant pain at rest that increases in severity without ECG changes and has a normal troponin level?

a) Unstable angina

502) What type of ECG changes can be seen with unstable angina?

a) Normal, ST depressions, or T wave inversions

503) What type of ACS involves a partial-thickness subendocardial ischemic injury with either no ECG changes or ST depressions, an elevated troponin, chest pain, nausea, diaphoresis, and shortness of breath?

a) Non-ST-segment elevated MI (Non-STEMI)

504) What type of ACS is a transmural infarction causing chest pain that radiates to the neck, jaw or arm, with diaphoresis, nausea, shortness of breath, and an elevated troponin?

a) ST-segment elevated MI (STEMI)

505) What is the earliest sign and ECG finding that can be seen with an acute MI?

a) Hyperacute T waves

506) List the ECG changes associated with ischemia and AMI.

a) T wave inversion, Hyperacute T waves, ST-segment elevation or depression, or Q waves

507) Does a completely normal ECG rule out an AMI?

a) No (up to 10% have an AMI)

508) List the ECG changes for diagnosing a STEMI.

a) ST-elevation > 1 mm in two continuous leads (except V2-V3 > 2mm Men and > 1.5 Women) with reciprocal changes

b) ST depression in 2+ leads V1-V4

c) Sgarbossa criteria

d) De Winter T wave

e) Wellens syndrome

509) What type of STEMI equivalent ECG change has ST depressions and a peaked T wave in the precordial leads V1-V3 and is predictive of an acute LAD occlusion?

a) De Winter's T waves

510) What syndrome is predictive of a LAD occlusion and has biphasic T wave ECG changes in the precordial leads?

a) Wellens syndrome

511) What is the definitive treatment for a STEMI?

a) Percutaneous catheter intervention (PCI) for coronary reperfusion

512) What is the target time frame for PCI treatment for a STEMI?

a) < 90 min door to balloon

513) If a patient arrives at a non-PCI capable hospital with a STEMI, what is the extended amount of time for PCI?

a) 120 min

514) If the 90 min PCI window is not possible for treating a STEMI what is the second-line treatment?

a) Tissue plasminogen activator (TPA)

515) What is the TPA dosing for a STEMI?

a) 100 mg

516) What are the most common side effects of the thrombolytic medication Streptokinase?

a) Allergic reaction and Hypotension

517) List the absolute contraindications of TPA administration.

a) CVA < 3 months
b) Hemorrhagic CVA history
c) Intracranial surgery or trauma < 3 months
d) Intracranial mass or AVM
e) Aortic dissection suspected
f) Active internal bleeding
g) Uncontrolled hypertension > 185/110
h) Major surgery < 14 days
i) Thrombocytopenia < 100,000
j) Pregnancy

518) What is the general medical treatment for all patients with STEMI, Non-STEMI and unstable angina?

a) Heparin (bolus and infusion) or Enoxaparin

519) Is it recommended to give heparin following TPA administration for patients being treated for a STEMI?

a) Yes

520) What is the Heparin bolus dosing for ACS?

a) 60 units/kg (4000 units max)

521) What is the Heparin infusion dosing for ACS?

a) 12 units/kg/hr (1000 units/hr)

522) What is the dosing for Enoxaparin for ACS?

a) 1 mg/kg BID

523) What medications can also be given before PCI in an acute MI?

a) Clopidogrel, GP IIb/IIIa inhibitors, Prasugrel, or Ticagrelor

524) In what situation is urgent PCI also recommended for a patient with a Non-STEMI or unstable angina?

a) Intractable symptoms despite medical therapy or Changing ECG

525) What medications can be given for a hypertensive emergency to bring down the BP with ACS?

a) Nitroglycerin infusion, Beta-blockers, or Calcium channel blockers

526) Above what heart rate is a beta-blocker recommended to be given in a Non-STEMI to prevent further injury?

a) > 90 bpm

527) Which medication is contraindicated in inferior and posterior MIs due to the risk of hypotension?

a) Nitroglycerin

528) What is the oxygen saturation target range during ACS?

a) 94-99%

529) What ECG findings are suggestive of a Posterior MI?

a) ST depression in V1, V2, and V3 with a large R wave

530) If a posterior MI is of concern, which ECG leads, need to be moved and where are they placed for a repeat ECG?

a) V4-V6 are moved to the back under the scapula and become V7-V9

531) What normal physiological ECG changes are typically seen in the younger patient population and can mimic a STEMI?

a) Early repolarization

532) What are the ECG changes that suggest benign early repolarization?

a) Early QRS peaking in precordial leads with a QRS notch and J point elevation of the ST segment

533) How do you determine if a patient has pericarditis or benign early repolarization on an ECG?

a) ST-segment / T wave ratio in V6

534) What is the ST segment / T wave ratio in V6 that suggests elevation from benign early repolarization?

a) < 0.25

535) What type of angina is caused by intermittent coronary artery spasms at rest causing chest pain and can cause ST-segment elevations on ECG?
a) Prinzmetal's angina

536) List early complications that can occur after an acute MI.
a) RBBB, LBBB, AV block, Cardiogenic shock, Inferior MI, and Mitral regurgitation

537) What is the most common cause of death in the hospital from an acute MI?
a) Cardiogenic shock

538) What cardiac complication can follow an acute MI or following a cardiac arrest that causes hypotension, and bradycardia?
a) Cardiogenic shock

539) Loss of what percent of the heart function post-MI can lead to cardiogenic shock?
a) ≥ 40%

540) Loss of what percentage of the heart function post-MI can lead to CHF?
a) ≥ 25%

541) New-onset CHF with pulmonary edema is more commonly due to what condition?
a) Acute MI

542) What are the ED treatments for cardiogenic shock?
a) Crystalloids, Inotropes, Cardiovascular consult for ECMO, CABG, or Intra-aortic balloon pump

543) What type of MI presents with hypotension, JVD, clear lungs sounds, and has ST elevations on right-sided chest leads (V4R)?
a) Right ventricular infarction

544) List the late complications that can occur after an acute MI.
a) Pericarditis, Dressler's syndrome, Mural thrombus, Myocardial rupture, Papillary rupture, Septal wall rupture, Ventricular wall aneurysm, or Arrhythmias

545) Acute mitral regurgitation and new systolic murmur with acute CHF that occurs 3-5 days after an MI are due to ischemia and rupture of what cardiac structure?
a) Papillary muscles

546) What imaging should be performed for suspected papillary muscle injury?
   a) Echocardiogram

547) What post-MI complication should be suspected with persistent ST-segment elevation or T wave inversions in the affected leads that can occur 6 weeks after a transmural MI?
   a) Ventricular wall aneurysm

548) What imaging should be performed if a ventricular wall aneurysm is suspected?
   a) Echocardiogram

549) What is the treatment of a ventricular wall aneurysm?
   a) Anticoagulant

550) What late post-MI complication presents with recurrent chest pain, fever, friction rub, and diffuse ST elevations with PR depression on ECG and occurs 2-8 weeks out?
   a) Dressler's syndrome

551) What coronary emergency seen in young women with hypertension and hormone therapy presents with chest pain and ST-segment ECG changes?
   a) Spontaneous coronary artery dissection

552) What is the ED treatment for a spontaneous coronary artery dissection?
   a) Supportive therapy, BP control, No anticoagulants, Cardiology consult (no PCI)

553) What cardiac etiology presents with chest pain that improves with leaning forward, dyspnea, diffuse ST elevations with PR depression on ECG, a cardiac rub on the heart sounds, and a history of a recent viral illness?
   a) Pericarditis

554) What is the typical time frame regular pericarditis can present post-MI?
   a) Usually 1-7 days

555) List the ECG changes that can be seen with pericarditis.
   a) Diffuse ST segment elevation (I,II, III, AVL, V2-V6)
   b) PR depression (I,II, III, AVL, V2-V6)
   c) PR elevation and ST depression in AVR

556) List the common causes of pericarditis.

a) Infectious (Viral, Bacterial, TB or Fungal)
b) Uremia
c) Post MI
d) Trauma
e) Paraneoplastic syndrome
f) Drug-induced
g) Post radiation
h) Immunological

557) What is the most common cause of pericarditis?
a) Viral

558) What is the most common infectious cause of pericarditis?
a) Coxsackievirus

559) List the ECG changes that can present in the four stages of pericarditis.
a) Stage 1: Diffuse ST-segment elevation and PR depression, with reciprocal changes in AVR (1-2 weeks)
b) Stage 2: Normalization of ST segments and T wave flattening (1 - 3 weeks)
c) Stage 3: Inverted T waves (3 + weeks)
d) Stage 4: ECG normalization

560) What is the treatment of pericarditis and Dressler's syndrome?
a) NSAIDs (1-3 weeks) or Steroids

561) What imaging is the best for the diagnosis of pericarditis?
a) Echocardiography

562) What type of post-MI cardiac complication presents with sudden onset pain, SOB, hypotension and is due to injury to the left ventricle wall?
a) Myocardial rupture

563) What is the definitive treatment for a post-MI myocardial rupture or septal wall rupture?
a) Cardiothoracic surgery

564) What medical condition presents with increasing peripheral edema, SOB, weight gain, rales on lung exam and a history of hypertension?
a) Congestive heart failure (CHF)

565) What imaging is done to diagnose CHF and quantify the severity?
   a) Echocardiography
566) What ejection fraction on echocardiogram helps classify if there is decreased cardiac function and possible heart failure?
   a) < 65%
567) What are the classic lung findings on chest X-ray with acute CHF?
   a) Pulmonary edema or Pleural effusions
568) What chest X-ray finding is defined by fluid in the costophrenic angles, and loss of pulmonary lung markings as it increases?
   a) Pleural effusion
569) What are the chest X-ray findings that suggest pulmonary edema?
   a) Kerley B lines
   b) Alveolar edema (Cephalization)
570) What chest X-ray finding with pulmonary edema is defined as short peripheral horizontal lines near the costophrenic angles?
   a) Kerley B lines
571) What values are considered to be normal BNP and NT-proBNP levels when evaluating CHF?
   a) BNP: < 100 pg/mL
   b) NT-proBNP: < 300 pg/mL
572) What BNP level suggests decompensated CHF?
   a) > 500 pg/mL (100-500 = uncertain)
573) What NT-proBNP levels suggest decompensated CHF?
   a) > 900 pg/mL
574) In what medical condition can BNP levels be falsely elevated?
   a) ESRD
575) In what medical condition can the BNP levels be falsely low?
   a) Obesity
576) What is the most common cause of heart failure?
   a) Hypertension
577) What are the two classification types of heart failure based on cardiac dysfunction?
   a) Systolic and Diastolic

578) What classification of heart failure is due to impaired contractility leading to a low ejection fraction and cardiac output with increased cardiac volumes, pressure, and afterload sensitivity?
   a) Systolic

579) What classification of heart failure is due to an impaired ventricular relaxation, decreased LV compliance and filling from LV hypertrophy and chronic hypertension?
   a) Diastolic

580) What type of heart failure is the most common?
   a) Systolic

581) What type of curve shows the relationship between preload, afterload, and heart contractility and helps describe the mechanism of heart failure?
   a) Frank-Starling curve

582) List the different types of acute heart failure.
   a) Hypertensive heart failure, Acute decompensated heart failure, High output failure, and Right heart failure

583) What type of heart failure presents with tachycardia, warm extremities, and pulmonary congestion with an increased cardiac output?
   a) High output heart failure

584) What medical conditions can lead to high output heart failure?
   a) Thyrotoxicosis, Arteriovenous shunts (in ESRD), Beriberi, and Paget's disease of the bones

585) Give the main causes of low output heart failure.
   a) Hypertension, PE, CAD, ACS, Cardiomyopathy, and Valvular disease

586) What type of heart failure is due to acutely increased blood pressure levels, and leads to pulmonary edema and SOB and develops in 1-2 days?
   a) Hypertensive acute heart failure

587) What characteristics help define decompensated heart failure differentiates it from acute hypertensive heart failure?
   a) Systolic BP < 140 mmHg and Gradual onset of symptoms + Peripheral edema

588) Which type of heart failure has a low cardiac output and leads to back up of venous flow, JVD, hepatomegaly, peripheral edema, and hypotension?
   a) Right-sided heart failure
589) What is the most common cause of right-sided heart failure?
   a) Left-sided heart failure
590) What type of heart failure presents with orthopnea, paroxysmal nocturnal dyspnea, tachycardia, dyspnea, and pulmonary edema?
   a) Left-sided heart failure
591) What type of heart gallop can be present with acute left-sided CHF?
   a) S3 gallop
592) What arrhythmias if new-onset or uncontrolled typically can lead to acute CHF?
   a) Atrial fibrillation or Atrial flutter
593) What is the pathophysiologic mechanism that leads to an increase in fluid retention in CHF?
   a) Reduced cardiac output leads to increased renin-angiotensin and secretion of antidiuretic hormone (ADH)
594) What are the treatments for an acute CHF exacerbation?
   a) Oxygen, IV Nitroglycerin, Morphine, ACE inhibitors, Nesiritide, Nitroprusside, Loop diuretics, +/- CPAP, BIPAP, or Intubation
595) What IV medications are used to increase contractility in a CHF exacerbation with low blood pressure or a patient with a history of a low EF?
   a) Dobutamine or Dopamine
596) What medication class has been shown to prolong survival in heart failure?
   a) ACE inhibitors
597) List common medications that cause edema.
   a) Calcium channel blockers, Pioglitazone, Gabapentin, Steroids, NSAIDs, Hydralazine, Nitrates, and Minoxidil
598) What cardiac condition in a 50 y/o IV drug abuser (IVDA) causes chest pain, fever, SOB, and a heart murmur, hemorrhagic plaques on the palms, and splinter hemorrhages on the fingernails on physical exam?
   a) Infective endocarditis

599) What is the most common cause of acute aortic regurgitation?
   a) Infective endocarditis
600) List the risk factors for infective endocarditis.
   a) IVDA, Mitral valve prolapse, Pacemaker, Prosthetic valves, Dialysis, or Prior history of Endocarditis, Rheumatic heart disease, or Congenital heart disease
601) List the classic physical exam findings with their descriptions that are seen with infective endocarditis.
   a) Osler nodes: Tender nodules on tips of fingers and toes
   b) Janeway lesions: Nontender, hemorrhagic plaques on the palms and sole
   c) Roth spots: Retinal hemorrhages with central clearing
   d) Splinter hemorrhages and Petechiae on the nails
602) How many blood cultures are recommended to be drawn when working up infective endocarditis?
   a) 3 or more
603) What imaging study is the diagnostic study of choice for infective endocarditis and can show valvular vegetations?
   a) Transesophageal echocardiography (TEE)
604) What lab is used to aid in the diagnosis of infective endocarditis?
   a) ↑ ESR
605) What is the most common clinical manifestation in infective endocarditis?
   a) Fever (80%)
606) What neurologic complication can occur due to infective endocarditis?
   a) Embolic stroke
607) What is the most common cause of mortality from infective endocarditis?
   a) CHF (severe)
608) What type of endocarditis usually involves younger patients with normal valves and has higher mortality due to a Staph. aureus infection?
   a) Acute endocarditis

609) What type of endocarditis is seen in older patients with abnormal valves and is with Strep. viridan infections?
   a) Subacute endocarditis
610) What is the most common valve involved in infective endocarditis?
   a) Mitral
611) What bacteria is most commonly involved in left-sided infective endocarditis?
   a) Strep. viridans
612) What type of emboli develops and is seen with left-sided infective endocarditis?
   a) Septic peripheral emboli with extremity and CNS infarcts
613) What valve is most commonly involved with infective endocarditis in IVDA?
   a) Tricuspid
614) What is the most common bacterium associated with right-sided infective endocarditis that affects the tricuspid valve in IVDA?
   a) Staph. Aureus and (less commonly gram negatives)
615) What is the suspected cause of multiple lobar patchy infiltrates seen on chest X-ray in a patient with right-sided endocarditis?
   a) Septic emboli causing pulmonary infarctions
616) Which bacteria most commonly infect prosthetic valves early postoperatively within the first 2 months?
   a) Staph. epidermidis and Staph. aureus
617) Which bacteria most commonly infect prosthetic valves late in the postoperative period?
   a) Strep. viridans, Enterococcus, Pseudomonas, or Serratia
618) What are the medications used to treat infective endocarditis?
   a) Penicillins + Aminoglycosides + Vancomycin (+/- Rifampin)
619) List the indications for surgical treatment in addition to medication treatment in infective endocarditis.
   a) Mycotic aneurysm, Multiple emboli, Valve ring abscess, or Worsening CHF
620) Patients with what specific medical history require prophylactic antibiotic treatment prior to surgery to prevent infective endocarditis?

a) Congenital heart disease (repaired and unrepaired), Cardiac transplant patients, History of endocarditis, or Prosthetic valves

621) Which specific surgical procedures require prophylactic antibiotics to decrease the risk of infective endocarditis from transient bacteremia?

a) Dental procedures, Respiratory surgery, and Procedures on infected skin (Abscesses)

622) How long before an invasive procedure are prophylactic antibiotics supposed to be given to prevent endocarditis in high-risk patients?

a) 60 min

623) What antibiotics are recommended for endocarditis prophylaxis in high-risk patients and those undergoing dental, respiratory, or skin procedures?

a) Amoxicillin 2 grams

b) Ceftriaxone 1 gram

c) Clindamycin 600 mg or Azithromycin 500mg (Penicillin allergic patients)

624) What heart condition should be suspected in a patient with a viral illness, chest pain, dyspnea, fever, tachycardia, elevated enzymes, AMS, and signs of CHF?

a) Myocarditis

625) Can there be elevated troponin levels with myocarditis?

a) Yes

626) What labs tests can be elevated with myocarditis?

a) ESR and CRP levels

627) List the ECG changes that can be seen with myocarditis.

a) ST-T segment changes, Inverted T waves, and Tachycardia

628) What are the most common infectious etiologies of myocarditis in the United States?

a) Enterovirus and Echovirus

629) What virus is the most common cause of myocarditis in pediatrics?

a) Coxsackie B virus

630) What are some other causes that lead to myocarditis?

a) Lyme, Rheumatic fever, Cocaine, HIV, Chemotherapy, and Adenovirus

631) How is myocarditis definitively diagnosed?

a) Cardiac biopsy or Cardiac MRI

632) What are the treatments available for myocarditis?

a) Supportive care, Admission, Inotropes, Fluids, ECMO (severe patients), +/- Antibiotics

633) What is the most common cause of valvular disease in the overall patient population?

a) Degenerative valvular disease

634) What type of valvular abnormality presents with chest pain and exertional syncope and has a hollow systolic murmur on the exam with a narrow pulse pressure?

a) Aortic stenosis

635) What locations can the murmur with aortic stenosis be heard?

a) Carotid arteries and Suprasternal notch

636) What type of ECG changes can be seen with aortic stenosis?

a) LVH or LBBB

637) Which symptoms seen with aortic stenosis are poor prognostic signs with a mortality rate < 5 years?

a) Angina, Syncope, and CHF

638) What are the causes of aortic stenosis?

a) Congenital (Bicuspid), Degenerative with age, or Rheumatic heart disease

639) What is the most common type of congenital aortic valve disease?

a) Bicuspid aortic valve

640) What is the most common cause of aortic stenosis in patients > 65 years old?

a) Degenerative / Calcification

641) What medications should be avoided in patients with an outflow obstruction from aortic stenosis due to a sudden drop in BP?

a) Nitrates or Vasodilators

642) What is the definitive treatment for severe aortic stenosis?

a) Valve replacement

643) What type of valvular abnormality caused by dissections, rheumatic disease, or endocarditis has a diastolic decrescendo murmur and leads to LV volume overload and CHF?
a) Aortic regurgitation

644) Is the pulse pressure wide or narrow with aortic regurgitation?
a) Widened pulse pressure

645) List the most common causes of acute aortic regurgitation.
a) Aortic Dissection and Endocarditis

646) List the most common cause of chronic aortic regurgitation.
a) Rheumatic heart disease

647) List the pathognomonic physical exam findings associated with aortic regurgitation.
a) Austin-Flint murmur
b) Diastolic decrescendo murmur
c) Duroziez's murmur
d) Quincke's sign
e) Water hammer pulses

648) What pathognomonic physical exam finding associated with aortic regurgitation is defined by bounding pulses?
a) Water hammer pulses

649) What pathognomonic physical exam finding with aortic regurgitation is defined by a diastolic murmur due to aortic regurgitation flow hitting the mitral valve?
a) Austin-Flint murmur

650) What pathognomonic physical exam finding with aortic regurgitation is defined by a murmur heard over the femoral artery?
a) Duroziez's murmur

651) What pathognomonic physical exam finding with aortic regurgitation is defined as pulsatile blushing of the nail beds?
a) Quincke's sign

652) What physical exam finding is commonly seen with aortic regurgitation during systole?
a) Head bobbing

653) What is the treatment for aortic regurgitation?
a) Afterload reduction and Inotropes

654)   What life-threatening condition needs to be ruled out in a patient who presents with an acute MI and aortic regurgitation?
   a)   Aortic dissection

655)   What is the most common symptom in patients with cardiac valve disease?
   a)   Exertional dyspnea

656)   What cardiac valve abnormality has a loud diastolic murmur with an opening snap, and leads to dyspnea on exertion and orthopnea over time?
   a)   Mitral stenosis

657)   What lung condition can develop gradually with severe mitral stenosis?
   a)   Pulmonary edema and Pulmonary hypertension

658)   What cardiac condition can develop gradually from the dilation of the atria with mitral stenosis or mitral regurgitation?
   a)   Atrial fibrillation

659)   What is the leading cause of mitral stenosis?
   a)   Rheumatic heart disease

660)   What finding on a chest X-ray can be seen with chronic mitral stenosis and is due to the appearance of a dilated atria?
   a)   Straightening of the left heart border

661)   What cardiac valve abnormality presents with acute dyspnea from pulmonary edema, a holosystolic murmur and is commonly seen in patients with a history of rheumatic heart disease?
   a)   Mitral regurgitation

662)   List the causes of acute mitral regurgitation.
   a)   Papillary muscle dysfunction and Chordae tendon rupture (Post MI)

663)   List the causes of chronic mitral regurgitation.
   a)   Rheumatic heart disease, Mitral valve prolapse, Dilated cardiomyopathy, and Valve calcification

664)   What is the treatment for mitral regurgitation?
   a)   Afterload reduction and Surgical repair

665)   Which cardiac valve abnormality has a mid-systolic click and late systolic murmur and can cause palpitations, dyspnea, and atypical chest pains?

a) Mitral valve prolapse

666) What positions increase the murmur heard with mitral valve prolapse?

a) Squatting and Leg raise (Increases left ventricle volume)

667) What patient population is mitral valve prolapse typically seen in?

a) Young females

668) What medications can be used to treat atypical chest pains and arrhythmias associated with mitral regurgitation?

a) Beta-blockers

669) What imaging modality is the study of choice for diagnosing cardiac valve abnormalities?

a) Echocardiogram

670) What is the most common valvular heart disease seen in industrialized countries?

a) Mitral valve prolapse

671) What type of cardiomyopathy is the most common and can follow a recent viral infection and presents with heart failure, intermittent arrhythmias, and has a globular heart chest X-ray?

a) Dilated cardiomyopathy

672) What is the most common type of cardiomyopathy seen in alcoholics?

a) Dilated cardiomyopathy

673) List causes of dilated cardiomyopathy.

a) Idiopathic, Infections, Pregnancy, Myocarditis, Sarcoidosis, Amyloidosis, and Heart failure

674) What is the most common cause of dilated cardiomyopathy?

a) Idiopathic

675) List the management options for dilated cardiomyopathy.

a) Diuretics, Afterload reduction, Inotropes, and Possible Transplant

676) What type of cardiomyopathy presents with CHF symptoms, pleural effusion on chest X-ray, and has a pathognomonic "square root sign" or "dip and plateau" defect on catheterization?

a) Restrictive/constrictive cardiomyopathy

677) What type of cardiomyopathy is familial, autosomal dominant, and presents with exertional syncope and sudden death in young athletes?
   a) Hypertrophic cardiomyopathy (HCM)
678) What is the genetic mutation that causes HCM?
   a) Beta myosin heavy chain mutation
679) What is the pathognomonic heart murmur associated with HCM?
   a) Mid-systolic murmur louder with Valsalva and Standing
680) Why does the systolic murmur with HCM increase with valsalva and standing?
   a) Decreased preload leading to the septum obstructing outflow from the left ventricle
681) What medications can lead to an increase murmur with HCM due to decreasing preload volumes?
   a) Nitrates and Beta-blockers
682) What things can decrease the murmur heard in HCM?
   a) Squatting, Trendelenburg, and Alpha and Beta-blockers
683) What are the structural cardiac changes seen with HCM?
   a) Asymmetric septal and mitral valve leaflet thickening, blocking the outflow from the left ventricle
684) What ECG changes can be seen with HCM?
   a) Septal LVH with deep narrow "Dagger-Like" Q waves inferiorly and laterally
685) What is the diagnostic study of choice for HCM?
   a) Echocardiogram
686) What is the treatment for HCM?
   a) Avoid exercise
   b) Beta-blockers
   c) Calcium channel blockers
   d) Myomectomy
687) What autosomal dominant life-threatening condition presents with non-exertional syncope and has ST elevations in V1 and V2 with an inverted T wave and leads to sudden cardiac death in young Asian patients from V. fib?
   a) Brugada syndrome

688) What is the etiology of Brugada syndrome?
   a) Sodium channelopathy
689) How many types of Brugada syndrome are there?
   a) 3
690) What type of Brugada has J point ST elevations with a down sloping ST-segment and an inverted T wave?
   a) Type 1
691) What type of Burgada has J point ST elevations with a "Saddleback" ST-T wave and an upright or biphasic T wave
   a) Type 2
692) What type of Brugada has J point ST elevations with a "Saddleback" ST-T wave and a positive T wave?
   a) Type 3
693) What is the treatment for Brugada syndrome?
   a) Automatic implantable cardiac defibrillator (AICD)
694) Give the JNC definition of benign essential hypertension.
   a) > 140 / 90 mmHg
695) Give the JNC criteria for pre-hypertension.
   a) 120-139 systolic / 80-89 diastolic
696) Give the JNC definition of stage 1 hypertension.
   a) 140-159 systolic / 90-99 diastolic
697) Give the JNC definition of stage 2 hypertension.
   a) > 160 / 100 mmHg
698) List some causes of chronic hypertension.
   a) Age, Smoking, Obesity, Hypercholesterolemia, Steroids, MAO inhibitors, Renal disease, and Pheochromocytoma
699) List some causes of acute hypertension seen in the ED.
   a) Alcohol withdrawal, Dehydration (early), Steroids (short course), Anxiety, Pain, Stroke, Epistaxis, Serotonin syndrome, Thyroid storm, and Drugs (cocaine or amphetamines)
700) What is the BP level that defines hypertensive urgency?
   a) BP > 180 / 110 mmHg
701) What is the JNC guideline for the treatment of asymptomatic hypertensive urgency?
   a) Decrease blood pressure over days to weeks
702) What makes hypertensive urgency a hypertensive emergency (malignant hypertension)?

a) Evidence of acute end-organ damage

703) What is the calculation for determining mean arterial pressure (MAP)?

a) MAP = DBP + (SBP – DBP) / 3

704) What conditions can be seen with hypertensive emergencies?

a) MI, CHF, Aortic Dissection, CVA (hemorrhagic and ischemic), Retinal hemorrhage, Papilledema, Pulmonary edema, Eclampsia, Preeclampsia, and Kidney or Liver failure

705) What blood pressure in the pediatric population qualifies as elevated for a hypertensive emergency?

a) > 95th percentile

706) What is the treatment of a hypertensive emergency?

a) Decrease MAP no more than 20% in the first hour followed by a decrease in BP over 24 hours

707) What medications can be administered in the ED for malignant hypertension?

a) Labetalol, Nicardipine, Esmolol, Nitroglycerin, or Nitroprusside

708) What areas of the brain do ischemic strokes occur with hypertensive emergencies and can be transient with symptom resolution after blood pressure control?

a) Watershed areas (border-zone regions between cerebral arteries)

709) Which antihypertensive medication used in hypertensive crises is a dual alpha-beta-blocker with a typical starting dose of 20-40mg?

a) Labetalol

710) What blood pressure medication if used chronically causes fever, fatigue, joint pains, joint swelling, and thrombocytopenia similar to lupus symptoms?

a) Hydralazine

711) What is the initial starting dose of Hydralazine?

a) 10 mg

712) Which antihypertensive medication decreases preload, dilates peripheral and pulmonary vasculature and can be used in CHF exacerbations and ACS?

a) Nitroglycerin

713) What is the initial starting dose for a Nitroglycerin infusion with ACS?
   a) 5-10 mcg/min
714) What antihypertensive medication centrally acts as an alpha-2-adrenergic agonist and has an initial starting dose of 0.1 mg?
   a) Clonidine
715) What is the initial starting dose of Phentolamine?
   a) 5-10 mg
716) What medical condition presents with a flushing, nausea, and diaphoresis followed by a transient loss of consciousness and spontaneous recovery without confusion?
   a) Syncope
717) What is the typical ED workup of syncope?
   a) CBC, BMP, EKG, Orthostatic Vitals, +/- (Urine pregnancy, CT brain, or Troponin) based on symptoms
718) List causes of syncope.
   a) Vasovagal, Neural mediated, Psychiatric, Orthostatic hypotension, Dehydration, Medications, Arrhythmias, Subclavian steal, Stroke, Infections, Aortic stenosis, AAA, Aortic dissection, PE, Ectopic pregnancy, HCM, Brugada, or MI
719) What ECG abnormalities should you look for after a syncopal episode?
   a) ST-segment change, T wave inversion, Prolonged QTc, LVH with Q waves (HCM), Saddle backed T waves (Brugada), AV blocks, and Arrhythmias
720) What is the most common cause of syncope?
   a) Vasovagal
721) Give the criteria for orthostatic hypotension based on the systolic and diastolic blood pressures.
   a) Systolic: > 20 mmHg drop
   b) Diastolic: > 10 mmHg drop
722) What positions are tested 1 min apart when performing orthostatic vitals?
   a) Lying, Sitting, and Standing
723) List the San Francisco syncope criteria for predicting high-risk patients and increased mortality.

a) CHF history
b) Hematocrit < 30%
c) EKG changes
d) Shortness of breath
e) Systolic BP < 90 mmHg at triage

724) What vascular condition presents with sudden onset extremity pain, decrease capillary refill, and pulses with skin pallor in a patient with atrial fibrillation?
a) Arterial limb ischemia

725) List the five P's associated with acute limb ischemia.
a) Pallor
b) Pain
c) Paralysis
d) Paresthesias
e) Pulselessness

726) List the different causes of arterial ischemia.
a) Embolus, Thrombus, Trauma, and Low flow states (hypovolemia, vasopressors, or heart failure)

727) What type of arterial limb ischemia presents suddenly and most commonly originates from the heart?
a) Embolism

728) What is the most common embolic cause of arterial limb ischemia?
a) Atrial fibrillation

729) What is the most common type of arterial limb ischemia that presents gradually over time due to decreased blood flow from atherosclerosis and blood vessel narrowing?
a) Thrombus

730) What physical testing can be done at the bedside to confirm peripheral arterial disease?
a) Ankle-brachial index (ABI)

731) List the definitions of the ABI for normal, moderate and severe peripheral artery disease.
a) Normal: > 0.9
b) Moderate: 0.4-0.9
c) Severe: < 0.4

732) List the vessel locations in order from most common to least common that arterial occlusions occur.
   a) 1) Femoropopliteal 2) Tibial 3) Aortoiliac 4) Brachial
733) What is the treatment for an acute arterial limb ischemia?
   a) Embolectomy (vascular consult) and Heparin
734) What treatment in addition to embolectomy and heparin is done for chronic atherosclerotic disease?
   a) Bypass
735) What are the clinical exam findings to suggest peripheral vascular disease?
   a) Hair loss on extremities, Nail thickening, Skin shimmer, Decreased pulses, and Hyperpigmented skin (hemosiderin deposits)
736) What are the triad of stasis, hypercoagulability, and endothelial damage called that leads to an increased risk of blood clot development?
   a) Virchow's triad
737) What physical exam findings suggest a deep venous thrombosis (DVT)?
   a) Calf or leg pain, Leg swelling, Erythema, or a Low-grade fever
738) What physical exam test, although insensitive, is often used for determining a DVT and is performed by squeezing the calf?
   a) Homan's sign
739) What is the clinical physical exam finding that suggests a large DVT when a patient's entire arm or leg is swollen and pale from arterial spasms?
   a) Phlegmasia alba dolens
740) What is the clinical physical exam finding that suggests a large DVT when a patient's entire arm or leg is swollen, cyanotic, and blue-purple?
   a) Phlegmasia cerulea dolens
741) What syndrome can develop due to compression of the iliac vein from to a large DVT?
   a) May-Thurner syndrome
742) What criteria is used to help determine a patient's risk for a DVT?

a) Wells criteria

743) List the Well's criteria for DVT.
   a) Active cancer
   b) Previous DVT
   c) Bedridden > 3 days or major surgery < 12 weeks
   d) Calf swelling > 3 cm compared to the opposite leg
   e) Collateral superficial veins present
   f) Entire leg swelling
   g) Localized tenderness along with the deep venous system
   h) Pitting edema
   i) Paralysis, paresis, or recent immobilization
   j) Alternative diagnosis to DVT more likely (negative points)

744) What is the greatest risk factor for a blood clot?
   a) Previous DVT

745) What lab test is performed if the patient is determined to be at low risk for a DVT and is 99% sensitive?
   a) D-Dimer

746) What imaging is most commonly performed in the ED if the patient is moderate to high risk for a DVT based on the Well's criteria or clinical gestalt, or has an elevated D-Dimer?
   a) Venous duplex ultrasound of the lower or upper extremities

747) If the initial venous duplex US is negative in a patient that is high risk what is the suggested path for follow up?
   a) Repeat venous duplex US in 1 week

748) What are the abnormal findings on a venous duplex US that suggest a DVT?
   a) Thrombus visualization
   b) Non-compressible vein (most reliable finding)
   c) Abnormal Doppler flow

749) What is an alternative imaging study that can be performed to determine the extent of a DVT and should be done if there are signs of phlegmasia cerulea or alba dolens?
   a) CT Venogram

750) If a blood clot is seen to extend into the femoral venous system what imaging should be ordered next?
   a) CT abdomen and pelvis

751) What locations of DVTs the highest risk of propagation to a PE?
   a) Popliteal and Femoral areas
752) What is the most common location of a DVT?
   a) In or proximal to the Popliteal Vein (80%)
753) What are the most common veins involved with upper extremity DVTs?
   a) Axillary and Subclavian veins
754) What is the most common cause leading to an upper extremity DVT?
   a) Iatrogenic (Port or PICC placement)
755) What is the ED treatment for an upper or lower extremity DVT?
   a) Heparin bolus and infusion (inpatient) or Oral anticoagulant (outpatient)
756) What medications can be used for outpatient treatment of a DVT?
   a) Rivaroxaban (Xarelto), Enoxaparin (Lovenox), Apixaban (Eliquis), Clopidogrel (Plavix), Warfarin (Coumadin), Dabigatran (Pradaxa), Prasugrel (Effient), or Ticagrelor (Brilinta)
757) If a DVT is shown to extend into the IVC or presents with phlegmasia alba or cerulea dolens, what is the definitive treatment?
   a) Vascular consult for embolectomy plus catheter-directed thrombolytics
758) What procedure is performed to prevent migration of DVTs to the lungs in patients with recurrent lower extremity DVT's?
   a) IVC Greenfield filter
759) What extremity complication from a DVT can occur due to severe swelling that develops causing severe leg pain, taut skin, and pain out of proportion to the exam?
   a) Compartment syndrome
760) What type of vessel ischemia develops from cholesterol emboli from plaques traveling to distal vessels causing pain and cyanosis of the digits?
   a) "Trash foot" or "Blue toe syndrome"

761) What pacemaker malfunction leads to suppression of the pacemaker causing it not to fire leading to bradycardia and syncope?

a) Pacemaker oversensing

762) What is the treatment for a defibrillator misfiring?

a) Apply magnet over defibrillator

763) What mode does the pacemaker revert to when a magnet is placed over it?

a) Asynchronous mode

Thoracic-Respiratory Disorders

764) Give a differential for shortness of breath in the emergency department.
   a) Asthma exacerbation, Acute respiratory distress syndrome, Alveolar hemorrhage, Atelectasis, Bronchitis, Cardiac tamponade, COPD exacerbation, Congestive heart failure, Infection, Lung tumor, Myocardial Infarction, Pleural effusion, Pneumonia, Pneumomediastinum, Pneumothorax, Pulmonary infarct, Pulmonary emboli (PE), or Rib fracture

765) Give the typical workup for respiratory complaints.
   a) Chest X-ray, CBC (infection), BMP (fluid overload) D-Dimer (PE), +/- ECG (chest pain), ABG (hypoxia), CT Chest with or without IV contrast

766) What lung sounds can be heard with a foreign body aspiration in the airway?
   a) Wheezing

767) What X-ray findings can be seen with a foreign body in the lower airway?
   a) Air trapping or hyperinflation

768) What specific finding on lateral decubitus chest X-ray suggests the presence of a foreign body in the lung?
   a) Failure of the dependent lung (the lung that is down) to collapse or Hyperinflation on the side of the obstruction

769) What side of the mainstem bronchi is the most common site for a foreign body obstruction in the lower airway and why?
   a) Right main stem because it is usually straighter than the left.

770) What procedure is required for removing an aspirated foreign body in the lungs?
   a) Rigid bronchoscopy

771) Give the formula for calculating the arterial-alveolar (A-a) gradient.
   a) A-a = 150 - {$PaCO_2$ / 0.8}

772) What is the range for a normal A-a gradient?
   a) 10-15 mmHg

773) What two pathophysiologies affect the A-a gradient?

a) Shunting and V/Q mismatch

774) What cardiac pathology can cause a ↑ A-a gradient due to shunting?

a) ASD

775) List the pathologies that can cause a ↑ A-a gradient from V/Q mismatch.

a) COPD, PE, or Pneumonia

776) At what level of Hb desaturation does cyanosis become present on a physical exam?

a) > 5 g/dL

777) What are the two types of cyanosis?

a) Central and peripheral

778) What chronic inflammatory lung disease seen with obesity and smoking, leads to hypoxemia with hypercapnia, pulmonary hypertension, and eventual right-side heart failure?

a) Chronic obstructive pulmonary disease (COPD)

779) What is the genetic factor increasing the risk of COPD?

a) Alpha-1 antitrypsin deficiency

780) What is the criterion used to diagnose chronic bronchitis and COPD?

a) Productive cough > 3 months in each of two consecutive years

781) List the different obstructive lung diseases within the COPD diagnosis.

a) Emphysema, Chronic bronchitis, and Asthma

782) What type of COPD patient is usually an overweight patient with SOB, increased productive cough, and chronic cyanosis on an exam?

a) "Blue bloater"

783) What lung condition is usually associated with the blue bloater patient?

a) Chronic bronchitis

784) What type of COPD patient is SOB, barrel chest, thin body habitus, hyperinflated lungs on chest X-ray, with accessory muscle use and lip pursing on the exam?

a) "Pink puffer"

785) What lung condition is more consistent with the pink puffers?

a) Emphysema

786) Why do emphysema patients purse their lips?

a) To increase peak expiratory pressure and the expiratory time

787) What are the most common causes of acute COPD exacerbation?

a) Viral and bacterial infections, and respiratory irritants

788) List the common symptom changes from baseline suggesting a COPD exacerbation.

a) Dyspnea, cough, sputum production, sputum color, wheezing, and congestion

789) What is the most common symptom complaint with a COPD exacerbation?

a) Dyspnea

790) Do COPD patients have an increased risk of PE?

a) Yes

791) What heart condition develops in COPD patients due to pulmonary hypertension from chronic hypoxia?

a) Cor pulmonale

792) What are the only two disease altering interventions proven to decrease mortality in a COPD patient?

a) Smoking cessation and Home Oxygen

793) What chronic inflammatory respiratory disease is from bronchospasm, inflammation, and mucous plugs that cause acute shortness of breath (SOB)?

a) Asthma

794) List some precipitants that can cause an asthma exacerbation.

a) URI (most common), Allergies, Infection, Exercise, Beta-blockers, ASA or NSAIDS, or Aerosolized irritants

795) List the three conditions seen with atopic syndrome associated with asthma.

a) Atopic dermatitis, Allergic rhinitis, and Allergic asthma

796) What is Samter's triad?

a) Asthma, Aspirin/NSAIDs sensitivity, and Nasal polyps

797) What type of asthma presents after participating in a sporting activity?

a) Exercised induced asthma

798) List the different types of asthma.
   a) Adult-onset, Allergic Asthma, Asthma-COPD Overlap, Exercise Induced Asthma, Non-Allergic Asthma, and Occupational Asthma
799) What asthma classification is defined as < 2 episodes weekly, < 2 nightly episodes, and no symptoms between attacks?
   a) Intermittent
800) What asthma classification is defined as > 2 weekly attacks, 3-4 nightly attacks a month, interrupts daily activities, with a FeV1 > 80?
   a) Mild persistent
801) What asthma classification is defined as daily attacks, > 1 nightly attack a week, and daily rescue inhaler use, with a FeV1< 80?
   a) Moderate persistent
802) What asthma classification is defined as frequent attacks, daytime symptoms, rescue inhaler use > 1x daily, with a FeV1 < 60?
   a) Severe persistent
803) List factors associated with increased mortality/morbidity in asthma.
   a) Overuse of inhalers, Prior intubation, Prior ICU admissions, > 2 ED visits in a month, Poverty, Chronic use of steroids, Drug use, Poor follow up, and Recurrent exacerbations
804) What are the two pathognomonic pathology findings with asthma?
   a) Curschmann spirals and Charcot-Leyden crystals
805) What is the 1st line treatment for asthma and COPD exacerbations?
   a) Beta-2 agonists (Albuterol)
806) What are the side effects of using a beta-2 agonist?
   a) Tachycardia and Anxiety
807) What beta-2 agonist medication other that Albuterol can be given to limit reflex tachycardia for an asthma exacerbation with significant tachycardia?
   a) Levalbuterol (Xopenex)
808) What other inhaled medication can be combined with albuterol to treat in asthma or COPD exacerbations?
   a) Ipratropium bromide (anticholinergic)

809) What medication can be administered to decrease inflammation in asthma and COPD exacerbations and has a delayed effect?
a) Steroids

810) Is there any difference in the efficacy of oral verse IV steroid administration in asthma or COPD exacerbations?
a) No, they have similar effects

811) What medication, relaxes smooth muscle, and can be administered in refractor asthma or COPD exacerbations in the ED?
a) Magnesium (1-2 g over 10 min)

812) What gas can help in refractory asthma exacerbation?
a) Heliox (80:20 or 70:30)

813) Can epinephrine be used in asthma exacerbation?
a) Yes (0.3 mg of 1:1,000 IM)

814) What medications are used for long-term asthma treatment?
a) Long-acting beta-2 agonist (Salmeterol)

815) What Leukotriene receptor blockers are used for long-term asthma treatment?
a) Montelukast and Zafirlukast

816) What is the long-acting medication used to treat COPD and prevent exacerbations?
a) Tiotropium bromide

817) What is the recommended treatment plan for a COPD exacerbation at discharge?
a) Inhaled beta agonists, Steroids, and Antibiotics

818) Why are antibiotics recommended in COPD exacerbations?
a) To decrease inflammation and treat for possible bacterial causes

819) List the medication classes used in COPD exacerbations.
a) Fluoroquinolones, Macrolides, or Doxycycline

820) What type of shock can occur with an acute asthma exacerbation with air trapping leading to increased intrathoracic pressure and decreased venous return?
a) Obstructive shock

821) How do you correct obstructive shock, air trapping, and barotrauma in an asthmatic or COPD patient on a BIPAP or a ventilator?
   a) Remove ventilator, External chest compression, and Bilateral chest tubes

822) What ventilator settings can be adjusted to help prevent barotrauma and air trapping in asthmatic and COPD patients?
   a) Increased expiratory time/phase

823) What bedside testing can be used to help determine if the patient is safe for discharge?
   a) Peak flow (based on age, height, and sex)

824) What is the peak flow percent goal of improvement for the predicted values in adults and children after an asthma exacerbation?
   a) 40% in adults and 70% in children

825) What sedation medication is recommended in asthma or COPD exacerbations that may require conscious sedation and intubation?
   a) Ketamine

826) Give the non-invasive ventilation treatment that can be used for COPD and asthma patients who fail to improve with breathing treatments.
   a) BIPAP

827) List the contraindications to noninvasive positive pressure ventilation (BIPAP/CPAP).
   a) Arrest, Altered mental status, Facial trauma, Unable to protect the airway, Unable to clear secretions, Upper GI bleed, and Unstable vitals

828) What lab testing can be done to evaluate treatment failure in asthma or COPD exacerbations initially after starting BIPAP?
   a) Arterial blood gas (ABG)

829) What lab changes on ABG indicate BIPAP treatment failure and suggests the need for intubation and ventilator treatment?
   a) ↓PaO_2 or ↑$PaCO_2$

830) What acute lung condition develops due to sepsis, trauma, pulmonary edema, CNS depression, aspiration, and overdoses and is defined as respiratory failure, with hypoxia $PaO_2 < 60$ mmHg?

a) Acute respiratory distress syndrome (ARDS)

831) What are the typical findings on chest X-ray seen with ARDS?
   a) Diffuse bilateral interstitial infiltrates

832) List the PaO_2/FiO_2 ratios associated with the different levels of mild, moderate and severe ARDS.
   a) Mild: 200 - 300
   b) Moderate: 100 - 200
   c) Severe: < 100

833) What pediatric lung condition presents with diffuse wheezing, respiratory distress with a viral URI in a 2-year-old?
   a) Bronchiolitis

834) What is the main infectious cause of bronchiolitis?
   a) Respiratory syncytial virus (RSV)

835) What are the recommended treatments for RSV bronchiolitis?
   a) Steroids
   b) Beta-2 agonist (Now falling out of favor)

836) What is the most common cause of pneumonia?
   a) Aspiration

837) What bacteria is the most common cause of pneumonia?
   a) Streptococcus pneumoniae

838) Describe the findings of streptococcus pneumoniae on gram stain.
   a) Gram-positive diplococci

839) What kind of sputum is seen with Streptococcus pneumonia?
   a) Rust-colored

840) What bacteria typically causes pneumonia in alcoholics, and has brown "currant jelly" sputum with cough?
   a) Klebsiella pneumoniae

841) What are the common chest X-ray findings seen with Klebsiella pneumoniae?
   a) Upper lobe infiltrate with a bulging fissure

842) Described the findings of Chlamydia on gram stain.
   a) Gram-negative rods

843) What bacteria typically causes pneumonia in hospitalized patients and causes a patchy multi-lobar infiltrate with a sweet green odorized sputum?

a) Pseudomonas

844) Described the findings of Pseudomonas on gram stain.

   a) Gram-negative rods

845) What type of bacteria typically cause pneumonia in alcoholics and in a patient who aspirated?

   a) Anaerobes (oral bacteria)

846) What is the common chest X-ray finding seen with aspiration pneumonia in an upright patient?

   a) Right lower lobe infiltrate

847) What is the common chest X-ray finding seen with aspiration pneumonia in a recumbent patient (intubated or found down)?

   a) Right upper posterior lobe infiltrate

848) List the conditions that increase the risk of aspiration.

   a) Altered mental status, Drug and alcohol use, Mental retardation, Stroke, Seizure, or Poor dentition

849) What does ENT suggest to be the most common cause of chronic aspiration?

   a) GERD

850) What is the PH level found with bronchoscopy with aspiration pneumonia?

   a) < 2.5

851) What are typical antibiotics used for aspiration pneumonia and anaerobic coverage?

   a) Metronidazole, Clindamycin, Piperacillin/Tazobactam, Ampicillin/Sulbactam, Levofloxacin, and Carbapenems

852) What bacteria are commonly seen to cause lung abscesses?

   a) Fusobacterium, Bacteroides, Klebsiella, Staph aureus, and Pseudomonas

853) What is the antibiotic drug of choice for lung abscesses?

   a) Clindamycin

854) What type of bacteria commonly causes pneumonia in IVDU and post-viral infections, and leads to cavitary lung abscesses?

   a) Staphylococcus aureus

855) Described the findings of Staph. aureus on gram stain.

   a) Gram-positive cocci in clusters

856) What is the sputum like with lung abscesses?

a) Fetid and bloody

857) What antibiotics are recommended for a Staph induced pneumonia?

a) Vancomycin or Nafcillin

858) What pneumonia classification type should be suspected with bilateral infiltrates, treatment failure, and chronic cough for a 3-4 week period?

a) Atypical pneumonia

859) What bacteria are classified as causing atypical pneumonia?

a) Mycoplasma, Chlamydia pneumoniae, Chlamydia psittacosis, and Legionella

860) What bacteria typically causes walking pneumonia, with a chronic cough, bullous myringitis, and bilateral patchy infiltrates on chest X-ray?

a) Mycoplasma

861) What musculoskeletal condition can coincide with a Mycoplasma infection?

a) Guillain-Barre'

862) What type of specific antibodies/agglutinins develop in a Mycoplasma infection and can be tested?

a) Cold agglutinins

863) What typical bacteria is seen in elderly patients with cough, fever, diarrhea, vomiting, elevated liver enzymes who uses a window air conditioning unit?

a) Legionella pneumophilia

864) What pathognomonic electrolyte abnormality can occur in a Legionella infection?

a) Hyponatremia

865) How is Legionella typically transmitted?

a) Inhaling aerosolized water droplets containing the bacteria

866) What tests are available for confirming Legionella?

a) Urine antigen test, Serum antibody, and Sputum culture

867) What bacteria typically causes a chronic staccato cough, fever, and conjunctivitis in an infant?

a) Chlamydia pneumoniae

868) Describe the findings of Chlamydia on gram stain.

a)   Gram-negative and intracellular

869)   What type of bacteria is seen in a patient with chronic cough, intermittent epistaxis and failed antibiotic treatment, who works with birds?

a)   Chlamydia psittacosis

870)   What are the antibiotics used for treating outpatient atypical pneumonia?

a)   Macrolides and Doxycycline

871)   What is the lab finding on gram stain with Hemophilus influenza?

a)   Gram-negative encapsulated coccobacillus

872)   What bacteria is associated with severe recurrent paroxysmal coughs, followed by stridorous inspiration and coughing and elevated WBC 25-50,000?

a)   Bordetella pertussis (whooping cough)

873)   What are the three stages are associated with pertussis?

a)   Catarrhal, Paroxysmal, and Convalescent

874)   In what stage of pertussis is it recommended to treat?

a)   Catarrhal

875)   What antibiotics are recommended for pertussis treatment?

a)   Erythromycin or TMP-SMX

876)   What are other causes of atypical pneumonia?

a)   Viral, Coxiella burnetii, and Fungal

877)   What bacteria causes an atypical pneumonia with cough, fever, and shortness of breath in farmers working with animals and can lead to hepatitis?

a)   Coxiella burnetii (Q fever)

878)   What antibiotics are used for Q fever?

a)   Doxycycline or Macrolides

879)   What type of fungal infection is from dirt in the Southwest US and causes cough, fever, erythema nodosum, and bilateral infiltrates and hilar adenopathy on chest X-ray?

a)   Coccidioidomycosis

880)   What type of fungal infection is seen in caves with bat feces in the Mississippi River valley, and causes cough, fever, and bilateral infiltrates on chest X-ray?

a) Histoplasmosis

881) What type of fungal infection seen in the Southeast US and causes cough, fever, ulcers, blisters, and bilateral infiltrates on chest X-ray?

a) Blastomycosis

882) What is the medication treatment for fungal pneumonia?

a) Itraconazole

883) What bacteria is suspected with a right upper lobe cavitary lesion and infiltrate, with hematemesis and fever in an immunocompromised patient or immigrant?

a) Mycobacterium tuberculosis (TB)

884) Define which types of TB affects the upper lobes and the middle lobes?

a) Upper lobe infection: Reactivation TB

b) Middle lobe infection: Primary TB

885) List the most common infectious causes of pneumonia in patients < 4 weeks old and give the antibiotic treatment.

a) < 4 weeks: Group B streptococcus, E.coli, Listeria (Baby "B.E.L.")

b) Treatment: Ampicillin + (Gentamycin or Cefotaxime)

886) What are the most common infectious causes of pneumonia in patients 1 mon-4 years old?

a) RSV, Influenza, Parainfluenza, Strep pneumonia, Chlamydia trachomatis, and Chlamydia pneumonia

887) What is the inpatient antibiotic treatment for bacterial pneumonia in patients 1 mon-4 years old?

a) Ampicillin + Cefotaxime

888) What are the most common infectious causes of pneumonia in patients 5-18 years old?

a) 5-18 years: RSV, Step pneumonia, Mycoplasma, and Chlamydia

889) What is the outpatient treatment for bacterial pneumonia in patients 5-18 years old?

a) Macrolides

890) What are the most common infectious causes of pneumonia in patients 18-65 years old?

a) Step pneumonia, Mycoplasma, H. Influenza, and Viruses

891) What are the most common infectious causes of pneumonia in patients > 65 years old?
   a) Strep pneumonia, Influenza, Anaerobes, Gram-negative rods, and H. Influenza
892) Which antibiotics can be used for outpatient treatment for bacterial pneumonia in patients > 18 years old?
   a) Fluoroquinolones, Macrolides, or Doxycycline
893) List the criteria for diagnosing hospital-acquired pneumonia (HAP).
   a) > 48 hours after admission
894) List the criteria for diagnosing healthcare-acquired pneumonia (HCAP).
   a) Hospitalization > 48 hours in past 90 days, Received IV antibiotics in the last 30 days, Nursing home resident, or Chronic dialysis
895) What is the criteria for diagnosing ventilator-acquired pneumonia (VAP)?
   a) New infection > 48 hours after intubation
896) List the bacteria commonly associated with HAP and HCAP.
   a) MRSA, MSSA, Pseudomonas, Strep pneumoniae and Acinetobacter
897) Give the inpatient medication treatment recommendations for community acquired pneumonia.
   a) Third generation Cephalosporin (Ceftriaxone) + Macrolide (Azithromycin) or Fluoroquinolone (Levofloxacin)
898) Give the inpatient medication treatment recommendations for HAP and HCAP.
   a) Cefepime or Ceftazidime or Piperacillin/Tazobactam + Macrolide (Azithromycin) or Fluoroquinolone (Levofloxacin) +/- Vancomycin or Linezolid (MRSA coverage)
899) What alternative medications are used for hospital/healthcare-acquired pneumonia with a penicillin allergy?
   a) Aztreonam, Gentamycin, or Levofloxacin + Azithromycin +/- Vancomycin or Linezolid

900) What lung complication can occur with failed pneumonia treatment, or an infected pleural effusion, and presents with fever, chills, back pain, and dyspnea?
   a) Empyema
901) What bacteria is most commonly associated with empyema?
   a) Staphylococcus
902) What are the typical findings of empyema on chest X-ray?
   a) Air fluid level in effusion or crossing fissures, or a loculated effusion
903) What is the treatment for empyema?
   a) Drainage and Antibiotics
904) What is the chest X-ray finding seen with atelectasis from volume loss?
   a) Elevated diaphragm
905) What are the most common viruses that cause cold symptoms?
   a) Coronavirus and Rhinovirus
906) What common virus presents with cough, sore throat, rhinitis, and conjunctivitis?
   a) Adenovirus
907) What type of virus comes from mice feces in the Southwest US and causes pulmonary edema, cough, fever, and progresses to cardiac and renal failure?
   a) Hantavirus
908) What is the treatment recommended for Hantavirus pulmonary syndrome?
   a) Supportive
909) What type of Asian form of the Coronavirus from aerosolized fecal material can lead to death?
   a) Severe acute respiratory syndrome (SARS)
910) What is the most common lung infection seen in AIDS patients?
   a) Pneumocystis carinii pneumoniae (PCP)
911) What is the treatment for PCP infection in AIDS patients?
   a) TMP/SMX, Pentamidine, or Dapsone, +/- Steroids
912) What are the indications to treat PCP with steroids?
   a) PaO_2 < 70 mmHg or A-a gradient > 35

913) What are other infectious causes of common lung infections in AIDS patients?
   a) TB, CMV, Mycobacterium avium complex (MAC), Fungi (Cryptococcus)
914) What virus most commonly leads to pneumonia in transplant patients 1-3 months out?
   a) CMV
915) List the different decision tools for risk stratification for outpatient verse inpatient treatment for pneumonia.
   a) CURB-65 and Pneumonia severity index
916) List the criteria used in CURB-65.
   a) Confusion
   b) BUN > 19
   c) Respiratory rate > 30
   d) SBP < 90 or DBP < 60
   e) Age > 65
917) What lung emergency can occur suddenly from a ruptured bleb in a COPD patient causing hypoxia, shortness of breath and chest pain?
   a) Pneumothorax
918) List causes of spontaneous pneumothorax.
   a) Valsalva, COPD, Asthma, Neoplasm, Pneumonia, Cystic fibrosis, and Marfan's
919) List the imaging modalities that can diagnose a pneumothorax.
   a) Chest X-ray, Chest CT or Chest Ultrasound
920) What type of chest X-ray is the most sensitive to finding a pneumothorax?
   a) Expiratory chest X-ray
921) What is the recommended treatment for pneumothorax < 15 - 20%?
   a) Non Rebreather mask at 15 L oxygen and observation
922) What is the recommended treatment for pneumothorax > 15 - 20%?
   a) Chest tube with water seal suction or a Heimlich valve
923) What lung emergency can occur from a traumatic penetrating injury to the chest causing shortness of breath, dilated neck veins,

tracheal deviation, hypotension and a mediastinal shift on chest X-ray?

a) Tension pneumothorax

924) What is the immediate treatment for tension pneumothorax?

a) 16 or 18 gauge needle in 2nd rib space or 5th intercostal space

925) Is it recommended to wait for a chest X-ray to confirm a tension pneumothorax before needle decompression?

a) No

926) What is the recommended 2nd line treatment if needle decompression fails to immediately relieve a tension pneumothorax?

a) Insert a chest tube

927) What location is recommended for chest tube placement when treating a pneumothorax?

a) 4-5th intercostal space mid-to-anterior axillary line

928) Why is it recommended to make the opening skin cut for a chest tube over the rib bone and not on the inferior part?

a) Due to intercostal vessels and nerves

929) During respiratory distress due to a pneumothorax is it recommended to intubate or place a chest tube first?

a) Chest tube first followed by intubation

930) Why does a chest tube need to be placed for a pneumothorax before aeromedical transport?

a) Concern for expanding pneumothorax

931) What are the indications for obtaining cardiothoracic consult for a possible thoracotomy in a patient with a pneumothorax and a chest tube?

a) Persistent air leak or Unstable

932) What are the lung complications of a re-expanding pneumothorax?

a) Pulmonary edema, Bronchopleural fistula, and Pneumomediastinum

933) What type of lung complication needs to be evaluated with continuous bubbling seen in the chest tube after placement?

a) Bronchopleural fistula

934) Describe the chest X-ray findings with a pneumothorax.

a) Medially displaced visceral pleural line, Loss of peripheral lung vascular markings, and Deep sulcus sign when supine

935) Describe the chest ultrasound findings with a pneumothorax.

a) Loss of lung sliding, Loss of comet-tail artifact, and Barcode sign on M-mode

936) What lung condition if very large can mimic a pneumothorax on chest X-ray?

a) Bleb

937) What medical condition can occur from trauma or esophageal rupture and causes chest pain, dyspnea, and subcutaneous emphysema in the chest wall and neck?

a) Pneumomediastinum

938) What is the name of the crunching sound heard over the heart with each heartbeat and is associated with a pneumomediastinum?

a) Hamman's crunch

939) What is the chest X-ray finding with pneumomediastinum?

a) Gas outlining the pericardium, bronchial wall, pulmonary arteries, and aorta, or Subcutaneous air

940) What life-threatening condition can occur from a pneumomediastinum and presents with hypotension and JVD?

a) Tension pneumomediastinum

941) What can occur in the mediastinum with a spreading infection from the head or neck?

a) Mediastinitis

942) How much fluid is needed to be seen on a decubitus chest X-ray with a pleural effusion?

a) 150-200 cc

943) What size measurement of a pleural effusion on a lateral decubitus X-ray indicates a significant effusion?

a) > 1 cm

944) What is the name of the criteria to determine whether the pleural effusion is transudative or exudative?

a) Light's criteria

945) What type of pleural effusion has a pleural: serum protein ratio of < 0.5, pleural: serum LDH < 0.6, a pleural fluid LDH < 200 IU/ml, and pleural protein < 3 gm/dL?

    a) Transudate effusion

946) List the main causes of transudative effusions.
    a) CHF, Cirrhosis, Nephrotic syndrome, Myxedema, and Hypoproteinemia

947) What is the pathophysiology of a transudate effusion?
    a) ↑Hydrostatic pressure or ↓ Oncotic pressure

948) What is the most common cause of a transudative effusion?
    a) CHF

949) What type of pleural effusion has a pleural: serum protein ratio of > 0.5, pleural: serum LDH > 0.6 and a pleural fluid LDH > 2/3 upper normal (or > 200 IU/ml)?
    a) Exudate effusion

950) List the main causes of exudative effusions.
    a) Malignancy, Pneumonia, TB, PE, Pancreatitis, Esophageal rupture, Vascular disease, Uremia, or Hemothorax

951) What is the most common cause of an exudative effusion?
    a) Infection

952) What procedure can be performed to treat a malignant pleural effusion with respiratory distress, hypoxia, and hypotension?
    a) Thoracentesis or Chest tube placement

953) What is the maximum amount of pleural fluid that is suggested to be removed with a thoracentesis in the ED?
    a) 1500 ml

954) What is the most common cause of pleural effusions?
    a) CHF

955) List the five T's of mediastinal masses.
    a) Thymoma
    b) Teratoma
    c) T cell lymphoma
    d) Thyroid
    e) Thoracic Aorta (dilated or aneurysm)

956) What is the most common mediastinal mass?
    a) Bronchogenic carcinoma

957) List the causes of hemoptysis.
    a) Bronchitis, Pneumonia, Neoplastic, TB, Mycetoma, PE, hemopneumothorax, and Vasculitis

958) What is the most common cause of hemoptysis?
  a) Bronchitis
959) What lung condition should be suspected in a patient > 50 years old with a smoking history, who presents with hemoptysis, weight loss, and a chronic cough?
  a) Lung cancer
960) What amount of hemoptysis is classified as minor?
  a) < 20 mL in 24 hours
961) What amount of hemoptysis is classified as massive?
  a) > 500-600 mL in 24 hours
  b) > 100 mL of blood an hour
  c) > 50 mL per cough
962) What is the most common cause of death with massive hemoptysis?
  a) Asphyxiation
963) What is the first interventional treatment with massive hemoptysis?
  a) Intubation (protect the airway)
964) If there is left side hemoptysis what is recommended when intubating?
  a) Selective mainstem intubation on the right
965) What position do you lay the patient with massive hemoptysis?
  a) Bleeding side down
966) What procedures are required to treat massive hemoptysis?
  a) Bronchoscopy and artery embolization (interventional radiology)
967) What other sources of bleeding need to be considered with hemoptysis?
  a) GI and Nasopharynx
968) What lung emergency presents with pleuritic chest pain that is worse with breathing, and associated dyspnea, tachycardia, tachypnea, and a syncope episode in a post-operative patient?
  a) Pulmonary emboli (PE)
969) Where do most PE's arise?
  a) Deep venous system in the legs

970) List the three criteria of Virchow's triad associated with an increase in clotting risk.
   a) Stasis
   b) Endothelial damage
   c) Hypercoagulability
971) What is the most common complaint with PEs?
   a) Dyspnea
972) What is the most common physical exam finding with a PE?
   a) Tachypnea
973) List the risk factors for developing a PE.
   a) Cancer, Hormone therapy, Pregnancy, Lupus, HIV, Immobilization, CHF, COPD, Trauma, Surgery, Hypercoagulable disorders, and Smoking
974) List some hypercoagulable disorders that increase the risk of a PE.
   a) Factor V Leiden, Protein C, and S deficiency, Antithrombin III deficiency, Factor XII deficiency, Prothrombin 2021A mutation, Hyperhomocysteinemia, and Plasminogen deficiency
975) What are the four clinical criteria lists used to determine the probability of a PE?
   a) Well's, PERC, Geneva, and Charlotte
976) List the criteria that makeup Well's criteria for a PE.
   a) Signs of a DVT
   b) PE #1 diagnostic criteria
   c) HR ≥ 100
   d) Immobilization > 3 days
   e) Surgery within 4 weeks
   f) Previous PE or DVT
   g) Hemoptysis
   h) Malignancy
977) List the PERC criteria for a PE.
   a) Age ≥ 50
   b) HR ≥ 100
   c) Hormone use
   d) Prior PE or DVT
   e) Recent surgery or trauma

f) Hemoptysis

g) Unilateral leg swelling

h) SaO₂ on room air < 95%

978) What is the imaging of choice for diagnosing PE?

    a) CT pulmonary arteries (CTPA)

979) What is an imaging modality can be used to help diagnose a PE in pregnant patients and patients with a contrast or iodine allergy?

    a) Ventilation-perfusion lung scan (VQ scan)

980) What is the sensitivity of ruling out a PE with a normal VQ scan?

    a) 99%

981) What percentage of V/Q scans are non-diagnostic?

    a) 75%

982) What lab test is used to help rule out a PE and has a 99% negative predictive value in a low probability patient?

    a) D-Dimer

983) In what patient population is a D-Dimer used?

    a) Low pretest probability

984) List the pathologies that can give a false positive elevated D-Dimer.

    a) Trauma, Pregnancy, Recent surgery, Infection, Stroke, and MI

985) Is imaging required for a patient with a low pretest probability for a PE and a negative D-Dimer?

    a) No

986) What imaging is required for a patient with a low-moderate pretest probability for a PE and a positive D-Dimer?

    a) CTPA

987) What is the plan of care for a patient with a high pretest probability for PE?

    a) CTPA

988) What is the rate of false-positive PE's found on CTA?

    a) Around 40%

989) What is the most common EKG change seen with PEs?

    a) Tachycardia

990) List other EKG findings that can be seen with PE.

    a) Nonspecific ST-segment changes, S1Q3T3, Inverted T waves, RBBB, and Right axis deviation

991) What are the chest X-ray findings that can be seen with a PE?
   a) Pleural based wedge infarction (Hampton's hump)
   b) Decreased vascularity distal to PE (Westermark's sign)
   c) Cut off pulmonary arteries (Fleischner's sign)
992) What are the medications used to treat a PE?
   a) Heparin, Rivaroxaban, Apixaban, Warfarin, or Enoxaparin
993) Is it possible to have a recurrent PE while on anticoagulation?
   a) Yes
994) What are the IV Heparin bolus and infusion dosing for a PE?
   a) 80 units/kg bolus followed by 18 units/kg infusion
995) What is the Enoxaparin dosing for treating a DVT or PE?
   a) 1 mg/kg BID
996) What is the medication used for massive PE with hypotension, right heart strain on CT, elevated troponin, and EKG changes?
   a) Alteplase (TPA)
997) What is the TPA dosing for a massive PE?
   a) 100 mg IV
998) What surgical treatment options are available for PE?
   a) Catheter-directed thrombolysis or Embolectomy
999) What can be placed to prevent further PEs in a patient with recurrent PE's?
   a) Greenfield IVC filter
1000) Is it still possible to get a PE with a Greenfield filter?
   a) Yes
1001) What lung condition can develop in a patient working with chemicals such as ammonia or bleach and leads to dyspnea?
   a) Chemical pneumonitis
1002) What life-threatening condition can occur with a recently placed tracheostomy tube?
   a) Tracheoinnominate fistula
1003) What artery lies adjacent to the tracheostomy?
   a) Innominate artery

1004) What are the recommended 1st and 2nd line ways to stop a tracheoinnominate fistula bleed?

a) 1st line: Hyperinflate the tracheostomy balloon

b) 2nd line: Direct pressure with your finger against the back of the sternum

Gastroenterology

1005) Give a brief emergency medicine differential diagnosis for abdominal pain.

    a) Heart attack, Abdominal Aortic Aneurysm (AAA), Cholangitis, Choledocholithiasis, Cholecystitis, Biliary colic, Esophageal rupture, Esophagitis, Peptic ulcer disease (PUD), Gastritis, Pancreatitis, Hepatitis, Hepatic abscess, Splenic thrombosis/rupture, Mesenteric ischemia, Bowel obstruction, Bowel perforation, Diverticulitis, Appendicitis, Incarcerated hernia, Hepatitis, Hepatic abscess, Ectopic pregnancy, Ovarian torsion, Testicular torsion, Tuboovarian Abscess, Pelvic inflammatory disease, UTI, Acute Urinary Retention, Hydronephrosis, Kidney stone, Pyelonephritis, Inflammatory bowel disease, etc.

1006) Give the typical workup for a patient presenting with abdominal pain.

    a) CBC, BMP, LFTs, UA, Lipase, Lactate, Pregnancy test (all reproductive females), +/- Abdominal series X-ray, CT Abdomen & Pelvis with or without contrast, Renal US, Right Upper Quadrant US, or ECG (ACS)

1007) What type of abdominal pain is poorly localized, diffuse, and comes from nerve fibers in solid organs and intestinal walls?

    a) Visceral

1008) What type of abdominal pain is well localized and comes from nerve fibers in the peritoneum and is the primary type of pain contributing to rebound tenderness?

    a) Somatic

1009) List the alarming features in patients that warrant an endoscopy referral.

    a) Upper GI bleed, Anemia, Weight loss, Epigastric mass, Dysphagia, Early Satiety, Jaundice, Persistent vomiting, or Anorexia

1010) What lab is required for all childbearing aged females presenting with abdominal pain?

    a) Pregnancy test

1011)   What abdominal condition presents with RUQ abdominal pain that is worse after eating, fever, nausea, and vomiting with an elevated WBC?
   a)   Cholecystitis
1012)   What abdominal condition presents with RUQ and epigastric intermittent sharp stabbing pain abdominal pain that is worse after eating fried or fatty foods and causes nausea and vomiting?
   a)   Biliary colic
1013)   What is the most common cause of a surgical abdomen in an elderly patient?
   a)   Cholecystitis
1014)   What type of cholecystitis is more commonly seen in pregnant, pediatric, septic, trauma, or post-op patients, presents with biliary sludge and a distended gallbladder on US and can lead to a gallbladder rupture?
   a)   Acalculous cholecystitis
1015)   What bacteria are typically involved in gallbladder infections?
   a)   E. coli or Klebsiella (most commonly); also Streptococcus, Enterococcus, and Clostridia
1016)   What physical exam finding and sign is sensitive for cholecystitis and is RUQ pain with palpation causing a sudden cessation of inspiration?
   a)   Murphy's sign
1017)   What imaging modality is the most sensitive in diagnosing cholecystitis?
   a)   Ultrasound (right upper quadrant)
1018)   What ultrasound findings are indicative of cholecystitis?
   a)   Sonographic Murphy's sign with presence of gallstones are most sensitive findings
   b)   Gallbladder wall > 3 mm
   c)   Pericholecystic fluid
   d)   Sludge in the gallbladder
   e)   Distended gallbladder > 10 cm in length x 4 cm in width
1019)   What imaging studies need to be performed if there are signs of cholecystitis with elevated liver enzymes?
   a)   CT abdomen and pelvis with IV contrast, ERCP, or MRCP

1020) What imaging study is used to assess gallbladder function and is also sensitive for diagnosing acute cholecystitis?

a) Hepatobiliary scintigraphy (HIDA)

1021) What type of pathology does a calcified gallbladder found on US or CT suggest?

a) Gallbladder cancer

1022) What type of cholecystitis infection rapidly spread due to gas-forming bacteria and is diagnosed by gas seen in the gallbladder walls on CT or US?

a) Emphysematous cholecystitis

1023) What is the treatment of cholecystitis?

a) Antibiotics and Surgery (cholecystectomy)

1024) What are the two types of gallbladder stones?

a) Cholesterol stones (most common), and Pigment (bilirubin)

1025) What type of gallbladder stone is radiolucent?

a) Cholesterol

1026) What at the five F's associated with cholelithiasis?

a) Female, Fat, Forty, Fertile, and Fair

1027) What are the management options available for asymptomatic gallstones?

a) Clinical follow-up, Lithotripsy, Medication induced breakdown, or Prophylactic cholecystectomy

1028) What type of life-threatening infection spreads through the biliary tree and leads to fever, jaundice, and RUQ pain, with sepsis and shock?

a) Ascending cholangitis

1029) What is the triad called for fever, jaundice, and RUQ pain found with cholangitis?

a) Charcot's triad

1030) What five criteria make up Reynold's pentad with cholangitis?

a) RUQ pain, Fever, Jaundice, Shock, and Altered mental status

1031) What are the common etiologies leading to ascending cholangitis?

a) Malignancy, Sclerosis or stenosis, and Choledocholithiasis

1032) What is the most common etiology leading to ascending cholangitis?

a) Choledocholithiasis

1033) What imaging modalities are commonly used to diagnose ascending cholangitis?
a) ERCP, MRCP, CT with IV contrast, and US

1034) What is the management for cholangitis?
a) Broad-spectrum antibiotics, GI consultation for ERCP and possible biliary stenting, and Surgical consultation for cholecystotomy

1035) What imaging modalities can diagnose choledocholithiasis?
a) RUQ Ultrasound, CT abdomen and pelvis with IV contrast, ERCP, MRCP, and CT cholangiography

1036) What complications can occur with a passing gallstone?
a) Choledocholithiasis, Cholangitis, Gallstone ileus, and Pancreatitis

1037) What is the recommended treatment for choledocholithiasis?
a) ERCP

1038) What syndrome, causing an obstructive jaundice presentation, develops due to compression of the common hepatic duct by a gallbladder or cystic duct stone
a) Mirizzi syndrome

1039) What abdominal infection causes umbilical pain that migrates to the RLQ, fever, nausea, and vomiting, with a decreased appetite?
a) Appendicitis

1040) What is the most common cause of a surgical abdomen?
a) Appendicitis

1041) What is the study of choice to diagnose appendicitis in adults?
a) CT abdomen and pelvis with IV contrast +/- oral contrast based on body habitus.

1042) What findings on an abdominal X-ray can suggest appendicitis?
a) Appendicolith

1043) What abdominal pathology is the most common abdominal disorder requiring surgery in pediatrics?
a) Appendicitis

1044) What is the most common symptom of appendicitis?
a) RLQ pain

1045) What physical exam finding in the right lower quadrant has a high positive predictive value in appendicitis?

a) Tenderness (McBurney's sign)

1046) What physical exam finding with appendicitis is defined as referred RLQ pain with LLQ palpation?

a) Rovsing's sign

1047) What physical exam finding with appendicitis is defined as RLQ pain with right thigh extension while the patient is laying on the left side?

a) Psoas sign

1048) What physical exam finding with appendicitis is defined as RLQ pain when the right thigh is flexed and internally rotated?

a) Obturator sign

1049) Can appendicitis also present with diarrhea and or have pyuria on the UA?

a) Yes

1050) What patient may have atypical symptoms with appendicitis, such as RUQ pain and back pain?

a) Pregnant patients and Patients with a retrocecal appendix

1051) What is the management of appendicitis?

a) Antibiotics and surgical consultation for appendectomy

1052) What GI pathology presents with LLQ abdominal pain, nausea, vomiting, rectal bleeding, and constipation +/- a fever in patients with diverticulosis history.

a) Diverticulitis

1053) What is the imaging study of choice for diagnosing diverticulitis?

a) CT IV contrast abdomen and pelvis

1054) Is a colonoscopy recommended as part of the workup and treatment of diverticulitis?

a) No (contraindicated due to risk of perforation)

1055) What do you treat uncomplicated diverticulitis with?

a) Antibiotics (Ciprofloxacin and Metronidazole), Pain medications, +/- IV fluids

1056) List indications for admitting patients with diverticulitis.

a) Abscess, Anemia, Perforation, Unable to tolerate PO, Uncontrolled pain, or Failed outpatient antibiotic therapy

1057) What GI complications can occur with diverticulitis?

a) Abscess, Perforation, and GI bleed

1058) What is the treatment for diverticulitis with a colonic abscess?

a) Surgery and Broad-spectrum antibiotics

1059) What condition presents with sudden onset sharp intermittent colicky flank pains, with urinary urgency, blood in urine, nausea, and vomiting?

a) Kidney stone

1060) What abdominal emergency presents with sudden onset mid-abdomen and flank pain in a male patient > 60 years old with syncope, a pulsatile abdominal mass, and hypotension?

a) Abdominal Aortic Aneurysm (AAA)

1061) What is the most common location AAA's occur?

a) Infrarenal

1062) What is the most common misdiagnosis made for an AAA?

a) Renal colic

1063) List the risk factors for AAA.

a) Smoking, > 60 years old, Hypertension, Hyperlipidemia, Atherosclerosis, Diabetes, or Connective tissue disease

1064) What is the most common risk factor of an AAA?

a) Atherosclerosis

1065) What can be heard over the abdomen with the bell of the stethoscope in a patient with an AAA?

a) Bruit

1066) Rectal bleeding in a patient with an AAA repair history, is a concern for which abdominal emergency?

a) Aortoenteric fistula

1067) What blood vessel can an AAA also erode into?

a) IVC

1068) What bedside study can confirm an AAA in the ED in an unstable patient?

a) Abdominal US

1069) What are the findings on abdominal US that suggest an AAA?

a) Aorta > 3 cm

1070) What is the average rate of aneurysmal dilation in an AAA per year?

    a) 0.25-0.5 cm per year

1071) What is the preferred imaging study to diagnose an AAA in a stable patient?

    a) CT Angiogram of the abdomen and pelvis

1072) What diameter is an elective repair of the aorta recommended with an AAA?

    a) > 5 cm or > 1 cm increase per year

1073) What is the definitive treatment for a leaking AAA, ruptured AAA, or aortoenteric fistula?

    a) Surgery

1074) What abdominal emergency has a mortality rate of > 75% and causes abrupt diffuse abdominal pain out of proportion to the physical exam, in a patient with atrial fibrillation and cardiac disease?

    a) Mesenteric ischemia

1075) What are the etiologies leading to mesenteric ischemia?

    a) Arterial emboli (most common), Arterial thrombosis (atherosclerosis), Nonocclusive disease (low flows states), Mesenteric venous thrombosis

1076) What metabolic abnormality can be seen with mesenteric ischemia?

    a) Lactic acidosis

1077) What laboratory marker is the best marker for diagnosing mesenteric ischemia?

    a) Lactate

1078) What finding on rectal exam increases likely hood of bowel ischemia?

    a) Rectal bleeding or Positive hemoccult

1079) Which classes of medications should be used "with caution" in patients with suspected mesenteric ischemia?

    a) Beta-blockers, Calcium channel blockers, Digoxin; Use of vasopressors

1080) What is the best imaging modality to diagnose mesenteric ischemia?

a) CT Angiogram of the abdomen and pelvis

1081) What are the CT findings seen with mesenteric ischemia?

a) Bowel wall edema (thumb printing), Fat stranding, Pneumatosis, and Mesentery artery filling defects

1082) What are the treatments for mesenteric ischemia?

a) IV fluid, Antibiotics, Anticoagulants, and Surgery

1083) What gynecological condition causes abdominal pain in the pelvis and RUQ, vaginal discharge, and has cervical motion tenderness (chandeliers sign) on pelvic exam?

a) Pelvic inflammatory disease (PID)

1084) What condition can cause achy flank pain, urinary urgency, and frequency, dysuria, nausea, CVA tenderness with or without fever?

a) Pyelonephritis

1085) What abdominal pathology causes epigastric abdominal pain radiates to the back, nausea, vomiting, with a PMH of alcohol use, and gallbladder stones.

a) Pancreatitis

1086) What are the two types of pancreatitis?

a) Acute and Chronic

1087) List drugs that are associated with pancreatitis.

a) Estrogens, Salicylates, Thiazides, Acetaminophen, Statins, Valproic acid, Tetracyclines, Furosemide, Metronidazole, Isoniazid, and Enalapril

1088) List the etiologies of pancreatitis.

a) Biliary disease (gallstone), Alcohol, ERCP, Mumps, Hepatitis, EBV, DKA, Hyperlipidemia (hypertriglyceridemia), Uremia, Salmonella, Mycoplasma, Scorpion stings, and Hypercalcemia

1089) What are the two most common causes of pancreatitis?

a) Alcohol use and Biliary disease (gallstone)

1090) What is the most common cause of pancreatitis worldwide?

a) Biliary disease (gallstone)

1091) What is the most common cause of pancreatitis in the United States?

a) Alcohol

1092) Elevated liver enzymes with pancreatitis suggest what etiology of pancreatitis?

a) Gallstone

1093) What is bruising on the flank called?

a) Grey Turner's sign

1094) What is bruising around the umbilicus called?

a) Cullen's sign

1095) What abdominal diagnoses are associated with Cullen's and Turner's signs?

a) Pancreatitis, Retroperitoneal hemorrhage, or Ruptured ectopic pregnancy

1096) What lab is more specific to the diagnosis of pancreatitis? Amylase or lipase?

a) Lipase

1097) Are lipase levels typically elevated in patients with chronic recurrent pancreatitis?

a) No

1098) List the etiologies that can lead to increased amylase levels.

a) Tumors, Parotitis, SBO, Mesenteric ischemia, Ectopic pregnancy, Ovarian issues, Pancreatitis, Renal or Liver failure, or Gallbladder dysfunction

1099) List Ranson's ED criteria for pancreatitis that are associated with increased mortality.

a) Glucose > 200 mg/dL

b) LDH > 350

c) Age > 55

d) AST > 250

e) WBC > 16,000

1100) List Ranson's criteria for pancreatitis at 48 hours that are associated with increase mortality.

a) PaO_2 < 60 mmHg

b) ↓ HCT > 10%

c) ↑ BUN > 5 mg/dL

d) Ca < 8 mg/dL

e) Base deficit > 4 mEq/L

f) Rapid Fluids sequestration > 6L

1101) What are the two pathognomonic findings seen with acute pancreatitis on an abdominal X-ray?

a) Sentinel loop (small bowel over the pancreas)

b) Colon cutoff: (dilation over the pancreas)

1102) What findings on an abdominal X-ray can be seen with chronic pancreatitis?

a) Pancreatic calcifications

1103) What imaging study should be performed if there is pancreatitis with transaminitis?

a) RUQ US

1104) What treatment is suggested with gallstone-induced pancreatitis with transaminitis?

a) ERCP

1105) What imaging is the study of choice to rule out pancreatic complications with pancreatitis, such as pancreatic necrosis or abscess formation if the patient is not improving?

a) IV contrast CT abdomen and pelvis

1106) Are most pancreatic pseudocysts symptomatic or asymptomatic?

a) Asymptomatic

1107) What pancreatic complication can occur in patients with chronic recurrent pancreatitis?

a) Exocrine insufficiency

1108) What endocrine etiology can develop in patients with a chronic pancreatitis history?

a) Diabetes

1109) What is the management for pancreatitis?

a) Supportive therapy, NPO, IV Fluids, and Pain control

1110) What type of abdominal pathology develops due to decreased intestinal peristalsis without obstruction causing constant abdominal pain, distention, decreased bowel sounds, and constipation, and is commonly seen after surgery?

a) Ileus

1111) List some causes of paralytic (adynamic) ileus.

a) Surgery, Hypokalemia, Hypocalcemia, Medications (opiates, CCB), Trauma, Dehydration, and Infection

1112) What are the abdominal X-ray findings seen with an ileus?

a) Distended bowel and/or Air-fluid levels of intestine throughout the abdomen

1113) What is the management of an abdominal ileus?

a) Supportive therapy (usually self-limited), Medication adjustment, Stool softeners, and IV hydration, +/- NG tube

1114) What abdominal pathology causes diffuse colicky abdominal pain, distention, nausea, vomiting, high-pitched bowel sounds, and tympani to percussion with a history of abdominal surgery?

a) Small Bowel obstruction (SBO)

1115) List the causes of a SBO.

a) Hernias, Adhesions, Abscess, Intussusception, Stricture, Bezoar, Gallstone ileus, and Malignancy

1116) What is the most common cause of SBO?

a) Adhesions

1117) What is the second most common cause of SBO?

a) Hernia

1118) List common electrolyte imbalances that occur with a SBO.

a) Hypokalemia and Hypochloremia

1119) What is the most common electrolyte imbalance seen with an ileus or bowel obstruction?

a) Hypokalemia

1120) What are the X-ray findings from an abdominal series that suggest an SBO?

a) Air fluids levels

b) Distended small bowel with a "string of pearls" or "stepladder" appearance

1121) What imaging study is more specific than an abdominal X-ray to diagnosis a SBO, and can rule out complications, distinguish between an ileus versus obstruction, and show the transition point?

a) IV +/- Oral contrast-enhanced CT abdomen and pelvis

1122) What are the treatment options for an SBO?

a) Nasogastric tube with low intermittent suction, IV hydration, Analgesia, and Surgery (if not improving)

1123) List common causes of large bowel obstructions.

a) Neoplasm, Volvulus, Diverticulitis, Strictures, or Fecal impaction

1124) What is the most common cause of large bowel obstruction?

    a)   Neoplasms (colorectal adenocarcinoma most common)

1125)   What are the abdominal X-ray findings seen with a large bowel obstruction?

    a)   Distended colon with prominent haustrations

1126)   What diameter of large bowel distention is considered a high risk of morbidity in patients with bowel obstruction?

    a)   > 10 cm

1127)   What are two types of "closed-loop" large bowel obstruction that increases the risk of mortality and perforation?

    a)   Ileocecal valve competent and Ileocecal valve incompetent

1128)   What are the two types of volvulus that can occur?

    a)   Cecal and Sigmoid

1129)   What type of volvulus is often seen in the elderly, those with neuropsychiatric or developmental disorders, or those on anticholinergic medications, and has a "coffee bean" or "bent inner tube" shape dilated bowel pattern on X-ray?

    a)   Sigmoid

1130)   What type of volvulus is the most common?

    a)   Sigmoid volvulus

1131)   What is the treatment for a sigmoid volvulus obstruction?

    a)   Sigmoidoscopy for decompression and detorsion or Laparoscopy if sigmoidoscopy fails

1132)   What type of volvulus typically presents suddenly in younger patients due to a laxity or lack of normal retroperitoneal cecal attachments?

    a)   Cecal

1133)   What are the X-ray findings seen with a cecal volvulus?

    a)   Kidney shaped dilated loop in the LUQ

1134)   What type of volvulus is the most common type seen in obstetric patients?

    a)   Cecal

1135)   What is the treatment for a cecal volvulus?

    a)   Hemicolectomy

1136)   What are treatment options for a fecal impaction causing bowel obstruction and constipation?

a) Enema, Mineral oil, Polyethylene glycol, Docusate, Magnesium citrate, and Manual disimpaction

1137) List causes of constipation.

a) Medications, Decreased fiber and fluid intake, Bowel obstruction, Diverticulitis, and Hypothyroidism

1138) What medications can lead to acute constipation?

a) Narcotic, Iron, Antipsychotics, and Calcium channel blockers

1139) What physical exam procedure should be performed before giving an enema for constipation?

a) Rectal exam for fecal impaction

1140) What type of pseudo-obstruction commonly presents in the lower colon of elderly patients on anticholinergic medications and has a large amount of gas on abdominal X-ray without air-fluid levels?

a) Ogilvie syndrome

1141) What complications can develop in an intestinal obstruction when the intraluminal pressure exceeds capillary and venous pressure in the bowel wall?

a) Bowel ischemia or necrosis, Decreased lymphatic drainage, Sepsis, Shock, and Organ failure

1142) What does an elevated WBC > 20,000 with a bowel obstruction raise concern for?

a) Bowel gangrene, Peritonitis, or Abscess

1143) What do elevated BUN, Cr, and Hct levels with a bowel obstruction suggest?

a) Dehydration or Volume depletion

1144) What does an elevated lactate level suggest?

a) Ischemia or Dehydration

1145) What surgical abdominal emergency presents with sudden onset abdominal pain, hypotension, tachycardia, vomiting, and abdominal distention in a patient with a GERD or PUD history?

a) Bowel perforation

1146) What is the most common source leading to a GI perforation?

a) Peptic ulcer

1147) Which type of peptic ulcer, duodenal or gastric, causes 2-3 times of the amount of small bowel perforations?

a) Duodenal ulcer

1148) What is the first imaging study done in the ED for suspected GI perforation?
a) Acute abdominal series with upright chest XR

1149) What are the findings on an acute abdominal series that suggest a bowel perforation?
a) Air under the diaphragm

1150) What imaging study should be performed with a suspected GI perforation and a negative abdominal series?
a) CT abdomen and pelvis with contrast

1151) What abdominal condition presents with abdominal pain, distention, and an irreducible inguinal mass with swelling, nausea, and vomiting.
a) Incarcerated hernia

1152) What type of irreducible hernia presents with overlying erythema due to vascular compromise leading to ischemia and is treated surgically?
a) Strangulated hernia

1153) What complications can occur if a strangulated hernia is manually reduced in the ED?
a) Reintroduction of dead bowel into the abdomen can lead to sepsis, acidosis, and shock

1154) Give the two types of inguinal hernias.
a) Direct and Indirect

1155) What type of inguinal hernia is caused by an abdominal wall defect, lateral to the abdominal rectus muscle and superior to the inguinal ligament?
a) Direct hernia

1156) What is the triangle called where direct hernias occur, and is made up of the rectus abdominal muscle, inferior epigastric artery, and inguinal ligament?
a) Hesselbach's triangle

1157) What type of inguinal hernia presents through the inguinal canal and can extend into the scrotal sac?
a) Indirect hernia

1158) In males, what side of the body are most indirect hernias found on?
   a) Right
1159) What is the most common hernia in females?
   a) Indirect inguinal hernia
1160) What is the term for a direct and indirect hernia present at the same time?
   a) Pantaloon hernia
1161) What two types of hernia are more common in females?
   a) Obturator and Femoral hernia
1162) What type of hernia involves the aponeurotic layer between the abdominal rectus muscle and the semilunar line laterally?
   a) Spigelian hernia
1163) What type of abdominal wall abnormality is located between the abdominal rectus muscles and is due to a weakened aponeurosis and is seen with obesity, pregnancy, or after surgery?
   a) Diastasis recti
1164) What type of hernia is associated with weakness in the abdominal wall and is usually due to trauma or surgical incisions?
   a) Ventral (incisional) hernia
1165) What type of hernia is due to the incarceration of the mesentery not including the bowel?
   a) Richter hernia
1166) What are the criteria for general surgery referral for a pediatric umbilical hernia?
   a) > 4 yo or > 2 cm in length
1167) What is the study of choice for hernia diagnosis?
   a) IV contrast CT abdomen and pelvis
1168) What is the treatment for a reducible hernia?
   a) Symptom control, Reduction, and Outpatient surgery referral
1169) What is the treatment for an irreducible incarcerated hernia?
   a) General surgery consult and Symptom control
1170) What is the treatment for a strangulated hernia?
   a) Emergency surgery, Antibiotics, and Symptom control
1171) What physical exam sign can help with the diagnosis of abdominal wall pain?
   a) Carnett's sign

1172) List medications commonly used as antiemetics.
   a) Ondansetron, Metoclopramide, Promethazine, Diphenhydramine, Prochlorperazine, Meclizine, and Haloperidol
1173) What infection etiology is the most common cause of diarrhea?
   a) Viral
1174) List viruses associated with diarrhea.
   a) Norwalk virus (norovirus), Rotavirus, Enterovirus, and Adenovirus
1175) What type of viral diarrhea is associated with travelers on a cruise ship?
   a) Norwalk virus
1176) What are notable bacterial causes of diarrhea?
   a) E. coli, Salmonella, Shigella, Staphylococcus, Yersinia enterocolitica, Campylobacter jejuni, Vibrio, Bacillus cereus, Clostridum difficile, and Giardia
1177) Which patients with diarrhea should get testing for clostridium difficile?
   a) Recent antibiotic use, Immunocompromised, or Recently hospitalized
1178) What type of C. difficile can present around 6 weeks postoperatively?
   a) Pseudomembranous colitis (PMC)
1179) How is C. difficile diagnosed?
   a) C. difficile toxin on stool culture
1180) What are the medication options for treatment of C. difficile?
   a) Vancomycin (oral) or Metronidazole oral
1181) Which medication is used to treat mild C. difficile infections and is typically used for outpatient therapy?
   a) Metronidazole (oral)
1182) Which medication is used to treat patients with C. difficile infections who have more severe symptoms or are inpatient?
   a) Vancomycin
1183) What bacteria from unpasteurized milk, pets, and undercooked poultry, causes diarrhea, and may also cause bloody diarrhea and fever?
   a) Campylobacter jejuni

1184)	What autoimmune condition attacks the nerve cells causing weakness and is associated with a recent campylobacter infection?
	a)	Guillain-Barré syndrome
1185)	What are the management options for campylobacter jejuni diarrhea in a healthy patient versus a very ill/immunocompromised patient?
	a)	Healthy: symptom control
	b)	Very ill/immunocompromised: Macrolides or Fluoroquinolones
1186)	Which bacteria produce the Shiga toxin and are most associated with hemolytic-uremic syndrome?
	a)	E. coli 0157:H7 and Shigella dysenteriae
1187)	What hematologic condition can E. coli 0157:H7 cause in adults?
	a)	TTP
1188)	What lab test is used to diagnose invasive bacteria causing diarrhea and shows the presence of WBC's?
	a)	Fecal Wright stain
1189)	What bacteria is seen from uncooked eggs and poultry, as well as contact with amphibians?
	a)	Salmonella
1190)	What are the most common causes of traveler's diarrhea?
	a)	E. coli, Shigella, Salmonella, and Campylobacter
1191)	What time frame does bacterial toxins generally cause symptoms after inoculation in travels diarrhea?
	a)	Within a few hours
1192)	What antibiotics can be used for bacterial induced traveler's diarrhea?
	a)	Fluoroquinolones or Macrolides (Thailand/SE Asia)
1193)	Which bacteria is seen with oyster ingestion and causes severe watery diarrhea?
	a)	Vibrio species
1194)	What are the treatment options for vibrio induced diarrhea?
	a)	Supportive care—most cases of Vibrio diarrhea are self-limiting
	b)	If antibiotics are indicated or nondiarrheal Vibrio illness suspected: Doxycycline, Macrolides, or Fluoroquinolones

1195) What type of bacterium causes invasive diarrhea, fever, RLQ abdominal pain and can mimic appendicitis?
   a) Yersinia enterocolitica
1196) What is the treatment of Yersinia induced diarrhea?
   a) Fluoroquinolones TMP/SMX, 3rd generation Cephalosporins, or Aminoglycosides.
1197) What lab test is used to identify certain bacteria-causing diarrhea?
   a) Stool culture
1198) Which bacterium causes foul-smelling, floating watery diarrhea and is due to ingesting contaminate lake or river water with animal urine, and is associated with beavers?
   a) Giardia
1199) What is the treatment of Giardia protozoa infections?
   a) Metronidazole
1200) What type of parasitic infections is spread by fecal – orally, causing diarrhea, and can cause extra-intestinal abscesses of the liver, lungs, and brain?
   a) Entamoeba histolytica (Amebiasis)
1201) What is the treatment of Entamoeba protozoa infections?
   a) Metronidazole +/- Iodoquinol
1202) What type of parasitic protozoa infection is the most common cause of severe watery diarrhea in AIDS and immunocompromised patients?
   a) Cryptosporidium
1203) What type of stool culture can identify Giardia, Entamoeba, and Cryptosporidium?
   a) Ovum and Parasites stool culture
1204) What type frame due protozoal pathogens generally present with symptoms after inoculation?
   a) 1-2 weeks
1205) What is the treatment of cryptosporidium induced diarrhea in healthy and immunocompromised patients?
   a) Nitazoxanide or Paromomycin
1206) What are the findings on the ovum and parasite stool culture that suggest a cryptosporidium infection?

a) Oocysts present

1207) What bacteria causes diarrhea from undercooked rice?

a) Bacillus cereus

1208) Name the ingredients of the BRAT diet used for diarrhea.

a) Bananas, Rice, Apples, and Toast

1209) Name some anti-diarrheal medications.

a) Loperamide, Diphenoxylate/Atropine, and Bismuth subsalicylate

1210) What inflammatory bowel condition present in a bimodal age distribution, causes recurrent abdominal cramping pain, weight loss, diarrhea, and bloody diarrhea?

a) Crohn's disease

1211) What test can be done in the emergency department to help diagnose Crohn's disease?

a) CT abdomen and pelvis with contrast

1212) What type of inflammatory lesions are present on the colonoscopy exam with Crohn's disease?

a) Skip lesions

1213) What are the locations Crohn's disease can develop?

a) Mouth to anus

1214) What are the most common locations to see Crohn's disease develop?

a) Ileum and Ascending colon

1215) Which inflammatory bowel condition has a high risk of colon cancer?

a) Ulcerative colitis (UC)

1216) What is the most common site of the colon where ulcerative colitis develops?

a) Rectum

1217) What are the extra-intestinal manifestations that can occur with inflammatory bowel disease?

a) Erythema nodosum, Pyoderma gangrenosum, and Uveitis

1218) Name some emergency complications that can develop swith inflammatory bowel diseases.

a) Obstruction (strictures), Abscess, Perforation, Hemorrhage, Toxic megacolon, Fistulas, Electrolyte abnormalities, Dehydration, and Malignancy

1219) How are UC and Crohn's disease definitively diagnosed?
a) Colonoscopy with biopsy

1220) List maintenance medications used for induction of remission for inflammatory bowel diseases.
a) Prednisone, Sulfasalazine, Mesalamine, Azathioprine, 6-Mercaptopurine, and Infliximab

1221) What is the ED management of an acute exacerbation of inflammatory bowel disease?
a) Rule out complications, Fluid and electrolyte balance, Pain control, NPO, Antibiotics (Cipro + Metronidazole), and +/- Steroids

1222) What complication of ulcerative colitis is an emergency?
a) Toxic megacolon

1223) List different etiologies that cause toxic megacolon.
a) Crohns, UC, Medications that impair gut motility, Colonoscopy, Barium enema, Radiation, or Infection

1224) What are the treatment options for toxic megacolon?
a) General surgery consult, Steroids, Antibiotics, and IV Fluids

1225) What condition presents with flatulence or malodorous discharge or gross stool from the vagina, and can be caused by infections, malignancies, inflammatory bowel disease, or previous rectal or gynecological surgery?
a) Rectovaginal fistula

1226) What GI pathology can develop as a complication from constipation, anal fissures, Crohn's, bowel resections, and perirectal abscesses that presents with foul-smelling drainage, erythema, and pain?
a) Anorectal fistula

1227) What is the leading cause of anal fistulas?
a) Perirectal abscess

1228) What is the treatment for anorectal fistulas?
a) Surgery referral and Sitz baths, +/- Antibiotics (infections) and I&D of abscesses

1229)   What antibiotics can be used for outpatient treatment of an anorectal fistula until definitive treatment?
   a)   Ciprofloxacin + Metronidazole
1230)   What type of anorectal abscess is the most common?
   a)   Perianal abscess
1231)   What type of abscess presents with erythematous fluctuant mass, throbbing rectal pain, +/- a fever?
   a)   Perirectal abscess
1232)   List the four types of perirectal abscesses.
   a)   Perianal, Supralevator, Ischiorectal, and Intersphincteric
1233)   What type of perirectal abscess can transverse the deep postanal space into the contralateral side forming a horseshoe abscess?
   a)   Ischiorectal abscess
1234)   What type of inflammatory bowel disease are perirectal abscesses more common in?
   a)   Crohn's disease
1235)   Give the treatments for each type of the following perirectal abscesses: perianal, supralevator, ischiorectal, and intersphincteric.
   a)   Perianal: I&D (without rectal verge involvement)
   b)   Supralevator: Surgery for I&D in OR
   c)   Ischiorectal: Surgery for I&D in OR
   d)   Intersphincteric: Surgery for I&D in OR
1236)   What type of abscess is due to an infected hair follicle in the natal cleft over the rectum or sacrum and is more common in males?
   a)   Pilonidal abscess
1237)   What is the treatment of a pilonidal abscess?
   a)   I&D and Surgical referral
1238)   What type of malignancy is the most common in the colorectal region?
   a)   Adenocarcinoma
1239)   What is the most common GI symptom that increases suspicion of colon cancer?
   a)   GI bleeding

1240) What procedure should be recommended to rule out malignancy as an outpatient workup for GI bleeding with an unknown cause?
a) Colonoscopy

1241) What is the most common cause of intussusception in an adult?
a) Tumors

1242) What is the criterion for diagnosing chronic diarrhea?
a) > 4 weeks

1243) List the different types of diarrhea.
a) Watery, Fatty (malabsorption), Infectious, and Inflammatory

1244) What GI malabsorption condition is due to damage to the intestinal villi due to an immune response to gluten and leads to diarrhea, abdominal cramping, and bloating?
a) Celiac disease

1245) What is the treatment for celiac disease?
a) Gluten-free diet

1246) What GI malabsorption condition is due to the inability of the gut to absorb dairy products, due to the lack of the enzyme lactase, leading to diarrhea, abdominal bloating, and flatulence?
a) Lactose intolerance

1247) What is the treatment for lactose intolerance?
a) Avoiding lactose products and Lactase replacement

1248) What infectious cause of malabsorption is seen in travelers and decreases absorption of B12, fat, and folate causing abdominal cramping, bloating, and nutritional deficiencies?
a) Tropical sprue

1249) What is the treatment of tropical sprue?
a) Antibiotics (tetracycline) and Nutrient replacement (folic acid, B12, iron)

1250) What can be done to help the cramping and bloating, symptoms after an acute diarrhea episode?
a) Probiotics

1251) What GI complication can be induced due to the overuse of stool bulking softeners if not enough water is ingested?
a) Laxative induce constipation

1252) What GI condition presents with a history of epigastric burning that radiating into the chest and is worse after eating spicy food, drinking alcohol or caffeine products and laying flat?
a) Gastroesophageal reflux disease (GERD)

1253) What anatomic dysfunction leads to GERD?
a) Lower esophageal sphincter weakness

1254) How is GERD diagnosed?
a) Endoscopy or 24 hr PH monitoring

1255) What medication classes are used for treating GERD?
a) Proton pump inhibitors (PPI)
b) H2 blockers (Ranitidine)
c) Metoclopramide
d) Sucralfate

1256) Give some treatment remedies that can be used to help with GERD after starting medication.
a) Elevated head of the bed, Smaller meal ingestion, Avoid triggers (spicy foods, alcohol, and caffeine), Lower esophageal banding

1257) List causes of esophagitis.
a) GERD, Radiation, Pill induced (bisphosphonates), Infectious (candida, herpes, CMV), and Crohn's

1258) What GI complication in a patient with a history of reflux causes epigastric achy, burning pain that radiates to the back, is worse at night, and exacerbated with eating?
a) Peptic ulcer disease (PUD)

1259) What are the two types of PUD?
a) Gastric and Duodenal

1260) What type of ulcer is the most common?
a) Duodenal

1261) What type of ulcer presents with pain 15 - 30 minutes following eating and is exacerbated with eating?
a) Gastric

1262) What type of ulcer presents with pain > 1-3 hours following eating and is sometimes relieved with eating?
a) Duodenal

1263) What bacteria is most commonly associated with PUD?
a) Helicobacter pylori (30-70% of patients)

1264) What future complications can occur with untreated H. pylori?
   a) Gastric cancer
1265) Overuse of what class of medication is commonly seen with the diagnosis of PUD?
   a) NSAIDs
1266) List the predisposing factors of PUD.
   a) Alcohol, Smoking, NSAID's, Steroids, and Zollinger-Ellison syndrome
1267) List the complications from untreated PUD.
   a) GI hemorrhage, Perforation, Cancer, and Gastric outlet obstruction
1268) What is the most common complication of PUD?
   a) Hemorrhage
1269) How sensitive is an upright chest radiograph in diagnosing perforated viscus?
   a) 80%
1270) How are peptic ulcers definitively diagnosed?
   a) EGD
1271) What medication classes are used for treating PUD?
   a) Proton pump inhibitors (PPI)
   b) H2 blockers (Ranitidine)
   c) Sucralfate
1272) What are the medication regimens used to treat H. pylori?
   a) PPI + Amoxicillin + Clarithromycin
   b) PPI + Metronidazole + Clarithromycin
1273) What are the two types of hiatal hernia?
   a) Sliding and Paraesophageal
1274) What type of hiatal hernia is the most common, leads to reflux symptoms due to the gastroesophageal junction and stomach fundus herniating into the thoracic cavity?
   a) Sliding
1275) What type of hiatal hernia does the stomach herniating through a diaphragmatic defect with a fixed gastroesophageal junction define?
   a) Paraesophageal

1276) What anatomic structure distinguishes between an upper or lower GI bleeds based on if the bleed is proximal or distal to it?
   a) Ligament of Treitz
1277) What physical exam finding on the rectal exam suggests an upper versus lower GI bleed?
   a) Color of the stool
1278) What color is the stool with most upper GI bleeds?
   a) Black tarry or Melena
1279) Can massive upper GI bleeds present with bright red blood per rectum?
   a) Yes (brisk upper GI bleed or increased GI transit)
1280) A patient who has coffee ground hematemesis and a positive gastroccult on an NG aspirate has what type of GI complication?
   a) Upper GI bleed
1281) List causes of upper GI bleeding.
   a) PUD, Gastritis, Mallory-Weiss tear, Esophagitis, Duodenitis, Esophageal varices, and Gastric cancer
1282) What is the most common cause of an upper GI bleed?
   a) PUD
1283) What diagnostic modality is the most accurate tool for evaluating and treating upper GI bleeding?
   a) Endoscopy
1284) What is the treatment for upper GI bleeding?
   a) 2 large bore IV's, PPI's, IV fluid, +/- PRBC, Vasopressors, and Endoscopy
1285) What type of upper GI bleed source should be suspected in an alcoholic, with jaundice, distended abdomen, and hepatomegaly with hypotension?
   a) Esophageal varices
1286) What is the most common cause leading to varices?
   a) Alcohol abuse
1287) What medication is used to treated variceal bleed by decreasing the splanchnic blood flow?
   a) Octreotide
1288) What vasopressor medication can be used to decrease bleeding from varices?

a) Vasopressin

1289) What mechanical structure should be used to prevent exsanguination from a variceal upper GI bleed if emergent EDG is not available?

a) Sengstaken–Blakemore tube

1290) What definitive procedure is performed by GI to treat portal hypertension and decrease varices?

a) Transjugular intrahepatic portosystemic shunt (TIPS)

1291) What type of GI bleed does hematochezia or bright red blood per rectum suggest?

a) Lower

1292) List causes of lower GI bleeding.

a) Upper GI bleed, Diverticulosis, Angiodysplasia (AV malformations), Upper GI bleed, Cancer, Polyps, Ulcerative colitis, Crohn's, or Aortoenteric fistula

1293) What is the most common cause of a lower GI bleed?

a) Upper GI bleed

1294) What is the second most common cause of a lower GI Bleed?

a) Diverticulosis

1295) What two conditions are most commonly associated with bright red blood per rectum and pain?

a) Anal fissures and External hemorrhoids

1296) What type of lower GI bleed is due to a tear in the skin causing pain with defecation, pruritis, and bright red blood when wiping and blood-streaked stool?

a) Anal fissure

1297) What is the most common source of painful rectal bleeding?

a) Anal fissure

1298) Where is the most common location on the rectum for an anal fissure to occur?

a) Posterior midline

1299) What type of medical conditions cause non-midline fissures and should be referred when diagnosed for further workup?

a) Inflammatory bowel disease, Tumors, and Leukemia

1300) What complications can occur with anal fissures?

a) Infection, Strictures, and Fistulas

1301) What medications can treat rectal spasms with anal fissures?
   a) Topical Nitroglycerin or Botulinum toxin

1302) What is the treatment for anal fissures?
   a) Stool softener, Laxatives, Sitz baths, and Surgical referral

1303) What medications can cause black tarry stools or melena?
   a) Bismuth and Iron tablets

1304) What food or liquids can cause red stool and a negative hemoccult test?
   a) Red food-coloring, Fruit juices, or Beets

1305) What lab test detects microscopic blood in the stool or emesis?
   a) Hemoccult and Gastroccult

1306) What lab within the BMP is usually elevated due to the breakdown of heme products from blood?
   a) BUN

1307) What are the most common sites for AV malformations?
   a) Cecum and Ascending colon

1308) What imaging study is the gold standard for diagnosing angiodysplasia/AV malformations causing lower GI bleeding?
   a) Mesenteric angiography

1309) What is the treatment of AV malformations causing a lower GI bleed in stable and unstable patients?
   a) Stable: Colonoscopy with coagulation or Interventional radiology for embolization
   b) Unstable: Surgery consult for hemicolectomy

1310) What are the management and treatment options for lower GI bleeding?
   a) 2 large bore IV's, PPI's, IV fluid, +/- PRBC, Vasopressors, +/- Surgery, Angiography (embolization), or Colonoscopy

1311) What type of GI pathology causes bright red blood per rectum, can be painful or painless with blood in the toilet, on the toilet paper, or streaking on the stool?
   a) Internal and External hemorrhoids

1312) What anatomical "line" differentiates between internal and external hemorrhoids?
   a) Pectinate (dentate) line

1313) List common risk factors leading to internal and external hemorrhoids
   a) Constipation, Narcotic use, Liver disease, Alcohol use, and Pregnancy
1314) Do non-prolapsed internal hemorrhoids cause pain?
   a) No
1315) Do you incise internal hemorrhoids?
   a) No
1316) Describe the findings of the four grades of internal hemorrhoids.
   a) Grade 1: No prolapse
   b) Grade 2: Prolapse that spontaneously reduces
   c) Grade 3: Prolapse that needs manual reduction
   d) Grade 4: Prolapse that requires surgery
1317) What is the treatment of a prolapsed internal hemorrhoid?
   a) Manual reduction or Surgery (for failed reduction)
1318) What are the treatment options for uncomplicated external and internal hemorrhoids?
   a) Stool softeners, Sitz baths, and Laxatives
1319) What physical exam findings with an external hemorrhoid suggest thrombosis?
   a) Pain, Blue/Purple, and Hard (non-fluctuant)
1320) What is the ED treatment of a thrombosed external hemorrhoid?
   a) Elliptical excision
1321) What rectal pathology can develop due to weakened pelvic floor muscles and constipation and presents with a "bulge" after defecation with prolapsed bowel tissue?
   a) Rectal prolapse
1322) Name the three types of rectal prolapse that can occur.
   a) Rectal mucosa prolapse
   b) Rectal prolapse of all 3 layers
   c) Intussusception (upper segment prolapse)
1323) What are the common causes of rectal prolapse in children?
   a) Constipation and Absent rectal mesentery

1324)   What congenital condition is associated with infant rectal prolapse and needs a further evaluation?
   a)   Cystic fibrosis

1325)   What are the treatment options for rectal prolapse?
   a)   Topical sugar application, Manual reduction, Stool softeners, and +/- Surgical consult (failed reductions or ischemia)

1326)   What is the most common congenital abnormality of the GI tract that presents with painless rectal bleeding (hematochezia)?
   a)   Meckel's diverticulum

1327)   What remnant of the embryonic GI tract makes up most Meckel's diverticulum?
   a)   Vitelline duct (omphalomesenteric duct)

1328)   What are the characteristics of a Meckel's diverticulum?
   a)   2 feet from the ileocecal valve
   b)   < 2 years old
   c)   2 inches long
   d)   2 cm wide
   e)   2% of the population
   f)   2 mucosal types

1329)   What is the most common tissue found in a Meckel's diverticulum?
   a)   Gastric tissue

1330)   What is the study of choice for diagnosing Meckel's?
   a)   Technetium-99m scan (Meckel's scan)

1331)   What is the definitive treatment option for a Meckel's diverticulum?
   a)   Surgery

1332)   What GI emergency can occur after vomiting and presents with sudden onset severe chest pain, hematemesis, subcutaneous emphysema, and dyspnea?
   a)   Boerhaave syndrome (full-thickness tear)

1333)   Perforation of what GI structure has the highest associated mortality?
   a)   Esophageal perforation

1334)   What imaging studies can diagnose an esophageal perforation?

a) Chest X-ray, CT chest, Esophagoscopy, or Esophagram (with water-soluble contrast)

1335) What is the most common anatomic location of an esophageal tear in Boerhaave syndrome?
a) Left posterior lateral wall of the lower third of the esophagus

1336) What are the findings on a chest X-ray that can be seen with an esophageal tear?
a) Mediastinal air (pneumomediastinum), Pleural effusion (left), Pneumothorax, or Widened mediastinum

1337) What is the term that defines the synchronous crunching sound heard with each heartbeat due to the mediastinal air after an esophageal rupture?
a) Hamman's crunch

1338) Presence of what specific product in the pleural fluid suggests effusion from an esophageal rupture?
a) Amylase

1339) What is the most common cause of esophageal perforation?
a) Iatrogenic (endoscopy)

1340) What is the most common location of an iatrogenic esophageal rupture?
a) Pharyngoesophageal

1341) What is the treatment for an esophageal tear?
a) Surgical repair and Antibiotics

1342) What type of esophageal injury is defined as a partial thickness tear and presents with hematemesis without pain after vomiting?
a) Mallory-Weiss tear

1343) What is the most common location of a Mallory-Weis tear?
a) Gastroesophageal junction

1344) What is the treatment of a Mallory-Weiss tear?
a) Symptom control (spontaneous resolution)

1345) What type of dysphagia has difficulty passing solids?
a) Mechanical

1346) What type of dysphagia has difficulty passing solids and liquids?
a) Neurosensory

1347) What type of neurosensory dysphagia is due to the loss of Auerbach's plexus?

a) Achalasia

1348) What kind of dysphagia is a problem at the start of swallowing and is commonly seen in post-stroke patients?

a) Transfer dysphagia

1349) List causes of mechanical dysphagia.

a) Scleroderma, Cancer, MS, Myasthenia gravis, Thyroid goiter, Zenker's diverticulum, Webs, Schatzki ring, Food bolus, and Strictures

1350) What type of mechanical dysphagia is due to a pharyngoesophageal outpouching and causes bad breath?

a) Zenker's diverticulum

1351) What type of mechanical dysphagia is due to anterior esophageal webs and is associated with iron deficiency and nail spooning?

a) Plumber Vinson syndrome

1352) What type of distal mechanical obstruction occurs after eating meat products and presents with esophageal spasms, drooling, and inability to swallow one's saliva?

a) Food bolus

1353) What are the medication options used for an impacted food bolus?

a) Glucagon, Atropine, or Nifedipine

1354) Are meat tenderizers a recommended therapy for a meat food bolus?

a) No

1355) What is the definitive treatment for an impacted food bolus that has failed medication treatment?

a) Emergent EGD

1356) What type of mechanical dysphagia is caused by the narrowing of the lower esophagus by a ring of mucosal tissue?

a) Schatzki ring

1357) What is the workup for dysphagia?

a) Esophagram, Endoscopy, and Swallow study

1358) What is the most common cause of esophageal cancer?

a) Squamous

1359) What is the most common cause of obstructive dysphagia?

a) Squamous cell cancer

1360) What medication may be used to manage persistent hiccups?
   a) Chlorpromazine
1361) List the anatomical structures associated with narrowing and foreign bodies at C6, T4, T6, and T11.
   a) C6: Cricopharyngeus muscle
   b) T4: Aortic arch
   c) T6: Tracheal bifurcation
   d) T11: Gastroesophageal junction
1362) What is the most common site of esophageal foreign body obstruction in adult patients?
   a) Distal (GE junction T11)
1363) Is neutralization of an ingested caustic agent generally recommended for treatment?
   a) No (excess heat production)
1364) What type of caustic agent leads to liquefaction necrosis?
   a) Alkali
1365) What type of caustic agent leads to coagulation necrosis?
   a) Acid
1366) What complications can occur from caustic agent ingestion?
   a) Perforation, Burns, or Strictures
1367) What procedures or actions are contraindicated in an esophageal burn from caustic ingestion?
   a) NG tube placement, Inducing emesis, or Charcoal use
1368) What procedure can be done to help determine the extent of esophageal damage from an ingested caustic agent?
   a) EGD
1369) What autosomal dominant condition leads to diffuse hemangiomas in the GI tract and mucous membranes, recurrent GI bleeds, and epistaxis, with a positive family history?
   a) Osler-Weber-Rendu Syndrome
1370) What type of GI pathology presents with RUQ abdominal pain, fatigue, jaundice, nausea, vomiting, anorexia and possible fever?
   a) Hepatitis
1371) List the causes of hepatitis.
   a) Viral, Alcoholic, Toxic drug ingestion, Autoimmune, and Infectious mononucleosis

1372) What labs are typically elevated in the thousands with acute hepatitis?
   a) AST and ALT

1373) What type of hepatitis can develop in patients with alcoholic fatty liver disease, and presents with fever, nausea, jaundice, and abdominal pain?
   a) Alcoholic hepatitis

1374) What is the progression of end-stage liver disease in patients with alcohol abuse?
   a) Fatty liver → Hepatitis → Cirrhosis → Liver failure

1375) What is the AST to ALT ratio of transaminases that suggests an alcohol-induced cause of hepatitis?
   a) 2:1

1376) List drugs and medications that commonly lead to toxin-induced hepatitis and liver failure.
   a) Acetominophen, Isoniazid, Chlorpromazine, Phenytoin, Amanita mushrooms, Steroids, and Hormone-replacement therapies

1377) What labs are typically elevated in cases of autoimmune hepatitis?
   a) ANA and Gamma globulin (> 1.5x)

1378) What are the treatment options for autoimmune hepatitis?
   a) Corticosteroids or Azathioprine

1379) What type of endemic hepatitis is transmitted by the fecal-oral route and is commonly seen in children and travelers?
   a) Hepatitis A

1380) What is the management of a hepatitis A infection?
   a) Supportive therapy

1381) What is the management for postexposure prophylaxis of hepatitis A in an unvaccinated patient?
   a) Hepatitis A vaccine or Immunoglobulin

1382) What type of hepatitis is the most common blood-borne infection, with an incubation period of 35-50 days and may be contracted through sexual, parenteral, and perinatal contact?
   a) Hepatitis C

1383) What is the most common transmission route of HCV?
   a) Parenteral (transfusions, IVDU, needle sticks, or tattoos)

1384) What type of hepatitis is the most common cause of chronic hepatitis?
   a) Hepatitis C

1385) What type of virus is hepatitis C?
   a) Single-strand RNA

1386) What is the risk of developing hepatitis C virus (HCV) after a needle stick?
   a) 1.8%

1387) What type of cancer is most associated with HCV chronic carriers?
   a) Hepatocellular carcinoma

1388) What are the new treatment options for acute and chronic HCV infections?
   a) Antiviral combo medications (i.e. elbasvir/grazoprevir, or ledipasvir/sofosbuvir)

1389) What is a definitive treatment option for a patient with chronic HCV and cirrhosis?
   a) Liver transplant

1390) Are there prophylaxis vaccines for HCV?
   a) No

1391) What type of hepatitis is life threatening in pregnancy and is transmitted fecal-orally and through contaminated water sources, and is seen in travelers to Asia and Africa?
   a) Hepatitis E

1392) Are there any treatment options or prophylaxis vaccines for a hepatitis E infection?
   a) No

1393) What type of hepatitis virus has a 30-day incubation period, requires hepatitis B for replication, and is seen more commonly in persons engaging in IV drug use and high-risk sexual activity?
   a) Hepatitis delta virus (HDV)

1394) What is the appropriate prophylaxis for HDV?
   a) Hepatitis B vaccine

1395) What serologic marker indicates immune protection from a hepatitis B vaccination?
   a) Hepatitis B surface antibody (HBsAb)

1396) What serologic markers indicate immune protection from having a previous hepatitis B infection?
   a) Hepatitis B surface antibody (HBsAb) + Hepatitis B core antibody (anti-HBc))

1397) What serologic markers indicate an acute infection in a hepatitis B patient?
   a) IgM anti-HBc + hepatitis B surface antigen (HBsAg)

1398) What serologic markers indicate a chronic infection in a hepatitis B patient?
   a) IgG anti-HBc + HBsAg

1399) What serologic marker indicates increased infectivity in a hepatitis B patient?
   a) Hepatitis B e antigen (HBeAg)

1400) Give the tests required in the ED for each the source and exposed patient for a needle stick with possible hepatitis B.
   a) Test source for HB surface antigen
   b) Test exposed for HB surface antibody

1401) What is the post-exposure prophylaxis (PEP) treatment for the unvaccinated HBV exposed patient from a positive source for HBV?
   a) HBV vaccine series (3 shots) and Hepatitis B immunoglobulin (HBIG)

1402) What is the PEP treatment for each of the vaccinated, incomplete vaccine series, and inadequate response to vaccine history HBV exposed patients from a positive source for HBV?
   a) Vaccinated (adequate HB antibodies): No treatment
   b) Incomplete HBV vaccine series: HBV vaccine booster
   c) Inadequate HB antibodies: HBV vaccine booster and Hepatitis B immunoglobulin (HBIG)

1403) What are the treatment options for a chronic hepatitis B infection?
   a) Lamivudine or Interferon alpha

1404) What type of virus is hepatitis B?
   a) Double-stranded DNA

1405) What is the average incubation period of hepatitis B?
   a) 75 days

1406) What abdominal pathology is expected with the physical exam findings of hepatomegaly, abdominal distention, collateral circulation of the abdominal wall, jaundice, and asterixis?
   a) Liver failure

1407) What is the most common medication that leads to liver failure?
   a) Acetaminophen

1408) What compound produced in the body is commonly elevated in liver failure and causes encephalopathy?
   a) Ammonia

1409) What is the treatment of hyperammonemia?
   a) Lactulose, Neomycin, and Low protein diet

1410) What lab test, if elevated, is also concerning for liver injury or liver failure?
   a) PT/INR

1411) What type of bilirubin is typically seen with hepatitis, liver disease, and obstruction of the common bile duct?
   a) Direct bilirubin

1412) What conditions can lead to increased indirect bilirubin levels?
   a) Hemolysis, Gilbert syndrome, and G6PD deficiency

1413) What complication of liver failure and ascites can develop with increased abdominal pain, distention, fever, sepsis, altered mental status, and vomiting?
   a) Spontaneous bacterial peritonitis (SBP)

1414) What bacteria is most commonly associated with SBP?
   a) E. Coli

1415) How do you diagnose SBP?
   a) Paracentesis

1416) What lab counts suggest SBP from the peritoneal fluid collected?
   a) Neutrophil count > 250 cells/μL
   b) WBC > 500 cells/ μL

1417) What are the treatments for SBP?
   a) IV 3rd generation cephalosporin (ceftriaxone or cefotaxime)
   b) Albumin (lowers mortality and renal failure if given within six hours)

1418) What is the treatment of spontaneous peritonitis in a peritoneal dialysis patient?

a) Intraperitoneal antibiotics (3rd generation cephalosporin)

1419) What medication can be used as SBP prophylaxis after resolution?

a) Fluoroquinolones

1420) What medication can be given prophylactically prior to performing a large volume paracentesis to reduce complications?

a) Albumin

1421) What GI pathology presents with a history of alternating diarrhea and constipation episodes with nausea, bloating, and abdominal pain, and a normal ED workup?

a) Irritable bowel syndrome (IBS)

1422) Is IBS a functional or organic condition?

a) Functional (no pathology found)

1423) List the Roma criteria for IBS diagnosis.

a) Abdominal pain 3 days a month for 3 months + 2 or more of the following: Change in form and frequency of stools, or Improvement with defecation

1424) What are the treatment options for IBS?

a) Depends on type and dominant symptoms: Laxatives, Antispasmodics, Antidiarrheals, High fiber diet, and Probiotics

1425) What GI condition can present similarly to IBS and has chronic reoccurring cramping diffuse abdominal pain, distention, nausea, and vomiting without signs of obstruction?

a) Pseudo-obstruction

1426) What medical conditions increase the risk for pseudo-obstruction?

a) Diabetes, Thyroid disease, Lupus, and Scleroderma?

1427) What are the treatment options for a pseudo-obstruction?

a) Bowel rest, NG or rectal tube placement, Analgesia, IV hydration, Surgical consultation, and +/- Consideration of neostigmine

1428) What complications can occur with rectal foreign bodies?

a) Constipation, Obstruction, Bowel perforation, Infection, and Bowel ischemia

1429) What is suggested in a patient traveling from another country, with tachycardia, altered mental status, vomiting, and abdominal pain with multiple foreign bodies on X-ray?
a) Body packing of drugs

1430) What are the management options for intestinal foreign bodies?
a) Sedation with manual removal, Monitoring until passed, or Surgical consult for removal

1431) What type of colitis should be suspected in patients with cancer in the abdominal or pelvic areas undergoing radiation treatment, having diarrhea and rectal bleeding?
a) Radiation proctocolitis

1432) What is the treatment option for radiation proctocolitis?
a) Supportive therapy

1433) What rectal condition is due to inflammation to the rectal mucosa and presents with rectal pain, bleeding, lesions, and rectal discharge generally associated with anal intercourse?
a) Sexually-transmitted infectious proctitis

1434) List causes of proctitis.
a) Infectious, HIV, Cryptitis, Radiation, Traumatic, and Inflammatory bowel disease

1435) What is the most common sexually transmitted cause of infectious proctitis?
a) Neisseria gonorrhea

1436) How is sexually transmitted infectious proctitis treated?
a) Treat the identified or suspected cause (i.e. antibiotics or antivirals, antiprotozoals)

1437) What type of proctitis is due to infection of the intestinal crypts and can lead to anal fissures, fistulas, and abscesses?
a) Cryptitis

1438) What are the treatment options for cryptitis?
a) Stool softeners, Sitz bath, Rectal irrigation, and Targeted treatment for specific cause

Resuscitation

1439)	Define the new "CAB" 2010 BLS resuscitation guidelines for adults, children, and infants (excluding newborns)?
   a)	Compressions
   b)	Airway
   c)	Breathing

1440)	Explain the reasoning behind the BLS guideline changes from "A-B-C" to "C-A-B"?
   a)	Due to the increased survival rate from compressions alone

1441)	What factors predict a difficult airway?
   a)	Mallampati score, Beard, Micrognathia, Facial trauma, Obesity, Short neck, Limited oral opening, Previous neck surgery or radiation, Neck masses, Angioedema, Burns, and Limited neck mobility (ROM)

1442)	What are the 3-3-2 rules that indicate a difficult airway for intubating?
   a)	Mouth opening < 3 fingers
   b)	Hyoid-chin distance < 3 fingers
   c)	Thyroid cartilage-mouth floor distance < 2 fingers

1443)	Define each of the three classes of the American Society Anesthesiologist's (ASA) classification for risk of an adverse event during intubation or sedation.
   a)	Class 1: Normal healthy patient
   b)	Class 2: Mild systemic disease
   c)	Class 3: Severe systemic disease

1444)	List the different criteria for the four classes of the Mallampati score used to determine a difficult airway.
   a)	Class 1: Complete visualization of the soft palate
   b)	Class 2: Complete visualization of the uvula
   c)	Class 3: Visualization only of the base of the uvula
   d)	Class 4: Soft palate is not visible

1445)	What is a relative contraindication to rapid sequence intubation (RSI)?
   a)	Anticipated difficulty ventilating or intubating

1446) What back up measures are used for a failed intubation with a laryngoscope?
   a) Glidescope, Crithyrotomy, LMA, and Gum elastic bougie
1447) Is it suggested to pre-oxygenate before intubating?
   a) Yes
1448) Which medication class during rapid sequence intubation is given first, sedation or paralytic?
   a) Sedation
1449) Why do you want to give the sedation medication before a paralytic?
   a) You do not want to paralyze a patient you cannot intubate
1450) List the medications used for RSI and conscious sedation.
   a) Etomidate, Propofol, Ketamine, Midazolam, Lorazepam, Nitrous oxide, and Fentanyl
1451) What complications that can occur with the use of two medications such as propofol and ketamine verses one when used in conscious sedation?
   a) Increased risk of side effects (apnea)
1452) Which agent used for sedation causes less hypotension and is the agent of choice for ASA 3 and higher?
   a) Etomidate
1453) What is the dosing of Etomidate sedation during RSI?
   a) 0.3 mg/kg IV
1454) What is the Etomidate dosing for conscious sedation?
   a) 0.1 mg/kg IV
1455) How long is the duration of action for Etomidate?
   a) 10-20 min
1456) What is a well-documented side effect of Etomidate?
   a) Adrenal suppression
1457) What patient populations is Etomidate not recommended to be used in due to adrenal suppression?
   a) Elderly and Septic patients
1458) What is the dosing for Propofol with conscious sedation and RSI?
   a) 0.5-2 mg/kg IV
1459) How else can Propofol be used outside of RSI and conscious sedation?

a) Antiemetic, Anticonvulsant, to ↓ ICP, and Intractable migraine

1460) What type of allergy is contraindicated for the use of Propofol

a) Egg allergy

1461) What is the dosing for Ketamine with RSI and conscious sedation?

a) 1-2 mg/kg IV

1462) What are the side effects of Ketamine?

a) Laryngospasm, Bronchorrhea, ↑ Intraocular pressure, and Emergence reaction

1463) How long is the duration of action for Ketamine?

a) 10-20 min

1464) List the paralytic drugs used for RSI.

a) Succinylcholine, Vecuronium, and Rocuronium

1465) What is the duration of action of Rocuronium?

a) 30-45 mins

1466) What is the dosing of Rocuronium?

a) 1 mg/kg

1467) What is the duration of action of Vecuronium?

a) 60-120 min

1468) What is the dosing of Vecuronium?

a) 0.1 mg/kg

1469) What is the dose for Succinylcholine for RSI?

a) 1-1.5 mg/kg IV

1470) What is the duration of action of Succinylcholine?

a) 2-3 min

1471) Give the side effects that can occur with Succinylcholine.

a) Hyperkalemia, Bradycardia, Masseter spasm, Malignant hyperthermia, and Increased ICP

1472) What conditions are relative contraindications to using Succinylcholine for RSI?

a) Burns > 5 days, Crush injuries, Rhabdomyolysis, Myasthenia gravis, Suspected ↑ ICP, and Severe infections > 5 days

1473) What are the 1st and 2nd line medications recommended to be given prior to intubating a patient with suspected elevated ICP?

a) 1st line: Defasciculating agents or Opioids

b) 2nd line: Lidocaine or Atropine

1474) During a respiratory or cardiac arrest, is it recommended to pre-oxygenate a patient before intubating, or should you just intubate?
   a) Intubate
1475) How do you confirm the placement of an endotracheal tube (ET)?
   a) Visualization, Bilateral breath sounds, No stomach sounds, CO_2 monitor, and Chest X-ray
1476) How far should the ET tube be placed from the carina?
   a) 4 cm
1477) How should the bag-mask be held with a one-person technique?
   a) C shaped
1478) What laryngoscope blade is straight?
   a) Miller
1479) What laryngoscope blade is curved?
   a) MAC
1480) What endotracheal tube sizes are recommended for adult female and male patients?
   a) Female: 7.0-8.0
   b) Male: 7.5-8.0
1481) What head position is recommended for intubation?
   a) Head extended and neck flexed
1482) What maneuvers can be done to visualize the cords during intubation?
   a) Backward, Upward, and Rightward pressure (BURP maneuver)
1483) What airway alternatives are available to help ventilate patients with a difficult airway before intubating?
   a) Nasal trumpet and Oral airway
1484) What is required during intubation in a patient with a c-spine injury?
   a) Inline cervical stabilization
1485) What medication is best for RSI with a difficult airway?
   a) Ketamine
1486) What cm H_2O do you set the PEEP at on the ventilator post-intubation?

    a) 5

1487) Why is PEEP not recommended in asthmatic patients?

    a) Barrow trauma due to decreased ability to exhale

1488) What is the maximum inspiratory peak pressure to stay below to prevent barotrauma?

    a) < 35

1489) What is the formula for calculating the tidal volume for the ventilator?

    a) 5-7 ml/kg of ideal body weight

1490) Is the tidal volume based on the patients actual weight or expected BMI for height and weight?

    a) BMI

1491) List the common causes of deterioration of an intubated patient that make up the "DOPE" pneumonic.

    a) Displacement of tube

    b) Obstruction of tube

    c) Pneumothorax

    d) Equipment failure

1492) List the drugs that can be given the endotracheal route.

    a) Naloxone, Atropine, Valium, Epinephrine, and Lidocaine

1493) During ACLS of pediatric patients, what are you supposed to do if you witness a sudden collapse?

    a) Provide 2 minutes CPR, then activate EMS/AED

1494) During ACLS of pediatric patients, what are you supposed to do if you find a child unresponsive?

    a) Send someone to activate EMS or get an AED

1495) Where do you check the pulse on an infant?

    a) Brachial

1496) Where do you check the pulse on children?

    a) Femoral or Carotid

1497) What is the compression to ventilation ratio for pediatric resuscitation with a lone rescuer versus 2 rescuers?

    a) Lone: 30:2

    b) 2 Rescuers: 15:2

1498) What techniques are used for delivering chest compressions on infants with a lone rescuer versus 2 rescuers?

a) Lone: Two finger
b) 2 Rescuer: Two thumbs encircling method

1499) What rescue procedure should be ready for a difficult intubation?

a) Cricothyrotomy

1500) Describe the technique used to perform an emergent cricothyrotomy in the ED?

a) Palpate cricothyroid membrane inferior to the thyroid cartilage
b) Make a 4 cm vertical incision over cricothyroid membrane
c) Blunt dissect to cricothyroid membrane
d) Make a horizontal incision through the membrane
e) Dilate opening in cricothyoid membrane

1501) Why is a vertical incision made first on the skin and not a horizontal incision when performing a cricothyrotomy?

a) To avoid a superior thyroid artery injury

1502) What size tracheostomy and endotracheal-cuffed tubes are placed after an emergent cricothyrotomy?

a) Tracheostomy cuffed tube: Size 4
b) Endotracheal cuffed tube: Size 6

1503) What age is a cricothyrotomy contraindicated?

a) < 10 years old

1504) If a needle crichothyrotomy is performed in a pediatric patient what is the proper way to ventilate?

a) Tracheal jet insufflation

1505) What is the typical recommended time tracheal jet insufflation can be used until a definitive airway should be performed?

a) 30 min

1506) What vocal cord difference between the adult and pediatric patients should be considered when intubating?

a) The pediatric airway is more anterior

1507) What is the narrowest part of the pediatric airway?

a) Cricoid cartilage

1508) What techniques are recommended for the removal of a foreign body in a child who is choking in an infant < 1 and child > 1-year-old?

a) Infant (< 1 year): 5 Back blows and 5 Chest thrusts

b) Child (> 1 year): Abdominal thrusts

1509) Is it recommended to do a blind finger sweep of a choking child?

a) No (can cause further obstruction)

1510) Give the pediatric formula for calculating the appropriate endotracheal tube size.

a) (Age/4) + 4

1511) At what age do you use a cuffed endotracheal tube versus uncuffed?

a) > 8 years : Cuffed

b) < 8 years old: Uncuffed (air leaks are normal)

1512) What else can help estimate a good ET tube size for intubation, in a patient with an unknown age?

a) Measure the diameter of patients small finger

1513) Give the suggested ET tube size for newborns < 1kg, 1-2 kg, 2-3 kg, > 3 kg.

a) < 1 kg: 2.5 mm

b) 1-2 kg: 3.0 mm

c) 2-3 kg: 3.5 mm

d) > 3 kg: 3.5-4.0 mm

1514) What is the formula for calculating the depth of the ET tube in pediatric patients?

a) 3 x tube size

1515) What laryngoscope blade, Miller or Mac, is recommended to use when intubating a pediatric patient?

a) Miller

1516) What size miller blade is used for preterm and term infants?

a) Preterm: #0

b) Term: #1

1517) What are the rate per second and rate per minute rescue breaths to be administered with a bag-mask valve during PALS?

a) Every 3-5 seconds or 12-20 per minute

1518) What are the rate per second and rate per minute rescue breaths are supposed to be administered with an definitive/invasive airway during PALS?

a) Every 6-8 seconds or 8-10 per minute

1519) What is performed due to the size of the pediatric occiput to align the airway when intubating?
   a) Placing a blanket under the back
1520) How do you measure for the correct size oral airway?
   a) Mandible angle to Lip corner
1521) What is the tidal volume used for pediatrics?
   a) 8-12 mL/kg
1522) Give the average respiratory rate for newborns, infants, and toddlers.
   a) Newborn: 50
   b) Infant: 20
   c) Toddler: 15
1523) What medication has controversial evidence on preventing bradycardia if it is given before RSI in pediatric patients?
   a) Atropine
1524) What is the fluid bolus amounts mL/kg that can be given for resuscitation for neonates and pediatric patients?
   a) Neonate: 10 mL/kg
   b) Pediatrics: 20 mL/kg
1525) What is the amount ml/kg of PRBC given for the resuscitation of pediatric patients?
   a) 10 mL/kg
1526) How many fluid boluses should be given before starting blood for hypotension during pediatric trauma resuscitation?
   a) 3
1527) What are the treatments for pediatric, hyponatremia, hypocalcemia, hypomagnesemia?
   a) Hyponatremia = 3% NaCl
   b) Hypocalcemia = Calcium gluconate
   c) Hypomagnesemia = Magnesium sulfate
1528) What is the IV Epinephrine 1:10,000 dosing for pediatrics?
   a) 0.01 mg/kg or 0.1 mL/kg
1529) What is the pediatric Adenosine dosing?
   a) 0.1 mg/kg
1530) What is the pediatric Atropine dosing?
   a) 0.02 mg/kg

1531) What is the pediatric Amiodarone dosing?

   a) 5 mg/kg (max 15 mg/kg)

1532) What is the pediatric Bicarbonate dosing?

   a) 1 mEq/kg

1533) What is the pediatric Naloxone dosing?

   a) 0.1 mg/kg

1534) What is the most common cause leading to pediatric arrest?

   a) Respiratory failure

1535) What is the most common rhythm seen in a pediatric arrest?

   a) Asystole

1536) What is the amount of energy J/kg used for pediatric synchronized cardioversion?

   a) 0.5-1 J/kg

1537) What is the amount of energy J/kg used for the starting and repeat dosing in pediatric defibrillation?

   a) Start 2 J/kg, Repeat dose: 4 J/kg

1538) What percent of dextrose is used to treat hypoglycemia in a neonate?

   a) 10% Dextrose

1539) What is the dose and percent of dextrose used to treat hypoglycemia in pediatric patients?

   a) 2-4 ml/kg of 25% Dextrose

1540) Within what period of time is the initial decision to begin neonatal resuscitation to be determined?

   a) First 30 seconds

1541) What are the initial measures that need to be taken immediately after birth for neonatal resuscitation?

   a) Dry, Warm, Tactile Stimulation, and Suction the mouth and nose

1542) Which do you suction first on a newborn infant after delivery, mouth or nose?

   a) Mouth

1543) Define APGAR score testing in newborns at 1 and 5 minutes post-birth.

   a) Appearance, Pulse, Grimace, Activity, and Respirations

1544) At what heart rate are you supposed to start positive pressure ventilation in a neonate?
   a) < 100 bpm
1545) At what heart rate are you supposed to begin chest compressions in a neonate?
   a) < 60 bpm
1546) What is the ventilation to compression rate for neonates?
   a) 3:1
1547) What is the best measure of appropriate ventilation during neonatal resuscitation?
   a) Increase in heart rate
1548) How do you differentiate between the two umbilical arteries and the umbilical vein during the placement of the umbilical catheter?
   a) The umbilical vein has a thin wall and looks like the mouth of a smiley face
1549) What medication can be given for apnea in preterm neonates < 27 weeks?
   a) Surfactant
1550) What type of fluids are suggested for trauma, sepsis and DKA patients?
   a) Crystalloid fluids (Lactated ringers or 0.9% Normal saline)
1551) In dehydration what two specific labs are the most reliable?
   a) Urine and Plasma osmolality
1552) What is the formula for pediatric maintenance fluid resuscitation?
   a) 4-2-1 rule mL/kg/hr (4 x 1st 10kg, 2 x 2nd 10 kg, and 1 x > 20kg)
1553) What is the recommended amount of fluid rehydration used in pediatrics for each % of dehydration per 24 hours?
   a) 10 mL/kg
1554) What is the calculation for determining the amount of fluid deficit?
   a) Kg x % Dehydration = Fluid deficit (L)
1555) What is the definition of shock?
   a) Circulatory insufficiency creating an imbalance of tissue oxygen supply and demand
1556) List the four types of shock.

a) Hypovolemic, Cardiogenic, Distributive (Neurogenic and Anaphylactic), and Obstructive

1557) After how many liters of resuscitation is the diagnosis of shock suggested if hypotension is still present?

a) After 2 L Normal saline

1558) In hemorrhagic shock when are blood products recommended?

a) After 2 L of Normal saline

1559) What type of blood is the universal donor and is given during trauma and hemorrhagic shock resuscitation?

a) O negative

1560) What is the target urine output with fluid resuscitation during shock resuscitation?

a) > 0.5 mL/kg/hr

1561) What is the target mean arterial pressure (MAP) during shock resuscitation?

a) MAP of 65-90 mmHg

1562) What medication can be given during shock resuscitation for severe acidosis of a PH < 7.1-7.2?

a) Bicarbonate

1563) What is the life-threatening reaction that typically occurs within 15-30 min of allergen exposure and leads to cardiovascular collapse?

a) Anaphylaxis

1564) What is the diagnostic criteria for anaphylaxis?

a) Involvement of two body systems: Skin, Respiratory, Cardiovascular, or GI

1565) List the medications used for an allergic reaction that does not meet anaphylaxis criteria.

a) Steroids, Diphenhydramine, and H2 blockers (Ranitidine)

1566) Why are steroids and antihistamine recommended for treatment home for an allergic reaction following the first dose?

a) Delayed reoccurrence or Biphasic reactions

1567) What specific medication is indicated for anaphylaxis in addition to steroids, Diphenhydramine, and an H2 blocker?

a) Epinephrine

1568) What is the adult IM Epinephrine dose used for anaphylaxis?
   a) 0.3 Mg of 1:1000, repeat every 5 minutes
1569) What is the pediatric IM Epinephrine dose used for anaphylaxis?
   a) 0.01 mg/kg max 0.5 mg of 1:1000, repeat every 5 minutes
1570) What is recommended for continuous treatment for anaphylaxis refractory to IM administration of Epinephrine?
   a) Epinephrine IV infusion 1-4 mcg/min
1571) What is the recommended observation time for patients who received Epinephrine for an allergic reaction before discharge?
   a) 4 hours without symptoms
1572) What medication can be given for wheezing and shortness of breath from an allergic reaction?
   a) Beta-agonist
1573) What medications and fluids can be given through interosseous (IO) lines?
   a) All
1574) List the areas of the body that IO lines can be placed.
   a) Proximal and Distal Tibia, Proximal Humerus, Distal Femur, Distal Radius and Ulna, Iliac spine, and Sternum
1575) List the contraindications to placing an IO in a chosen location.
   a) Fracture, Previous orthopedic procedure at the site, Overlying skin/soft tissue infection, Unable to palpate anatomy, Previous IO within last 48 hours, Burns, Osteogenesis Imperfecta, or Osteomyelitis
1576) What is the proportional rate of tachycardia associated with each degree of temperature elevation in a fever?
   a) ↑ 10 beats per ↑ of 1° C

Toxicology

1577) List the indications for the use of gastric decontamination with an overdose.
   a) Ingestion within 1 hour, No altered mental status, and a Toxic substance ingestion

1578) List the different methods of gastric decontamination.
   a) Activated charcoal, Whole bowel irrigation, and Gastric lavage (less favorable)

1579) List the contraindications for using gastric decontamination with overdoses.
   a) Caustic agent ingestion, Hydrocarbons ingestion, Bleeding disorder, Seizures, Altered mental status, Unprotected airway, Bowel obstruction or perforation, Xenobiotic with limited toxicity or low ingested dose, or Late presentation (many hours post-ingestion).

1580) What is the dose of activated charcoal?
   a) 1-2 g/kg (max 100 g)

1581) What products are poorly bound by activated charcoal?
   a) Lithium, Iron, Caustics, Cyanide, Hydrocarbons, Alcohol, Alkali, and Acids

1582) What gastric decontamination method and medication can be useful in the treatment of toxic ingestions of Iron, enteric-coated medications, Lithium, and for body packers or foreign body ingestions?
   a) Whole bowel irrigation (Polyethylene glycol)

1583) What imaging modality is recommended for ruling out foreign body ingestion in a body stuffer (packer)?
   a) CT abdomen & pelvis

1584) Overdose of which drugs is urine alkalization used for treatment?
   a) Salicylates, Phenobarbital, and INH

1585) What two drug levels are the most important labs to order in an overdose workup?
   a) Salicylate and Acetaminophen

1586) Which drug overdoses can hemodialysis be helpful for drug elimination?
   a) Salicylates, Lithium, Methanol, Isopropanol, Ethylene glycol, Theophylline, Caffeine, Metformin, Valproic acid, and Phenobarbital
1587) List the drugs and alcohol products that can lead to metabolic acidosis with toxicity.
   a) Methanol, Metformin, Paracetamol (Acetminophen), Iron, Isoniazid (INH), Ethylene glycol, and Salicylates
1588) Give the formula for calculating the anion gap in metabolic acidosis.
   a) $AG = Na^+ - (Cl + HCO3)$
1589) Give the calculation for determining the osmolar gap.
   a) $OG = 2(Na^+) + BUN/2.8 + Glucose/18$
1590) Which drug overdoses lead to an increased osmolar gap?
   a) Acetone, Isopropanol, Methanol, Ethylene glycol, Propylene glycol, Mannitol, and Ethanol
1591) What drug overdose is the most common cause of an increased osmolar gap?
   a) Ethanol
1592) What synthetic opiate is not screened on common drug panels?
   a) Synthetic Fentanyl
1593) What medications are best for delirium, agitation, and seizures with drug overdose?
   a) Benzodiazepines
1594) What is the acronym of drugs used for an agitated delirious psychotic patient on drugs?
   a) B52 (50 mg Benadryl, 5mg Haldol, 2 mg Ativan)
1595) What type of drug elimination is a constant percentage per unit of time and is dependent on the drug concentration?
   a) First-order elimination
1596) What type of drug elimination occurs with ETOH metabolism?
   a) Zero-order elimination
1597) What drug toxidrome causes hyperthermia, blurry vision, dry skin, absent bowel sounds, urinary retention, flushing, and altered mental status?

    a) Anticholinergic

1598) What drug overdoses can lead to an anticholinergic toxidrome?

    a) Atropine, Antihistamines (Benadryl), Jimsonweed, Belladonna, Cyclic Antidepressants (TCA), Phenothiazines, and Antiparkinson drugs

1599) What medication is used for the treatment of wide complex tachycardia (widened QRS >100 ms) with a drug overdose?

    a) Sodium bicarbonate

1600) What cholinergic drug is the last resort for treatment for anticholinergic toxidrome symptoms?

    a) Physostigmine (contraindicated in TCA overdose)

1601) What toxidrome causes dilated pupils, agitation, hypertension, tachycardia, diaphoresis, normal bowel sounds, and hyperthermia?

    a) Sympathomimetic

1602) What common drugs cause a sympathomimetic effect?

    a) Cocaine, Amphetamines, and PCP

1603) Does PCP show up on a urine drug screen?

    a) No

1604) What is the treatment for a sympathomimetic toxidrome?

    a) Benzodiazepines

1605) What specific alpha-1-antagonist can be used for a resistant hypertensive emergency in a cocaine overdose?

    a) Phentolamine

1606) What antihypertensive medication class should be avoided in a hypertensive crisis due to cocaine use?

    a) Beta-blocker

1607) What lung conditions can occur with a deep forceful valsalva during inhalation while smoking causing sudden chest pain and shortness of breath?

    a) Pneumothorax or Pneumomediastinum

1608) What specific toxin is formed when cocaine and ethanol are mixed and has a longer duration of action that increases the risk of MI and stroke?

    a) Cocaethylene (ethyl cocaine)

1609) What is the treatment of cocaine or amphetamine-induced MIs due to drug-induced coronary vasospasm?

    a) Oxygen, Benzodiazepines, Phentolamine, Nitrates, and Heparin

1610) What condition can be seen with PCP, Amphetamine or Cocaine overdoses in a psychotic hyperactive patient, with hyperthermia, brown urine, and muscle cramps?
   a) Rhabdomyolysis

1611) What drug use causes pathognomonic rotatory nystagmus, agitation, muscle rigidity, hyperthermia, and altered mental status?
   a) Phencyclidine (PCP)

1612) What medication do you want to avoid in an agitated patient on PCP (acid) due to the theoretical risk of worsening symptoms?
   a) Ketamine

1613) What sympathomimetic drug enhances the effects and blocks the reuptake of catecholamines, causing hyperactivity, tachycardia, hyperthermia, diaphoresis, MI, and hypertension?
   a) Amphetamines

1614) What is the most common reason for death with MMDA (Ecstasy) abuse?
   a) Dehydration: leads to renal failure and hyponatremia

1615) What xanthine medication is typically used in asthma and COPD, and can cause tachycardia, tremors, and seizures from an increased catecholamine release, and metabolic acidosis with an overdose?
   a) Theophylline

1616) What are the theophylline levels associated with toxicity?
   a) > 20 mg/L

1617) What treatment is indicated in theophylline poisoning with severe hypotension, seizures, and arrhythmias?
   a) Hemodialysis

1618) What acute and chronic theophylline levels is hemodialysis recommended with theophylline poisoning?
   a) Acute level: > 80 mg/L
   b) Chronic level: > 40 mg/L

1619) What amount (mg/kg) is a lethal dose of theophylline?
   a) 150-200 mg/kg

1620) What is the most commonly used psychoactive drug in the world?
   a) Caffeine

1621) What caffeine serum concentration can cause life-threatening signs?
   a) > 120 micrograms/ml
1622) What toxidrome from drug overdose causes salivation, lacrimation, urination, diarrhea, gastrointestinal upset, emesis, bradycardia, and bronchospasm?
   a) Cholinergic
1623) What are the pupil changes seen with a cholinergic toxidrome?
   a) Miosis (pinpoint)
1624) List the drugs that can cause a cholinergic toxidrome.
   a) Organophosphates, Carbamates, Mushrooms, and Nerve agents
1625) List the cholinergic toxidrome symptoms in the acronym DUMBBELS.
   a) Diarrhea, Urination, Miosis, Bronchorrhea, Bronchospasm, Bradycardia, Emesis, Lacrimation, and Salivation
1626) What cholinergic substance typically used in pesticides for farming causes muscle weakness, bradycardia, bronchospasm, salivation, and vomiting?
   a) Organophosphate
1627) List some organophosphates pesticides.
   a) Parathion, Malathion, and Diazinon
1628) List some nerve agents that can cause a cholinergic toxidrome.
   a) Sarin, Soman, and Tabun
1629) What are the muscarinic, nicotinic, and CNS clinical effects of organophosphate/nerve agent poisoning?
   a) Muscarinic: salivation, lacrimation, urination, defecation, GI cramping, and emesis.
   b) Nicotinic: muscle fasciculation, weakness, and paralysis.
   c) CNS: loss of consciousness, seizures, and respiratory depression
1630) What medications are used to treat organophosphate and nerve agent poisoning?
   a) Atropine and Pralidoxime (2-PAM)
1631) What paralytic drug should you avoid when intubating an organophosphates poisoned patient?
   a) Succinylcholine
1632) What is the treatment of poison hemlock ingestion?

a) GI decontamination
1633) What class of medications causes respiratory depression, altered mental status, and coma with pinpoint pupils during an overdose?
a) Opioids
1634) What is the treatment for opioid overdose?
a) Naloxone
1635) What is the typical duration of Naloxone and time frame re-administration may be needed?
a) 30-60 minutes
1636) List the different ways Naloxone can be administered.
a) SC, IN, ET, IM, IV, and Nebulizer
1637) What are the cardiac side effects of Naloxone administration?
a) New-onset arrhythmias (a-fib, atrial flutter)
1638) What type of opioid overdose requires repeat doses of naloxone and larger amounts?
a) Fentanyl analogues
1639) What antihypertensive medication can mimic an opioid overdose, with the addition of hypotension and bradycardia and is used to help treat opioid withdrawal symptoms?
a) Clonidine (alpha 2 agonist)
1640) Give the symptoms of Clonidine withdrawal.
a) Hypertension, anxiety, tachycardia, and diaphoresis
1641) What medication can be used for alcohol cessation by reducing cravings and for Clonidine overdoses?
a) Naltrexone
1642) What medication class can be used for alcohol, barbiturate, and benzodiazepine withdrawal symptoms?
a) Benzodiazepines
1643) What are the symptoms of alcohol/benzodiazepine withdrawal?
a) Nausea/vomiting
b) Tremor
c) Anxiety
d) Inattention and impairment in cognitive and perceptual function (Tactile, Auditory and Visual hallucinations)

e) Delirium tremens: Acute and fluctuating disturbances in consciousness, confusion, psychomotor agitation

f) Life-threatening fluid, metabolic, electrolyte imbalances and unstable vitals

g) Seizures

1644) What medication overdose is the number one leading cause of drug induced liver failure, and causes nausea, vomiting, and abdominal pain?

a) Acetaminophen

1645) What is the toxic dose of acetaminophen?

a) 150 mg/kg

1646) Describe the physiologic mechanism of how acetaminophen toxicity can cause liver damage?

a) Saturation of glucuronidation and sulfonation pathways leading to toxic metabolite accumulation via cytochrome 2E1 pathway

1647) What is the toxic metabolite produced in acetaminophen toxicity?

a) NAPQI

1648) Depletion of what liver metabolite leads to liver toxicity in acetaminophen overdose?

a) Glutathione

1649) What is the antidote for acetaminophen overdose that inhibits the toxic metabolite NAPQI from binding hepatocytes?

a) N-acetylcysteine

1650) List the 4 symptom stages with their time frame in acetaminophen overdose.

a) Stage 1 < 24 hours: Nausea, Vomiting, Diaphoresis

b) Stage 2 24-48 hours: RUQ pain, ↑ liver enzymes and ↑ PT

c) Stage 3 72-96 hours: Hepatic and Renal failure

d) Stage 4 3-7 days: Resolution of hepatic toxicity, Organ failure, and Death

1651) What graph is used to follow toxicity levels of acetaminophen?

a) Rumack-Matthew nomogram

1652) What is the acetaminophen toxic blood level at 4 hours to suggest treatment with N-acetylcysteine?

a) > 150 mcg/ml

1653) What are the other criteria to suggest antidote treatment before having a 4-hour level with an acetaminophen overdose?
   a) Ingestion of > 150 mg/kg or > 7 grams in adults

1654) What is the initial dosing of N-acetylcysteine IV and oral?
   a) IV: 150 mg/kg
   b) Oral: 140 mg/kg

1655) What drug causes GI symptoms, tinnitus, hyperventilation, hypoglycemia, vomiting, seizures, renal failure and an anion gap metabolic acidosis with an acute overdose?
   a) Salicylates

1656) What are the classic metabolic and respiratory changes that occur with salicylate overdose?
   a) Anion gap metabolic acidosis and Respiratory alkalosis

1657) Does a normal anion gap with a metabolic acidosis rule out salicylate poisoning in patients with unknown ingestion?
   a) No

1658) What common house agent contains salicylates and can cause severe toxicity and death if ingested?
   a) Oil of wintergreen

1659) What ophthalmic medication used for glaucoma can lead to chronic salicylate poisoning?
   a) Carbonic anhydrase inhibitors

1660) What are the mg/kg salicylate doses that correlate with mild, moderate, and severe ingestion and symptoms?
   a) Mild: > 150 mg/kg
   b) Moderate: 150-300 mg/kg
   c) Severe: > 300 mg/kg

1661) Give the treatments used for salicylate overdose.
   a) Blood and Urine alkalization (HCO3), Admission, IV fluids, +/- Hemodialysis, Glucose, and Potassium replacement

1662) What is the target PH level for urine alkalization treatment in salicylate poisoning?
   a) > 7.5

1663) What medication is used for urine alkalization and how is it administered?

a) NaHCO₃ bolus (1-2 meq/kg), followed by infusion of 3 amps of NaHCO₃ in 1L of D5W at 1.5-2x maintenance rate

1664) What salicylate drug level is hemodialysis recommended with acute and chronic overdoses?
a) Acute: > 100 mg/dL
b) Chronic: > 60-80 mg/dL

1665) What level of chronic Aspirin (salicylate) ingestion can lead to an increased PT time?
a) > 60 mg/dL

1666) How often are ASA (Aspirin) levels checked until the level is non-toxic?
a) Every 2 hours until there is a steady decline in levels

1667) List the criteria for hemodialysis therapy for salicylate toxicity that are not based on the salicylate level.
a) Altered mental status, Refractory acidosis, Renal or Cardiac failure, Cerebral edema, Seizures, or Pulmonary edema

1668) What GI symptoms can occur with chronic NSAID use and ingestion?
a) Peptic ulcer disease

1669) What type of alcohol ingestion causes an increased osmolar gap, an anion gap metabolic acidosis, with seizures, vomiting, and blindness?
a) Methanol

1670) What is the toxic component of methanol poisoning?
a) Formic acid

1671) When is dialysis the recommend treatment in methanol poisoning?
a) Levels > 50 mg/dL, Vision changes, Severe acidosis, impaired renal functions, Coma, or Seizure

1672) What methanol and ethylene glycol levels are considered toxic?
a) > 20 mg/dL

1673) Poisoning from what type of alcohol can lead to a coma, anion gap acidosis, increased osmolar gap, renal failure, hematuria, and hypocalcemia?
a) Ethylene glycol

1674) What is the toxic component produced in ethylene glycol poisoning?
   a) Oxalic acid
1675) What can be seen in the urine in ethylene glycol poisoning?
   a) Calcium oxalate crystals
1676) What bedside test can be performed on the urine collected in the ED, to rule in ethylene glycol poisoning from antifreeze?
   a) Woods lamp (fluorescent urine)
1677) What are the treatments for ethylene glycol and methanol poisoning?
   a) Fomepizole, IV Alcohol/Ethanol, Folic acid, and +/- Dialysis
1678) How do you dose fomepizole?
   a) 15 mg/kg bolus, then 10 mg/kg every 12 hours till the level <20
1679) When is dialysis recommended for ethylene glycol poisoning treatment?
   a) Refractory acidosis
   b) Levels > 50 mg/dL
   c) Renal failure
1680) How does ethanol work in preventing further methanol and ethylene glycol poisoning?
   a) It occupies ADH and prevents methanol and ethylene glycol breakdown
1681) Which alcohol poisoning causes CNS depression, pulmonary edema, hypoglycemia, and hemorrhagic gastritis with an increased osmolar gap?
   a) Isopropyl alcohol
1682) What is the recommended treatment for isopropyl alcohol poisoning?
   a) Supportive
1683) What medication can be given to prevent alcohol ingestion in alcoholics, and causes flushing, diaphoresis, nausea, vomiting, hypotension, and seizures?
   a) Disulfiram
1684) What drug reaction occurs with the combination of alcohol and Metronidazole leading to flushing, diaphoresis, nausea, vomiting, hypotension, and seizures?

a) Disulfiram reaction

1685) What metal poisoning in weed killers, and pesticides, causes GI symptoms, hypotension, delirium, peripheral neuropathy in a stocking-glove pattern, and leads to hepatic and renal failure?

a) Arsenic

1686) What physical exam finding on the fingers is seen in arsenic and thallium poisoning?

a) Mee's lines (white lines in the fingernails)

1687) What is the treatment for arsenic poisoning?

a) Chelation with BAL (Dimercaprol) and DMSA (Dimercaptosuccinic acid or Succimer)

1688) What metal drug overdose causes gastroenteritis symptoms, metabolic gap acidosis, liver damage and can be seen on an abdominal X-ray?

a) Iron

1689) What is the antidote for Iron overdose/toxicity?

a) Deferoxamine (10-15 mg/kg/hr)

1690) What is the toxic dose of iron?

a) > 20-60 mg/kg of elemental iron

1691) List the indications for Deferoxamine administration.

a) Iron level > 500 mcg/dl, Metabolic Acidosis, Shock, or Severe GI symptoms

1692) What color does Deferoxamine change the urine with excretion of the iron complex?

a) "Vin rose" (reddish-brown)

1693) Give the 5 stages of iron toxicity and their time frames.

a) Stage 1 0-6 hours: GI symptoms and Dehydration

b) Stage 2 6-24 hours: Latent phase

c) Stage 3 6-72 hours: Shock, Acidosis, and Coma

d) Stage 4 2-3 days: Liver failure

e) Stage 5 2-8 weeks: Symptom recovery and Gastric outlet obstruction (Gastric stricture and scaring)

1694) What chronic metal poisoning is commonly seen in children living in old inner-city homes causes headaches, anorexia, abdominal pain, and darkening of their gums?

a) Lead

1695) What upper extremity physical exam finding is classic for lead poisoning and is due to peripheral neuropathy?
   a) Wrist drop

1696) What lead levels do symptoms start to present with chronic toxicity?
   a) 10 mcg/dL

1697) What levels of lead poisoning are classified as severe?
   a) > 70 mcg/dL

1698) What are the findings of lead poisoning on a blood smear?
   a) Basophilic stippling

1699) What chelating agents can be used to treat lead poisoning?
   a) Chelation with Dimercaprol (BAL), Succimer (DMSA, Dimercaptosuccinic acid), and Calcium sodium Ethylenediaminetetraacetic acid (CaNa$_2$EDTA)

1700) What chelating agent is used for asymptomatic lead poisoning with levels > 50 mcg/dL?
   a) Oral Succimer (DMSA)

1701) What chelating agents are used for lead toxicity with levels > 100 mcg/dL causing encephalopathy?
   a) IM Dimercaprol (BAL) + CaNa$_2$EDTA

1702) What are the pathognomonic findings found on extremity X-rays that can be seen with lead poisoning?
   a) Lead lines

1703) What metal toxicity causes GI symptoms, altered mental status, and renal injury that is diagnosed with a 24-hour urine collection after ingestion?
   a) Mercury

1704) What are the treatment options for mercury poisoning?
   a) Dimercaprol (BAL) or Succimer

1705) What chelating medication is used to treat inorganic elemental mercury poisoning?
   a) Dimercaprol (BAL)

1706) What chelating medication is used to treat organic mercury poisoning?
   a) Succimer

1707) What antipsychotic and antiepileptic medication overdose leads to confusion, slurred speech, tremor, ataxia, seizure, renal injury, coma, and arrhythmias?

a) Lithium

1708) What specific renal disease can develop with chronic Lithium use?

a) Nephrogenic diabetes insipidus

1709) What ECG changes can occur with Lithium toxicity?

a) Prolonged QT, ST-segment depression, and T-wave inversions

1710) What are the treatments for Lithium toxicity or poisoning?

a) IV Fluids, Admit, and +/- Dialysis

1711) What serum Lithium level is hemodialysis recommended for the treatment in an acute overdose or poisoning?

a) Lithium level > 5-6 mEq/L

1712) What serum Lithium level is hemodialysis recommended for the treatment in a chronic toxicity or poisoning?

a) Lithium level > 4.0 mEq/L

1713) Give the symptom indications for treatment with dialysis in a Lithium overdose/poisoning that are not based on the Lithium level.

a) Coma, Seizures, Shock, Renal failure, and Dysrhythmias

1714) What antihypertensive medications can cause hypotension, bradycardia, and AV block in an overdose?

a) Beta-blocker, Calcium channel blocker (CCB), and Digoxin overdose

1715) Give the treatments used for a beta-blocker overdose.

a) Glucagon (5-10mg) and high-dose insulin and glucose infusion (0.5-1 unit/kg)

1716) What metabolic abnormality can occur with a beta-blocker overdose and differentiates it from a CCB overdose?

a) Hypoglycemia

1717) Give the treatments used for a calcium channel blocker overdose.

a) Calcium chloride or gluconate, Insulin infusion/glucose, or Intravenous lipid emulsion

1718) What type of insulin and dosing of insulin is used in a calcium channel blocker overdose?

a) Regular insulin 1 U/kg bolus followed by infusion

1719) What metabolic abnormality can occur with a calcium channel blocker overdose?
   a) Hyperglycemia

1720) Which antiarrhythmic medication overdose causes paroxysmal atrial tachycardia with an AV block, nausea, vomiting, dizziness, and confusion?
   a) Digitalis

1721) What is the toxic dose of digitalis that can cause symptoms in adults and pediatrics?
   a) Adult: 3 mg
   b) Pediatric: 1 mg

1722) What is the most common EKG finding in digoxin overdose/toxicity?
   a) PVCs

1723) What pathognomonic EKG finding can occur with digoxin toxicity?
   a) Bidirectional (positive and negative) V-tach

1724) What ocular distortion occurs with digoxin toxicity?
   a) Yellow halos around lights

1725) What type of cell pump does digitalis inhibit to limit cardiac activity?
   a) Na^+- K^+- ATPase pump

1726) What type of plants is digitalis derived from?
   a) Foxglove, Lily of the Valley, and Oleander

1727) What herbal substance when combinded with digoxin causes an additive effect leading to bradycardia?
   a) Hawthorne

1728) What is the antidote used in digoxin toxicity?
   a) Digoxin immune Fab (suggested to start with 1-2 vials until level returns)

1729) What is the suggested treatment for chronic digoxin toxicity?
   a) IV hydration, Potassium and Magnesium repletion, and Digoxin immune Fab

1730) What electrolyte deficiencies can lead to chronic digoxin toxicity along with dehydration?

a) Hypokalemia, Hypomagnesemia, and Hypercalcemia

1731) What is the formula to determine the number of vials for a full reversal of digoxin toxicity if the steady-state digitalis level is known?

a) # of vials = [serum digoxin (ng/ml) x body weight (kg)]/ 100

1732) What are the two suggested antiarrhythmic medications used for ventricular dysrhythmias in a digoxin overdose or toxicity?

a) Lidocaine or Phenytoin

1733) What are the vitamin K dependent clotting factors inhibited with the use of Warfarin?

a) II, VII, IX, and X

1734) What are the treatment options for Warfarin (Coumadin) overdose with an elevated INR?

a) Hold Warfarin dose, Vitamin K, or FFP

1735) What antiepileptic medication overdose causes miosis, hypotension, CNS depression, and cutaneous bullae?

a) Barbiturates

1736) Which antiepileptic medication overdose has a classic triad of dizziness, ataxia, and nystagmus with slurred speech and CNS depression?

a) Carbamazepine (Tegretol)

1737) What are the treatment options for Carbamazepine overdose?

a) Charcoal, Supportive care, +/- Dialysis

1738) What anti-epileptic medication can cause nystagmus, vomiting, coma, dystonia, and ataxia from increase drug levels or overdose?

a) Phenytoin and Fosphenytoin

1739) What is the treatment for Phenytoin overdose?

a) Charcoal and Airway control

1740) Which medication overdose causes coma, ataxia, hypotension, and respiratory depression and is treated with observation and supportive care?

a) Benzodiazepine

1741) What is the antidote for a benzodiazepine overdose?

a) Flumazenil

1742) What complication can occur if Flumazenil is given to patients with a history of chronic benzodiazepine use?

a) Intractable seizures

1743) Which industrial toxic gas with a bitter almond odor, leads to nausea, bradycardia, acidosis, and cardiovascular collapse with a normal PaO_2 and O_2?

a) Cyanide

1744) Give the treatments for cyanide poisoning.

a) Hydroxocobalamin (B12), Sodium Thiosulfate, Sodium Nitrite, or Amyl nitrite

1745) What type of poisoning can occur with the ingestion of too many fruit seeds from cherries, apricot, and peaches?

a) Cyanide toxicity

1746) What hypertensive medication can lead to cyanide poisoning if used for a long period?

a) Sodium Nitroprusside

1747) What is the chemical substance in pits that leads to cyanide poisoning?

a) Amygdalin

1748) What condition leads to oxidation of Fe^{++} to Fe^{+++} causing hypoxia, cyanosis that is unresponsive to oxygen therapy and chocolate brown blood?

a) Methemoglobinemia (MetHgb)

1749) At what MetHgb levels do cyanosis and hypoxia usually present?

a) MetHgb > 10% (1.5 g/dL)

1750) List some drugs that commonly lead to methemoglobinemia.

a) Benzocaine, Phenazopyridine (Pyridium), Dapsone, Nitrates, and Nitrites

1751) What is the antidote for methemoglobinemia?

a) Methylene blue

1752) What is the usual dose of methylene blue?

a) 1-2 mg/kg IV over 5 min. If cyanosis doesn't resolve within 60 min, a second dose can be given.

1753) What are the second-line treatment options for an unstable patient with methemoglobinemia who failed to improve from Methylene blue treatment?

a) Exchange transfusion or Hyperbaric oxygen (HBO)

1754) What type of gas present in farming silos can cause pulmonary edema, and methemoglobinemia with poisoning?
   a) Nitrogen dioxide

1755) What type of hemoglobinopathy can develop due to Metoclopramide, Sumatriptan, or Trinitroluene (TNT) use and shows up as dark greenish-black blood on blood draw?
   a) Sulfhemoglobinemia (SulfHb)

1756) What is the treatment of sulfhemoglobinemia?
   a) Supportive and Stop offending medication

1757) What is the recommended treatment for severe sulfhemoglobinemia?
   a) Exchange (blood) transfusion

1758) What drug used in date rape, presents with respiratory depression, lethargy, depressed mental status in a patient who has sudden recovery of consciousness after a few hours of observation?
   a) Gamma Hydroxybutyric Acid (GHB)

1759) Does GHB show up on drug screens?
   a) No

1760) What is the treatment for GHB toxicity?
   a) Observation and Airway protection

1761) What antidepressant medication leads to headaches, hypertension, and tachycardia with overdose or with co-ingestion of amphetamines, fava beans, wine, or cheese?
   a) Monamine Oxidase Inhibitors (MAOI)

1762) List some hallucinogenic drugs.
   a) LSD (acid), Mushrooms, Mescaline, and Morning glory seeds

1763) List symptoms typical of a hallucinogen ingestion.
   a) Tachycardia, Hyperthermia, Dilated pupils, Altered mental status, and Psychosis

1764) Which drug ingestion causes combative bizarre behavior, hallucinations, tachycardia, mydriasis, hypertension, and hyperthermia?
   a) LSD (acid)

1765) What is the recommended treatment for LSD?
   a) Supportive care and Benzodiazepines

1766) What type of mushroom ingestion leads to nausea, vomiting, diarrhea, followed by a latent symptom period and then liver and renal failure 24-48 hours after ingestion?

a) Amanita phalloides

1767) What is the suggested treatment for Amanita phalloides toxicity?

a) Supportive therapy, N-acetylcysteine and Silibinin (milk thistle)

1768) Which type of mushroom is a GABA agonist, has a red cap with white polka dots, and causes mental status changes, hallucinations, and delirium?

a) Amanita muscaria

1769) What type of mushrooms commonly used for a psychedelic trip, have small round brown caps and cause hallucinations, euphoria, and vomiting?

a) Psilocybin

1770) What type of mushrooms are mistaken by Morel mushroom hunters during the spring, and can cause vomiting, headaches, liver failure, and seizures if ingested?

a) Gyromitrin (false morel)

1771) What is the toxin in the Gyromitrin mushrooms?

a) Monomethylhydrazine

1772) What is the suggested treatment for seizure activity from a toxic Gyromitrin mushroom ingestion?

a) Pyridoxine (Vitamin B6)

1773) What side effects can occur with ingestion of the muscarine containing mushrooms Inocybe and Clitocybe?

a) Lacrimation, Salivation, Diarrhea, Urination, and Emesis (muscarinic effects)

1774) Which medication class's side effects cause dystonia, akathisia, tardive dyskinesia, QT prolongation, and decreased mental status with chronic use or overdose?

a) Antipsychotic medications

1775) What side effect from neuroleptics and antipsychotic medications cause, altered mental status, hypertension, severe hyperthermia, tachycardia, muscle rigidity, and opisthotonos?

a) Neuroleptic malignant syndrome (NMS)

1776)   What is the treatment for NMS?
   a)   Dantrolene, Bromocriptine or Amantadine + Benzodiazepines
        and Antipyretics
1777)   What hyperthermic condition is similar to NMS but occurs after
   the administration of inhaled anesthetics before surgery?
   a)   Malignant hyperthermia
1778)   How is malignant hyperthermia distinguished from NMS?
   a)   By history
1779)   What is the treatment of malignant hyperthermia?
   a)   Dantrolene
1780)   What medical condition is due to increased medication levels or
   overdose in a patient on antidepressants, and presents with altered
   mental status, hyperthermia, tachycardia, and muscle clonus?
   a)   Serotonin syndrome
1781)   What is the treatment for Serotonin syndrome?
   a)   Cyproheptadine and Stop drug
1782)   Give the medication classes that can increase serotonin levels
   when combined or taken in overdose.
   a)   SSRI, Tricyclic antidepressants, MAOI, and Tramadol
1783)   List the two diagnostic criteria that can help with the diagnosis
   of serotonin syndrome.
   a)   Hunter and Sternbach's criteria
1784)   List the Hunter diagnostic criteria for serotonin syndrome.
   Requires 1 of the following:
   a)   Spontaneous clonus
   b)   Inducible clonus with agitation or diaphoresis
   c)   Ocular clonus with agitation or diaphoresis
   d)   Tremor and hyperreflexia
   e)   Hypertonia, fever with ocular or inducible clonus
1785)   List the Sternbach's criteria that requires 3 of 10 symptoms, to
   help diagnose serotonin syndrome.
   a)   AMS, Myoclonus, Ocular clonus, Rhabdomyolysis, Shivering,
        Tremor, Tonic-clonic seizure, Hyperreflexia, Fever, Diaphoresis,
        Diarrhea, or Agitation
1786)   What are the ECG findings seen with a Citalopram overdose?
   a)   QRS widening and QTc prolongation

1787) What drug levels in a Bupropion overdose is it recommended to admit for 24-hour monitoring?

a) > 450 mg

1788) What type of antidepressant medication overdose leads to depressed mental status, flushing, dry mouth, delirium, seizures, and tachycardia with QRS widening on ECG?

a) Tricyclic antidepressants (TCA)

1789) What are the 7 mechanisms of TCA toxicity?

a) Na Channel Blockade

b) Potassium channel blockade

c) α1-receptor Blockade

d) Antihistamine

e) Anticholinergic (Antimuscarinic)

f) Amine reuptake inhibition

g) GABA receptor blockade

1790) What medication decreases cardiac toxicity and is used in a TCA overdose with a widened QRS > 100ms?

a) Sodium bicarbonate

1791) Which type of caustic ingestion agent leads to liquefaction necrosis?

a) Alkali

1792) Which type of caustic ingestion agent leads to coagulation necrosis?

a) Acids

1793) Is it recommended to treat liquid caustic agent ingestion by diluting?

a) No

1794) What acidic yellow-green gas chemical can cause a respiratory exacerbation, nausea, lightheadedness in a person cleaning their bathroom?

a) Chlorine

1795) How do you treat a hydrofluoric acid burn?

a) Cover with Calcium gluconate 2.5% gel or Local injection of 10% calcium gluconate

1796) Give the mechanism of action for calcium gluconate in a hydrofluoric acid burn.
   a) Calcium binds the fluoride ion stopping the burn
1797) What is the etiology leading to death in a patient with > a 2.5% total body surface burn from hydrofluoric acid?
   a) Hypocalcemia leading to a prolonged QT
1798) List a common hydrocarbon of abuse.
   a) Toluene
1799) What lung condition can develop with huffing hydrocarbons from glues, inks, paint removers, or pesticides?
   a) Chemical pneumonitis
1800) What cardiac side effect occurs from sniffing hydrocarbons?
   a) Ventricular dysrhythmias
1801) What is the recommended managment for patients huffing hydrocarbons who are symptomatic?
   a) Decontamination and Admit if symptomatic
1802) What toxic gas from oil, sewage, and mines, has a rotten egg smell and inhibits cytochrome oxidase leading to anaerobic metabolism, causing headaches, nausea, vomiting, and watery eyes and loss of consciousness?
   a) Hydrogen Sulfide (H_2S)
1803) Give the lethal dose of hydrogen sulfide that causes death.
   a) > 500 ppm
1804) List the treatments for H_2S toxicity.
   a) Supportive therapy, Remove victim from source, 100% oxygen, and Antidote
1805) What is the antidote for hydrogen sulfide toxicity?
   a) Cyanocobalamin or Sodium nitrite
1806) What tuberculosis drug overdose leads to coma, metabolic acidosis, and seizures from depleted vitamin B6?
   a) Isoniazid (INH)
1807) What is the treatment of INH overdose or toxicity?
   a) Pyridoxine (Vitamin B6)
1808) What is the treatment for a sulfonylurea medication overdose causing hypoglycemia?
   a) Octreotide

1809) List some sulfonylurea drugs.
   a) Glyburide, Glipizide, Glimepiride, and Chlorpropamide
1810) What therapy is used to control reoccurring hypoglycemia after a sulfonylurea or insulin overdose?
   a) Dextrose IV drip 5% or 10%
1811) What diabetic medication causes lactic acidosis with normal use and overdose and should also be held after IV contrast dye administration?
   a) Metformin
1812) What type of plant with purple berries inhibits mucosal regeneration and if ingested causes nausea, vomiting, diarrhea, hemorrhagic enteritis, leukocytosis and respiratory failure with a severe toxicity?
   a) Pokeweed
1813) What type of common red houseplant flower causes dermatitis, and vomiting if ingested?
   a) Poinsettia
1814) What type of green leafy houseplant ingestion causes, cramping vomiting, and immediate pain and burning in the mouth?
   a) Philodendrons
1815) What type of plant ingestion causes vomiting with pathognomonic calcium oxalate crystals seen in the urine?
   a) Dieffenbachia
1816) Give the symptoms that can occur with the ingestion of a large dose of tobacco.
   a) Vomiting, Diarrhea, Miosis, Altered mental status, and Seizures
1817) What is the reversal agent used specifically for a dabigatran overdose?
   a) Idarucizumab
1818) What are the antidotes for a Methotrexate overdose?
   a) Leucovorin or Glucarpidase
1819) What is the antidote for a Valproic acid overdose with mental status changes?
   a) L-carnitine
1820) What is the treatment for red squill poisoning?
   a) Digoxin

1821) What is the treatment of Thallium toxicity?
   a) Prussian blue

1822) What is the treatment for toxicity of the organochlorine pesticide Chlordecone?
   a) Cholestyramine

1823) List the vitamin names associated with each of B1, B2, B3, and B6.
   a) B1: Thiamine
   b) B2: Riboflavin
   c) B3: Niacin
   d) B6: Pyridoxine

1824) What vitamin deficiency causes diarrhea, dermatitis, and dementia?
   a) Niacin (B3) also known as "Pellagra"

1825) List the fat-soluble vitamins.
   a) D, E, A, and K

1826) Toxicity of what vitamin causes headaches, hypercalcemia, increased intracranial pressure, and hepatotoxicity?
   a) Vitamin A

1827) List the uses of the following herbal substances in medicine: Black cohosh, Nutmeg, Hawthorne, Sabah, and Juniper.
   a) Black cohosh: Abortifacient, menstrual irregularity, and menopause
   b) Nutmeg: Hallucinogen, abortifacient, aphrodisiac, GI disorders, and dyspepsia
   c) Hawthorne: Heart failure, HTN, and cardiac disorders
   d) Sabah: Weight loss
   e) Juniper: Hallucinogen or diuretic

1828)   Give the antidote for each drug overdose for the following: acetaminophen, arsenic, aspirin, beta-blocker, barbiturate, benzodiazepine, calcium channel blocker, carbamate, carbon monoxide, cyanide, digitalis, ethylene glycol, heparin, hydrofluoric acid, iron, isoniazid (INH), lead, mercury, methanol, methemoglobin, methotrexate, opiates, organophosphates, oral hypoglycemic, TCA's, and warfarin.

a)   Acetaminophen: N-Acetylcysteine
b)   Arsenic: BAL, DMS
c)   Aspirin: $NaHCO_3$ and dialysis
d)   Beta-blocker: Glucagon, Insulin/glucose
e)   Barbiturate: Hemodialysis
f)   Benzodiazepine: Flumazenil
g)   Calcium channel blocker: Calcium, Glucagon, Insulin/glucose
h)   Carbamate: Atropine
i)   Carbon monoxide: 100% O_2, Hyperbaric O_2
j)   Cyanide: Sodium nitrite, Sodium thiosulfate, Hydroxocobalamin
k)   Digitalis: Digibind
l)   Ethylene glycol: Ethanol, Fomepizole, Dialysis, Thiamine
m) Heparin: Protamine
n)   Hydrofluoric acid: Calcium gluconate, magnesium
o)   Iron: Deferoxamine
p)   Isoniazid (INH): Pyridoxine
q)   Lead: BAL, DMSA, EDTA
r)   Mercury: BAL, DMSA
s)   Methanol: Ethanol, Fomepizole, Dialysis, Folic acid
t)   Methemoglobin: Methylene blue
u)   Methotrexate: Glucarpidase, Leucovorin
v)   Opiates: Naloxone
w)   Organophosphates: Atropine, Pralidoxime (2-PAM)
x)   Sulfonylureas: Glucose, Glucagon, Octreotide
y)   Tricyclic antidepressants: Sodium bicarbonate
z)   Warfarin: Vit K

Pediatrics

1829)   Give the formula for determining infant and toddlers' average systolic blood pressure.

    a)   90 mmHg + (2 x age in years)

1830)   What is the formula used to determine if a pediatric systolic blood pressure meets hypotension criteria between 1-10 years old?

    a)   < 70 mmHg + (2 x age in years)

1831)   List the definition of hypotension for pediatric patients for each age group; neonate, infant, children 1-10 years old, and children > 10.

    a)   Neonate (0-28 days): < 60 mmHg

    b)   Infant (< 1): < 70 mmHg

    c)   Children (1-10): < 70 mmHg + (2 x age in years)

    d)   School-aged (> 10): < 90 mmHg

1832)   List the average respiratory rates for pediatric patients by age group for infants, toddler, preschooler, school-age, and adolescent.

    a)   Infant (< 1): 30-60

    b)   Toddler (1-4): 24-40

    c)   Preschooler (4-6): 22-34

    d)   School-aged (6-12): 18-30

    e)   Adolescent (> 12): 12-16

1833)   List the average heart rates for pediatric patients by age group, for newborns-3 months, 3 months-2 years, 2-10 years, and > 10 years.

    a)   Newborns-3 months: 85-205

    b)   3 months-2 years: 100-190

    c)   2-10 years: 60-140

    d)   > 10 years: 60-100

1834)   Give the modified Glasgow coma scale for eye opening in children and infants.

    a)   Spontaneous: 4

    b)   To speech: 3

    c)   To pain only: 2

    d)   No response: 1

1835) Give the modified Glasgow coma scale for verbal response in children and infants.
   a) Oriented/ Coos and babbles: 5
   b) Confused/ Irritable cry: 4
   c) Inappropriate words/ Cries to pain: 3
   d) Incomprehensible sounds/ Moans to pain: 2
   e) No response: 1

1836) Give the modified Glasgow coma scale for motor response in children and infants.
   a) Obeys commands/ Moves spontaneously: 6
   b) Localizes painful stimulus/ Withdraws to touch: 5
   c) Withdraws in response to pain: 4
   d) Flexion in response to pain: 3
   e) Extension in response to pain: 2
   f) No response: 1

1837) What is the calculation for estimating pediatric weight in kgs?
   a) (2 x Age) + 10 = Kg

1838) What percent of neonatal weight loss is expected after birth and regained by 2 weeks of life?
   a) 5-10%

1839) List the neonatal reflexes.
   a) Grasp, Root, Suck, and Moro reflex

1840) At what age do children start to grow teeth?
   a) 5-9 months

1841) At what age is the birth weight expected to double and triple?
   a) Double by 5 months and Triple by 1 year

1842) Around what age are children about double their birth height?
   a) 5 years

1843) At what age do children begin to roll?
   a) 4 months

1844) At what age do children begin to sit on their own?
   a) 6 months

1845) At what age do children begin to have stranger anxiety?
   a) 9-12 months

1846) At what age do children begin to walk?
   a) Earliest around 9 months

1847) What age range does the anterior fontanelle begin to close?

a) 12-18 months

1848) What is the first sign of female puberty?

a) Breast buds

1849) What is the first sign of male puberty?

a) Testicular enlargement

1850) What is the most common cause of death in pediatric patients?

a) Trauma

1851) What diagnosis should be suspected with an inconsolable crying infant and a pale toe?

a) Hair-thread tourniquet syndrome

1852) List signs and symptoms seen with pediatric heart disease.

a) Failure to thrive, Poor exercise tolerance, Respiratory failure or distress, Feeding difficulties, Poor growth, and Apnea

1853) How should the blood pressure be obtained in an infant with suspected CHF from heart disease?

a) BP in all four extremities

1854) What feature of the fetal circulation system helps blood to bypass the liver?

a) Ductus venosus

1855) What feature of fetal circulation allows blood to pass between the left and right atria?

a) Foramen ovale

1856) What feature of fetal circulation shunts blood away from the pulmonary circulation to enter the descending aorta?

a) Ductus arteriosus

1857) What condition should be suspected in an infant who presents ash grey, poor capillary refill, dyspnea, tachypnea, and tachycardia, with a heart murmur?

a) Congestive heart failure (CHF) with shock

1858) Give the classic triad seen in infants with CHF.

a) Hepatosplenomegaly, Tachypnea, and Tachycardia

1859) What medications should be given for pediatric patients who present in CHF?

a) Furosemide, Inotropes, Oxygen, +/- PRBC infusion for anemia, or Prostaglandin (for a congenital heart defect)

1860) What benign cardiac murmur is louder when lying supine and is commonly present in pediatric patients?
   a) Still's murmur
1861) Name the cyanotic congenital heart abnormalities.
   a) Tetralogy of Fallot, Truncus arteriosus, Transposition of the great vessels, Total anomalous pulmonary venous return, Tricuspid atresia, Hypoplastic left heart syndrome, Pulmonary atresia,and Ebstein's anomaly
1862) What is the most common cyanotic cardiac lesion < 1 year of age and presents with exertional dyspnea, cyanosis with feeding and crying in an infant?
   a) Tetralogy of Fallot
1863) What emergency bedside maneuver increases peripheral resistance and decreases venous return during a "Tet spell" seen with Tetralogy of Fallot and can improve symptoms?
   a) Knee to chest positioning
1864) What treatments are recommended for Tetralogy of Fallot stabilization in the ED?
   a) Knee-chest positioning, Oxygen, Bicarbonate, Propranolol, Phenylephrine, and Morphine
1865) What are the four anomalies of that makeup Tetralogy of Fallot?
   a) Pulmonary stenosis, Right ventricular hypertrophy, Overriding aorta, and Ventricular septal defect (VSD)
1866) What is the finding on a chest X-ray with Tetralogy of Fallot?
   a) Boot shaped heart
1867) What is the most common cyanotic heart disease present within the first week of life?
   a) Transposition of the great vessels
1868) What is the finding on a chest X-ray with transposition of the great vessels?
   a) Egg on a string
1869) List the heart defects that are ductal dependent.
   a) Hypoplastic left heart, Aortic coarctation, and Aortic stenosis

1870) What medication can treat heart failure from a ductal dependent heart defect and works by keeping the ductus arteriosus open?

a) Prostaglandin infusion PGE1

1871) What are the most common side effects of prostaglandin administration?

a) Apnea (most common), Hypotension, Bradycardia, and Seizures

1872) Which test is performed in patients with cyanosis to determine if the cause is central from a heart defect?

a) Hyperoxia test

1873) How is the hyperoxia test performed?

a) Administer 100% oxygen and evaluate for an increase in PaO2 of more than 20 mmHg

1874) Which type of cyanosis is present in a pediatric patient with discoloration of the skin and mucous membranes?

a) Central cyanosis

1875) What lab can help distinguish between cyanosis from a congenital heart defect and a lung condition?

a) Arterial blood gas (ABG)

1876) Name the different types of acyanotic congenital heart defects.

a) VSD, ASD, PDA, Aortic coarctation, Pulmonary valve stenosis, and Aortic valve stenosis

1877) What congenital defect is the most common heart abnormality?

a) Ventricular septal defect (VSD)

1878) What pediatric congenital heart anomaly involves an infant in distress with absent femoral pulses and poor perfusion without cyanosis?

a) Aortic coarctation

1879) What is the most common maternal cause of a 3rd-degree heart block in an infant?

a) Maternal Lupus

1880) What four conditions can cause a complete heart block in a newborn?

a) Lupus, Rocky Mountain spotted fever, Lyme disease, or Transposition of the great vessels

1881)   What medical condition should be suspected in a pediatric patient with a fever >5 days, non-exudative conjunctivitis, polymorphous rash, strawberry tongue, fissured lips, cervical lymphadenopathy, and desquamation of skin on the hands?

    a)   Kawasaki disease

1882)   How many diagnostic criteria for Kawasaki disease are required to make the diagnosis?

    a)   At least 4 of 5 met with a fever > 5 days.

1883)   What labs can help with the diagnosis of Kawasaki disease?

    a)   CRP and ESR

1884)   What is the most common cause of acquired heart disease in pediatrics?

    a)   Kawasaki disease

1885)   What cardiovascular complication can develop with untreated Kawasaki disease?

    a)   Coronary aneurysm

1886)   What imaging modality is recommended for patients with suspected Kawasaki disease?

    a)   Echocardiography

1887)   What gastrointestinal complication can develop with Kawasaki disease?

    a)   Gallbladder hydrops (Cholecystitis)

1888)   What are the medical treatments for Kawasaki disease?

    a)   Intravenous gamma globulin (IVIG)

    b)   High dose Aspirin

    c)   Steroids

1889)   What condition should be suspected in a child with a recent untreated pharyngitis who presents with fever, arthralgia, rash, and subcutaneous nodules on the extensor surfaces of the extremities?

    a)   Rheumatic fever

1890)   List the Jones 5 major diagnostic criteria for rheumatic fever.

    a)   Polyarthritis

    b)   Carditis

    c)   Subcutaneous nodules

    d)   Erythema marginatum

    e)   Sydenham's chorea

1891) List the Jones minor diagnostic criteria for rheumatic fever.
   a) Fever
   b) Arthralgia
   c) Elevated ESR or CRP
   d) Prolonged PR on ECG

1892) What are the Jones diagnostic criteria for rheumatic fever?
   a) 2 major criteria or 1 major and 2 minor criteria, with evidence of a prior streptococcal infection

1893) What bacteria if untreated in the pediatric population can lead to rheumatic fever?
   a) Group A beta-hemolytic streptococci

1894) What is the most common pediatric acquired heart disease in the world?
   a) Rheumatic fever

1895) What heart valve abnormality develops due to damage from rheumatic fever?
   a) Mitral stenosis

1896) What is the recommended treatment for rheumatic fever?
   a) Antibiotics (penicillin) and Aspirin

1897) What is the treatment for Supraventricular Tachycardia (SVT) in infants?
   a) Ice pack over closed eyes for 15-30 seconds

1898) What is the most common dysrhythmia in pediatrics?
   a) SVT

1899) What is the most common dysrhythmia in pediatric arrest?
   a) Asystole

1900) What is the pediatric dose of Epinephrine IV (1:10,000)?
   a) 0.01 mg/kg or 0.1ml/kg

1901) What is the maintenance fluid rule for pediatrics?
   a) 4 ml/kg/hr for first 10kg, 2 ml/kg/hr for second 10kg, 1 ml/kg/hr thereafter

1902) What type of maintenance fluids are used in pediatric patients > 15 kg and < 15 kg?
   a) > 15 kg: D5W + ½ NS
   b) < 15 kg: D5W + ¼ NS

1903) What is the most common cause of readmission of infants after delivery?
a) Neonatal jaundice

1904) What is the most common cause of indirect hyperbilirubinemia in a newborn and typically resolves within 5-7 days?
a) Physiologic jaundice

1905) Inhibition of what gene leads to breast milk related jaundice and can cause bilirubin levels between 10-20 mg/dL around 10-14 days after birth?
a) Glucuronyl transferase inhibitors

1906) At what bilirubin level in a neonate is light therapy recommended?
a) >20 mg/dL

1907) What test is performed in infants to determine if the cause of hyperbilirubinemia is due to maternal antibodies?
a) Direct Coombs test

1908) What autosomal disease can also present with asymptomatic elevated unconjugated bilirubin levels?
a) Gilbert's syndrome

1909) What type of autosomal disease leads to hyperbilirubinemia and kernicterus in the first few days of life after delivery and has two genetic types due to mutations with UDP glucuronyl transferase?
a) Crigler-Najjar syndrome

1910) What are the treatments for type 1 Crigler-Najjar syndrome?
a) Exchange transfusion, Phototherapy, and Liver transplant

1911) What medication can be used in the less severe type 2 Crigler-Najjar syndrome with lower bilirubin levels?
a) Phenobarbital

1912) What test is elevated in hemorrhagic disease of the newborn?
a) PT

1913) What is the leading cause of anemia in pediatrics?
a) Iron deficiency

1914) What is the most common cause of non-measurable water loss in pediatrics?
a) Fever

1915)   What side of the main stem bronchus does a swallowed foreign body usually lodge?

    a)   Right

1916)   What anatomical location is a swallowed foreign body (coin) when the coin's circular face is seen on a lateral soft tissue neck X-ray?

    a)   Trachea (sagittal plane-same as the vocal cords "coin slot")

1917)   Are most foreign bodies radiopaque?

    a)   No

1918)   What physical exam findings are associated with a foreign body in the airway?

    a)   Sudden-onset of stridor, Wheezing, or Coughing

1919)   What is the most common site for esophageal foreign body obstruction in pediatric patients?

    a)   Cricopharyngeus muscle (in upper third of esophagus)

1920)   What anatomical location is a coin that is swallowed, when the coin's circular face is anterior posteriorly oriented on an AP soft tissue neck X-ray?

    a)   Esophagus

1921)   Is a button battery in the esophagus an emergency to remove?

    a)   Yes

1922)   What complications can occur if a button battery is not removed from the esophagus?

    a)   Perforation or Acid burns

1923)   What are the characteristics of swallowed foreign bodies that require emergent removal?

    a)   Long objects > 5-6 cm, Wide objects > 2.5 cm, Sharp objects, Esophageal button batteries, and Multiple magnets

1924)   What is the treatment plan for a swallowed foreign body that has passed the pylorus or is in the stomach?

    a)   Serial X-rays

1925)   What procedure is used to remove a foreign body in the airway?

    a)   Rigid bronchoscopy

1926) What procedure is used to remove a foreign body in the upper gastrointestinal system?
   a) EGD

1927) What delayed infection can occur after an inhaled foreign body?
   a) Pneumonia

1928) What imaging study is the best to determine the presence of a swallowed foreign body if not present on X-ray films?
   a) CT

1929) What are the characteristic differences in a pediatric airway verse adult airway?
   a) Larger tongue, Increased vagal response, and the Larynx is more superior and anterior

1930) List common physical exam findings associated with respiratory distress in pediatrics.
   a) Nasal flaring, Intercostal retractions, Tracheal tugging, abdominal breathing, Grunting, and Tachypnea

1931) What form of chronic lung disease affects preterm newborns, previously intubated infants, or infants with chronic oxygen therapy?
   a) Bronchopulmonary dysplasia

1932) What respiratory illness presents in children between 2 months-2 years old with increased work of breathing, diffuse wheezing, and a viral syndrome?
   a) Bronchiolitis

1933) What is the most common cause of bronchiolitis?
   a) Respiratory syncytial virus (RSV)

1934) What is the medical treatment for bronchiolitis?
   a) Decadron

1935) What is the most common cause of laryngotracheobronchitis (croup)?
   a) Parainfluenza virus

1936) What type of stridor presents with croup?
   a) Inspiratory stridor (upper airway)

1937) What is the pathognomonic finding on the anterior view of a soft tissue cervical X-ray with croup?
   a) Steeple sign

1938) What is the treatment of croup without resting stridor?

a) Steroids

1939) What specific treatment is added to steroids for croup with resting stridor or respiratory distress?

a) Racemic epinephrine

1940) What is the recommended observation time before discharge for children who receive racemic epinephrine treatment for croup?

a) 2-4 hours

1941) What severe respiratory condition can present with high fever, dyspnea, inspiratory and expiratory stridor, and drooling after an upper respiratory infection?

a) Bacterial tracheitis

1942) What infection presents in children 6 months-3 years old with a fever, lateral neck swelling, muffled voice, and a sore throat?

a) Retropharyngeal abscess

1943) What is the most common pediatric abscess in the head and neck region?

a) Peritonsillar abscess

1944) What is the treatment of pertussis?

a) Azithromycin or Erythromycin

1945) What vaccine is recommended to be updated for those around newborns to prevent pertussis?

a) Tdap

1946) Is prophylactic antibiotic treatment recommend for household members exposed to pertussis?

a) Yes

1947) What is the most common site of infection in a neonate?

a) Lungs

1948) List the most common causes of neonatal pneumonia.

a) Group B strep, Strep pneumonia, and E. coli

1949) What antibiotics are recommended for outpatient pediatric pneumonia?

a) Amoxicillin or Azithromycin

1950) Is the high dose or low dose of Amoxicillin used for outpatient treatment of pneumonia in pediatrics?

a) High dose (90mg/kg/day)

1951) What antibiotics are recommended for inpatient treatment of pediatric pneumonia?
   a) Cefuroxime or Ceftriaxone (50 mg/kg)
1952) What bacteria causes walking pneumonia in school-aged children, and can cause bullous myringitis?
   a) Mycoplasma
1953) What antibiotic is recommended for treating walking pneumonia?
   a) Azithromycin
1954) What genetic lung condition is autosomal recessive and leads to recurrent respiratory infections, pancreatic deficiency and leads to loss of chloride?
   a) Cystic fibrosis (CF)
1955) What gene is defective in CF?
   a) CFTR gene
1956) What bacteria is commonly associated with pneumonia in CF patients?
   a) Pseudomonas
1957) What GI symptoms present at birth can suggest possible CF?
   a) Meconium ileus or Malabsorption
1958) What tests are used to diagnose CF?
   a) Sweat chloride test, IRT, and Mutation testing
1959) What is the treatment for CF exacerbations?
   a) Bronchodilators, Antibiotics, Chest physiotherapy, Mucoactive agents, and Steroids
1960) What bacteria is associated with a staccato cough and conjunctivitis in an infant 1-3 weeks old?
   a) Chlamydia pneumoniae
1961) What airway emergency presents with fever, sore throat, and abrupt onset of dysphagia, drooling, and respiratory distress in the tripod position?
   a) Epiglottitis
1962) What are the pathognomonic radiographic findings seen with epiglottitis?
   a) Thumbprint sign

1963) What is the recommended treatment for epiglottitis?
a) Secure the airway

1964) What antibiotics are recommended for epiglottitis?
a) Vancomycin + Ceftriaxone

1965) What is the order set for a septic work up in a febrile neonate less than 28-90 days?
a) CBC, UA, CSF, Blood cultures, and +/- Chest X-ray

1966) What are the most common bacteria involved in ?
a) Listeria, E. coli, Group B Streptococcus, or Herpes

1967) What antibiotics are recommended for newborn sepsis < 28 days?
a) Ampicillin + (Cefotaxime or Ceftriaxone), +/- Vancomycin (for + CSF infection), +/- Acyclovir (for viral CSF infection)

1968) What antibiotics are recommended for infant sepsis 28-90 days?
a) Ceftriaxone, +/- Vancomycin (for + CSF infection), +/- Acyclovir (for viral CSF infection)

1969) What are the most common bacteria involved in infant sepsis?
a) Neisseria meningitides, Strep pneumoniae, and Staph aureus

1970) What age range is used for a cut off to obtain a U/A in a febrile female infant?
a) < 12 month

1971) What age range is used for a cut off to obtain a U/A in febrile uncircumcised and circumcised male infants?
a) Uncircumcised: < 12 months
b) Circumcised: < 6 months

1972) What bacteria is the most common cause of a UTI in neonates?
a) Klebsiella

1973) What bacteria is the most common cause of a UTI in children > 1?
a) E. coli

1974) What is the most common extracranial malignancy of a child?
a) Neuroblastoma

1975) What toxicological items are the most commonly ingested by children?
a) Cosmetic and Personal care items

1976) What is the most common opportunistic infection seen in pediatric HIV patients?
a) Pneumocystis carinii

1977) What is the most common route of HIV transmission in children?
a) Maternal during birth

1978) What pediatric illness follows a recent viral infection with arthralgia, abdominal pain, and palpable purpura on the legs and buttocks?
a) Henoch-Schonlein Purpura (HSP)

1979) What is the most common cause of vasculitis in children?
a) HSP

1980) What abnormalities can be found on urinalysis with HSP that suggest renal involvement?
a) Proteinuria and Hematuria

1981) What gastrointestinal complication can occur with HSP and can present with abdominal pain and blood in the stool?
a) Intussusception

1982) What is the treatment for HSP?
a) Observation, +/- Steroids

1983) What condition presents with abdominal pain, bloody diarrhea, acute renal failure, hematuria, rash, and proteinuria in children?
a) Hemolytic uremic syndrome (HUS)

1984) What type of red blood cells are seen on a blood smear with HUS?
a) Schistocytes (Helmet cells)

1985) What foodborne bacterium often leads to HUS?
a) E. coli 0157:H7

1986) Does the PT, PTT, or fibrinogen levels change with HUS?
a) No

1987) What type of generalized seizure occurs in children 6 months-5 years old with a fever, lasts no more than 15 minutes, has minimal postictal period with a return to baseline and resolves without treatment?
a) Simple febrile seizure

1988) What is the recommended treatment and workup for a simple febrile seizure?
   a) Antipyretics and Supportive therapy
1989) List the findings that suggest a complicated febrile seizure.
   a) > 5 years old, < 6 months old, > 15 min duration, Reoccurrence within 24 hours, or Focal seizure
1990) What is the work up for a complex febrile seizure in a child?
   a) Septic work up (Labs, UA, +/- LP, and chest X-ray)
1991) List causes of seizures in pediatric patients.
   a) Fever, Hypoglycemia, Hyponatremia, Hypocalcemia, Hypomagnesemia, Isoniazid ingestion, Traumatic brain injury, or Hypertension encephalopathy
1992) What is the most common cause of recurrent seizures?
   a) Medication non-compliance
1993) What type of seizure is the most common in the pediatric population?
   a) Generalized seizure
1994) What medications are used for seizure treatment?
   a) Fosphenytoin, Phenytoin, Phenobarbital, Levetiracetam, Lorazepam, Diazepam, Midazolam, and Propofol
1995) What medication class is used as the first-line treatment to break seizure activity?
   a) Benzodiazepines
1996) What type of seizure commonly in school-aged children presents with staring episodes, eyelid flickering, and blank stares without a postictal phase?
   a) Absence seizure
1997) What is the medication treatment for absence seizures?
   a) Ethosuximide
1998) What pediatric condition commonly in 3-9-month-olds presents with sudden muscle spasms, lasting a few seconds that can reoccur multiple times a day?
   a) Infantile spasms
1999) What neurological condition should be ruled out in the emergency department with a new-onset neonatal seizure?
   a) Traumatic brain bleed

2000) Is seizure prophylaxis recommended with severe traumatic brain injury (TBI)?
 a) Yes

2001) What is the most common cause of a pediatric seizure from an electrolyte abnormality?
 a) Hyponatremia due to watered down formula

2002) What is the term used for a child who is crying vigorously and in between cries holds their breath leading to a brief syncope event?
 a) Breath-holding spell

2003) What diagnosis is given for the sensory deficits or extremity weakness found after a seizure episode that resolves with time?
 a) Todd's paralysis

2004) Is it recommended to perform a head CT for a first time generalized tonic-clonic seizure lasting < 5 mins in length in children > 2 years old?
 a) No

2005) List the indications for ordering a CT brain with a pediatric seizure.
 a) New focal seizure, Prolonged seizure activity or postictal phase, < 6 months of age, Post-traumatic seizure, Abnormal neurological exam finding, or Presence of a VP shunt

2006) Give the criteria defining status epilepticus.
 a) Multiple seizures without return to baseline within 30 mins
 b) Seizure lasting > 5 mins

2007) What pediatric neurological condition presents with a large head, large fontanelles, dilated scalp veins, vomiting, headache, and papilledema?
 a) Hydrocephalus

2008) List the two types of hydrocephalus.
 a) Communicating and Non-communicating

2009) What is the brain CT finding with hydrocephalus?
 a) Enlarged ventricles

2010) List common causes of hydrocephalus.
 a) Congenital fusion of cranial sutures, Meningitis, Intracranial hemorrhage, and Tumors

2011) What is the treatment for hydrocephalus?

a) Shunt

2012) What type of cranial shunt complication presents with headache, bradycardia, trouble breathing, vomiting, blurry vision, and altered mental status?

a) Obstruction

2013) What physical exam findings can be found with hydrocephalus from an obstructed VP shunt?

a) Non-compressible shunt bladder, Encephalopathy, Papilledema, and Irregular respiratory pattern

2014) What symptoms makeup "Cushing's triad" seen with increased intracranial pressure?

a) Bradycardia, Hypertension, and an Irregular respiratory pattern

2015) What imaging is done for the workup of a shunt malfunction?

a) Shunt series (X-rays: head, neck, chest, and abdomen) and CT head

2016) What is the emergent treatment for an obstructed shunt with mental status changes?

a) Tap the shunt

2017) What are the most common bacterial causes of meningitis in < 1-month-old?

a) E. coli, Group B strep, and Listeria

2018) What antibiotics are recommended for bacterial meningitis < 1-month-old?

a) Ampicillin + Gentamycin or Cefotaxime

2019) What are the most common bacterial cause of meningitis in > 1 month?

a) Strep. pneumoniae, Neisseria meningitides, and H. influenza

2020) What antibiotics are recommended for bacterial meningitis > 1 month old?

a) Vancomycin + Cefotaxime or Ceftriaxone

2021) How is meningitis diagnosed?

a) Lumbar puncture (LP) and CSF analysis

2022) What level of opening pressure on LP is considered abnormal in pediatrics?

a) > 28 cm H_2O

2023) What labs are ordered on the CSF when ruling out meningitis?

a) Protein, Cell count, Glucose, Culture, and Gram stain

2024) What is the most common gastrointestinal emergency in neonates and consists of a feeding intolerance, diarrhea, abdominal distention, bloody stools, and shock?

a) Necrotizing enterocolitis

2025) What abdominal X-ray finding is seen with necrotizing enterocolitis and consists of intramural air and double density layering of the abdominal walls?

a) Pneumatosis intestinalis

2026) What is the most common viral cause of pediatric diarrhea?

a) Rotavirus

2027) List the leading causes of blood in the stool of infants.

a) Anal fissures, Swallowed maternal blood, and Cow's milk intolerance

2028) What bacteria is associated with daycare, bloody diarrhea, and seizure activity?

a) Shigella

2029) What is the most common medical condition that causes pediatric electrolyte and fluid disturbances??

a) Gastroenteritis

2030) List causes of pediatric bowel obstructions.

a) Intussusception, Meconium ileus, Hirschsprung, Malrotation with volvulus, Duodenal atresia, and Pyloric stenosis

2031) What is the most common cause of small bowel obstruction in neonates that presents with sudden onset abdominal pain, distention, and bilious emesis?

a) Malrotation with a volvulus

2032) What is the absent ligament that predisposes infants to malrotation of the bowel?

a) Ligament of Treitz

2033) How is a volvulus diagnosed?

a) Upper GI contrast study or Abdominal series X-ray

2034) What is the finding on an abdominal X-ray that can be seen with an intestinal malrotation with a volvulus?

a) Double bubble sign (air-fluid level in the stomach and duodenum)

2035) What is the treatment for pediatric malrotation with a volvulus?
   a) NG tube and Surgery
2036) What is the most common cause of neonatal large bowel obstruction?
   a) Hirschsprung's disease
2037) What are the findings and symptoms that suggest Hirschsprung's disease?
   a) Failure of the neonate to pass meconium or stool, Abdominal distention, or No presence of stool on rectal exam
2038) What rectal nerves are absent in Hirschsprung's disease leading to an obstruction?
   a) Parasympathetic ganglion cells
2039) How is Hirschsprung's disease diagnosed and what is the treatment?
   a) Rectal biopsy and Surgery consult
2040) What type of congenital abdominal wall defect is defined as intestine exiting through a hole beside the belly button at birth and is outside of the peritoneum?
   a) Gastroschisis
2041) What type of congenital abdominal wall defect has the intestines herniating through a hole by the umbilicus that is encased in the peritoneum?
   a) Omphalocele
2042) What abdominal emergency should be suspected in a 3-6 week old firstborn male, with projectile non-bilious emesis and olive-like epigastric mass on the exam?
   a) Pyloric stenosis
2043) What metabolic and electrolyte abnormality can be seen with pyloric stenosis?
   a) Hypochloremia hypokalemia metabolic alkalosis
2044) What imaging modality is used to diagnose pyloric stenosis?
   a) Ultrasound
2045) What specific sign is seen with an upper GI contrast study and pyloric stenosis?
   a) String sign (narrowed pyloric canal)
2046) What is the treatment for pyloric stenosis?

a) Surgery

2047) What is the most common anorectal disorder in pediatrics that presents with pain and blood with wiping and blood-streaked stool with bowel movements?

a) Rectal fissures

2048) What is the most common cause of severe upper GI bleeds in pediatrics patients > 2?

a) Varices

2049) What is a common cause of blood in the stool found in newborns and is confirmed with the Apt test?

a) Swallowed maternal blood

2050) What is the treatment plan for a pediatric patient with gross blood or coffee-ground emesis and blood on NG aspirate?

a) Endoscopy

2051) What condition can develop in newborns not given a vitamin K shot before discharge that develop hematemesis?

a) Hemorrhagic disease of the newborn

2052) What lab abnormalities are seen in patients with hemorrhagic disease of a newborn?

a) Prolonged PT

2053) What etiology can also cause a lower GI bleed in a well-appearing infant > 1 with a new diet regimen?

a) Milk allergy

2054) What is the most common cause of bowel obstruction in pediatric patients 2 months - 6 years of age that presents with intermittent cramping abdominal pains, and currant jelly stools?

a) Intussusception

2055) What is the imaging modality of choice for intussusception diagnosis?

a) Ultrasound

2056) What is the classic abdominal exam finding with intussusception?

a) Right abdominal sausage-shaped mass

2057) List the four classic abdominal X-ray findings seen with intussusception.

a) Target sign, Crescent sign, Air fluid levels (bowel obstruction), and Absent live edge sign

2058) What medical conditions predispose children to intussusception?

a) Meckel's diverticulum, Cystic fibrosis, Polyps, Hypertrophy of Peyer's patches, and Henoch-Schonlein Purpura (HSP)

2059) What physical exam findings are consistent with Dance's sign suggesting an intussusception?

a) Scaphoid abdomen and Empty right lower quadrant

2060) What are the treatment options for intussusception?

a) Enema (water-soluble, barium, saline, or air) or Surgery (preferred if necrosis, reoccurrence, or contraindicated enema)

2061) What congenital condition presents with jaundice from elevated direct/conjugated bilirubin as well as hepatomegaly and acholic stools?

a) Biliary atresia

2062) What imaging study is used to diagnose biliary atresia?

a) DISIDA (Hepatobiliary) scan

2063) What congenital condition presents in infancy with choking, coughing, and cyanosis with feeding, and increased salivation?

a) Tracheoesophageal fistula (TEF)

2064) What type of TEF is the most common form?

a) Esophageal atresia with a distal tracheoesophageal fistula

2065) What infant GI issue may be present with an infant that is fussy and spits up frequently after feeds?

a) Gastroesophageal reflux disease (GERD)

2066) What is the treatment for infant GERD?

a) Smaller and more frequent feeds or Formula change

2067) What is the treatment for infant thrush?

a) Fluconazole

2068) What congenital defect leads to an increased incidence of inguinal hernias?

a) Patent tunica vaginalis

2069) Why do pediatric inguinal hernias need to be referred to general surgery within 24-72 hours?

a) High risk of incarceration

2070) What is the most common cause of inconsolable crying and is defined as 3 or more hours per day for 3 or more days over 3 weeks?
   a) Colic
2071) What is the treatment of colic in an infant?
   a) Decrease stimulation and Reassurance
2072) What type of kidney tumor in the abdomen rarely crosses the midline and is associated with a palpable tumor?
   a) Wilm's tumor
2073) What is the imaging modality of choice for diagnosing appendicitis in the pediatric population?
   a) Ultrasound
2074) What are the US findings suggesting appendicitis?
   a) Dilated noncompressible appendix > 6mm
2075) Do all patients with appendicitis have an elevated WBC and or Fever?
   a) No
2076) What type of appendicitis can present with RUQ abdominal pain and mimic gallbladder disease?
   a) Retrocecal
2077) What is the most reliable sign in pediatric patients with appendicitis?
   a) Rebound tenderness
2078) What diagnosis is used to explain a sudden, brief (< 1 minute) episode of cyanosis, with a change in breathing, change in muscle tonicity, or altered responsiveness that resolves spontaneously?
   a) Brief resolved unexplained event (BRUE)
2079) What was the previous term used for BRUE?
   a) Acute life threatening event (ALTE)
2080) List the criteria to determine if a patient is low-risk with a BRUE.
   a) Term infant, No CPR, < 1 min episode, 1st event, and Age > 60 days
2081) List suspected causes of BRUE.
   a) Seizure, Infections, Intracranial hemorrhage, Botulism, Airway obstructions, Hypoglycemia, Trauma, and Reflux
2082) Apnea events longer than how many seconds suggest alternative pathology instead of a BRUE?

a) > 20 seconds

2083) What is the recommended disposition for a BRUE event in a low-risk patient?
a) Discharge

2084) What is the most common cause of death < 1 year old, and is found to be a higher risk with younger mothers, fetal prematurity, maternal substance abusers, and the number of children?
a) Sudden infant death syndrome (SIDS)

2085) What is the recommended sleeping position for an infant to prevent SIDS?
a) Back to bed

2086) What is the most common bone fracture found in pediatrics?
a) Clavicle

2087) What infection needs to be ruled out in a child with a fever and hip pain?
a) Septic arthritis

2088) What is the most common bacterium that leads to pediatric septic arthritis?
a) Staph. aureus

2089) What is the most common route bacteria spreads that can lead to septic arthritis?
a) Hematogenous

2090) What labs are used to rule out septic arthritis?
a) CBC, ESR, and CRP

2091) What are the ultrasound findings seen with septic arthritis?
a) Joint effusion

2092) What type of joint infection presents similarly to septic arthritis and follows a recent viral infection with a normal ESR, CRP, and CBC?
a) Transient (toxic) synovitis

2093) What type of adolescent hip injury is seen in obese boys age 12-14 who present with knee pain and a lip?
a) Slipped capital femoral epiphysis (SCFE)

2094) What X-ray imaging view is recommended for the diagnosis of SCFE?
a) Frog leg pelvis view

2095) What type of arthritis is non-migratory and is seen after a recent strep infection, has a + strep ASO, and is treated with NSAIDs and Penicillin?
   a) Post-strep reactive arthritis
2096) Which common cause of pediatric hip pain involves avascular necrosis of the femoral head and presents with a lip in a child?
   a) Leg calve perthes
2097) Which chronic blood disease can lead to avascular necrosis of the hip?
   a) Sickle cell disease
2098) What type of congenital abnormality is seen with an asymmetry of the groin, limb shortening, and an Ortolani click?
   a) Congenital hip dislocation
2099) What is the most common cause of death in pediatrics?
   a) Trauma
2100) What infant rash has crusty, scaly, red areas on the face, scalp, and intertriginous zones, in infants < 3 months?
   a) Seborrheic dermatitis
2101) What type of diaper rash causes erythema of the groin area but spares the skin folds, unlike a candidiasis rash?
   a) Contact dermatitis diaper rash
2102) What congenital condition should be suspected in a child with ambiguous genitalia who develops hypotension, hypoglycemia, and lethargy with a minor illness?
   a) Congenital adrenal hyperplasia (CAH)
2103) What gene deficiency is the most common cause of CAH?
   a) 21-beta-hydroxylase deficiency
2104) What lab abnormalities are found with CAH due to 21-beta-hydroxylase deficiency?
   a) $\uparrow K^+$ and $\downarrow Na^+$
2105) What is the treatment for a patient with suspected adrenal suppression from CAH?
   a) Hydrocortisone, Fluids, +/- Dextrose
2106) What is the congenital defect that leads to hyperammonemia in a neonate?
   a) Urea cycle defect

2107) What are the treatment options for hyperammonemia?
   a) Sodium benzoate, L-arginine, +/- Dialysis for levels > 300
2108) What is the treatment for organic acidemias from inborn errors of metabolism?
   a) L-Carnitine
2109) What is the most common blood type combination of ABO incompatibility that is seen in a mother and an infant?
   a) Mother O and Infant A
2110) What is the most severe blood type combination of ABO incompatibility that is seen in a mother and an infant?
   a) Mother O and Infant B

Head, Ear, Nose & Throat Disorders

2111) Name the two diagnostic tests for determining the type of hearing loss present.
  a) Weber and Rinne

2112) Which test is done using a tuning fork on the mastoid to compare air vs. bone conduction?
  a) Rinne

2113) What is the most common cause of sudden hearing loss?
  a) Idiopathic

2114) Name the two types of hearing loss.
  a) Conduction and Sensory

2115) List the causes of sensorineural hearing loss.
  a) Viral infections, Leukemia, Diabetes, Temporal Arteritis, Loud noise, Acoustic neuroma, Age (presbycusis), and Drugs

2116) What drugs are ototoxic?
  a) Loop diuretics, Salicylates, NSAIDS, Quinine, Aminoglycosides, Erythromycin, and Neomycin

2117) List causes of conduction hearing loss.
  a) Cerumen impaction, Middle ear effusion, Foreign bodies, Benign tumors, and TM abnormality

2118) What is the most common cause of conduction hearing loss in each of the adult and pediatric populations?
  a) Cerumen impaction: Adults
  b) Otitis media: Pediatrics

2119) What type of ear infection involves the external canal, and causes pain, purities, hearing loss, and is associated with swimming?
  a) Otitis externa

2120) What bacteria most commonly cause otitis externa?
  a) Pseudomonas or Staph.aureus

2121) What is the treatment for Otitis Externa?
  a) Irrigation, Ofloxacin, Ciprofloxacin +/- a Corticosteroid, or Acetic acid/Hydrocortisone otic drops

2122) What preparation of antibiotic should be used in otitis externa with a TM perforation?
  a) Suspension

2123)   What infectious source typically causes external ear pain and discharge with grayish black or yellow dots surrounded by a cotton-like material in the external ear?
a)   Aspergillus niger

2124)   What are the two most common fungal pathogens that cause fungal otitis externa (otomycosis)?
a)   Aspergillus and Candida

2125)   What is the treatment for otomycosis?
a)   Antifungal drop (Clotrimazole or Fluconazole)

2126)   What is the complication of untreated otitis externa, consisting of osteomyelitis and fever?
a)   Malignant otitis externa

2127)   What imaging modality is the best for diagnosis and staging of malignant otitis externa?
a)   CT temporal bones

2128)   What bacteria is the most common cause of malignant otitis externa?
a)   Pseudomonas

2129)   What are the treatment options for malignant otitis externa?
a)   ENT consult and IV Antibiotics (Tobramycin + Piperacillin or Ciprofloxacin)

2130)   What is the most sensitive sign for diagnosing otitis media (OM)?
a)   Immobility of TM to insufflation

2131)   What developmental middle ear abnormality leads to an increased number of OM ear infections in children versus adults?
a)   The straitened middle ear canal

2132)   What bacteria is the most common cause of otitis media?
a)   Streptococcus pneumoniae

2133)   What is the recommended antibiotic and dosing for pediatric OM?
a)   Amoxicillin 90/mg/kg/day

2134)   What antibiotics are recommended for the treatment of OM?
a)   Amoxicillin, Azithromycin, or Cefuroxime

2135)   What is the length of time that antibiotics therapy is recommended for the treatment of OM?

a) 10 days (penicillins) or 5 days (macrolides)

2136) How long should the antibiotic therapy be for OM with effusion?

a) 3 weeks

2137) What antibiotics are recommended to treat recurrent or failed treatment of OM?

a) Clindamycin, Amoxicillin-Clavulanic acid, or IM Ceftriaxone

2138) What complications can occur from untreated OM?

a) Meningitis and Mastoiditis

2139) What is the definitive recommended treatment for recurrent or persistent OM?

a) Ear tubes (tympanostomy tubes)

2140) What is the diagnosis of OM with multiple fluid filled blisters on the TM?

a) Bullous myringitis

2141) What is the most common bacteria that causes bullous myringitis?

a) Streptococcus pneumoniae

2142) What is the second most common cause of bullous myringitis?

a) Mycoplasma

2143) What complication of extending OM presents with fever, erythema, protrusion of the auricle, swelling, and pain over the mastoid?

a) Mastoiditis

2144) What imaging is best to diagnose mastoiditis?

a) CT temporal bones

2145) What is the treatment for mastoiditis?

a) ENT consult, IV Antibiotics (Vancomycin or Ceftriaxone), and +/- Surgical drainage

2146) Which viral disease can cause Ramsay Hunt syndrome that is a vesicular rash, hearing loss, and a CN 7 paralysis?

a) Herpes zoster

2147) What is the treatment of an auricular hematoma?

a) Aseptic drainage or I&D with a pressure dressing

2148) What is the term for the complication that occurs from ear hematomas and is the development of asymmetric cartilage formation?
   a) Cauliflower ear
2149) What ear infection can develop after trauma?
   a) Perichondritis
2150) What is the treatment for a traumatic TM perforation from noise, diving, or altitude?
   a) ENT referral only, no antibiotics necessary
2151) What is the treatment of a TM perforation due to water entry or infection?
   a) Antibiotics
2152) What complication occurs from extension of an infection into the lateral or sigmoid cranial venous sinuses, causing headache, papilledema, 6th cranial nerve palsy, and vertigo?
   a) Lateral sinus thrombosis
2153) What is the treatment of a lateral sinus thrombosis?
   a) ENT consult and IV Antibiotics (Nafcillin + Ceftriaxone + Metronidazole)
2154) What medication is recommended to immobilize a live insect in the ear canal and help with removal?
   a) 2% Lidocaine
2155) Name the two types of vertigo and their onset.
   a) Peripheral (sudden) and Central (gradual)
2156) What type is more associated with tinnitus?
   a) Peripheral
2157) What test can help differentiate between the two vertigo types?
   a) Dix-Hallpike test
2158) What is the most common cause of sudden onset peripheral vertigo that is reoccurring and worse with positional change?
   a) Benign paroxysmal positional vertigo (BPPV)
2159) What middle ear abnormality causes BPPV?
   a) Impaired endolymph flow in the semicircular canal
2160) What maneuver can help treat BPPV?
   a) Epley Maneuver

2161) Is the nystagmus in BPPV fatigable?
   a) Yes
2162) What pathologies can cause peripheral vertigo?
   a) Labyrinthitis, Meniere's disease, Ototoxicity (drugs), Herpes zoster, Vestibular neuronitis, BPPV, Cholesteatoma, Perilymphatic fistula, and Cerumen impaction
2163) What are the first-line and second-line medication treatments of vertigo?
   a) 1) Meclizine
   b) 2) Benzodiazepines
2164) What disease causes unilateral sensorineural loss, vertigo, and tinnitus?
   a) Meniere's disease
2165) What inner ear pathology coincides with a viral upper respiratory infection, possible ear infection, and leads to vertigo?
   a) Labyrinthitis
2166) What familial condition is a tumor of the Schwann cells and leads to peripheral vertigo, tinnitus, hearing loss, and ataxia?
   a) Acoustic neuroma (schwannoma)
2167) What imaging study is the best to diagnose a Schwannoma?
   a) MRI
2168) Name the causes of central vertigo.
   a) Cerebellar or Brain stem hemorrhage/infarction, Vertebrobasilar insufficiency, Orthostatic dizziness, Hypertensive dizziness, Multiple sclerosis, Tumor (schwannoma's or central pontine angle tumor), Migraine, Cerebral concussion, Alcohol intoxication, or Medications
2169) What eye finding on physical exam suggests a central origin cause of vertigo?
   a) Vertical nystagmus
2170) What is the difference between lightheaded and dizziness (vertigo)?
   a) Lightheaded is near syncope
   b) Dizziness is the room is spinning
2171) What is the length of time used to diagnose chronic sinusitis?
   a) > 3 months duration

2172) Name some complications from sinusitis.
   a) Orbital cellulitis, Osteomyelitis, Brain abscess, and Cavernous sinus thrombosis
2173) Name the diagnosis, in a female patient on birth control, with a recent sinusitis, and fever, facial and periorbital edema, CN 6 palsy, and a headache.
   a) Cavernous sinus thrombosis
2174) What septal complications from nasal trauma consists of a large purple swelling of the septum?
   a) Septal hematoma
2175) What is the treatment of a septal hematoma?
   a) I&D, Penrose drain, and Antibiotics
2176) What nasal complications can occur from an untreated septal hematoma?
   a) Necrosis (saddle nose deformity), Infection, and Perforation
2177) List some techniques for removing a nasal foreign body.
   a) Positive pressure techniques, Suction, and Forceps
2178) What bone fracture post nasal injury can cause CSF rhinorrhea and is diagnosed on CT?
   a) Cribriform plate (ethmoid bone)
2179) What diagnostic sign confirms positive CSF fluid?
   a) Ring sign
2180) What is the area called that is the most common site for anterior nose bleeds?
   a) Kiesselbach's plexus (Little's area)
2181) What artery is usually involved in posterior nose bleeds?
   a) Sphenopalatine artery
2182) List the treatment options for an anterior nose bleed.
   a) Compression, Cautery, Topical hemostatic agents, and Nasal packing
2183) What topical medications can be used for vasoconstriction in anterior nose bleeds?
   a) Oxymetazoline, Epinephrine, Lidocaine, or Cocaine
2184) What is the treatment for a posterior nose bleed?
   a) Nasal packing with hospital admission and ENT consult
2185) What complications from nasal packing can be prevented with the addition of antibiotics?

a) Toxic shock syndrome and Sinusitis

2186) What airway emergency can cause dysphagia, dyspnea, drooling, and fever with URI symptoms?

a) Epiglottitis

2187) What pathognomonic X-ray finding is seen in epiglottitis?

a) Thumbprint sign or "Thumb shaped" epiglottis

2188) What is the most common bacterium that causes epiglottitis in adults?

a) H. influenza Type B

2189) What is the most common bacterium that causes epiglottitis in vaccinated pediatric patients?

a) S. pneumonia

2190) What is the most common cause of epiglottitis in unvaccinated pediatric patients?

a) H. influenza Type B

2191) What is the first step in the treatment of epiglottis in a pediatric patient with stridor and drooling?

a) Call anesthesia for intubation

2192) What bacterial infection of the supraglottic region causes cough, fever, inspiratory and expiratory stridor, drooling, and a toxic appearing patient with URI symptoms?

a) Bacterial tracheitis (membranous laryngotracheobronchitis)

2193) What are the common bacterial causes of bacterial tracheitis?

a) S. aureus, S. pneumonia, or H. influenza

2194) What can be seen on a lateral soft tissue neck X-ray with bacterial tracheitis?

a) Irregular tracheal margins

2195) What antibiotic coverage is recommended for bacterial tracheitis?

a) Ampicillin/Sulbactam or Cefotriaxone + Vancomycin

2196) What gland can be infected with a blockage of Stensen's duct that causes pain and swelling?

a) Parotid gland

2197) What type of infection is due to a blocked duct and presents with lateral facial swelling anterior to the ear and extending to the mandibular angle, with overlying erythema which is tender to palpation?

a) Parotitis

2198) What other facial gland can also present with pain and swelling under the mandible and is also due to a blocked duct?

a) Submandibular gland

2199) What viral infection can cause exudative pharyngitis like strep but is differentiated by fatigue and posterior cervical chain lymphadenopathy?

a) Epstein Barr mononucleosis (EBV)

2200) What diagnostic test for EBV mono?

a) Mono Spot test

2201) What is the recommend time to perform a mono spot test after symptoms start due to probability of a false negative?

a) 2 weeks

2202) What organ might show signs of an EBV infection with abnormal labs?

a) Liver (elevated LFT's)

2203) What organ can become enlarged and inflammed with EBV and is the main premise of restricting contact sports during the infection?

a) Spleen

2204) What is the treatment for Streptococcus A pharyngitis?

a) Penicillins or Azithromycin

2205) What complications can occur with an untreated streptococcus infection?

a) Glomerulonephritis and Rheumatic fever

2206) List the Centor criteria for diagnosis and treatment of Strep throat.

a) Fever, Tender cervical lymphadenopathy, no cough, and exudative tonsillitis

2207) What are the treatment guidelines with the Centor criteria and strep throat when 2 or more criteria are present and when all 4 are present?

a) 2 or more criteria: Strep Test (15% chance of infection)

b) All 4 criteria: Treat (56% chance of infection)

2208) What is a common deep neck infection in adults that causes a hot potato voice and is associated with URI symptoms?
a) Peritonsillar abscess

2209) What is the treatment for a peritonsillar abscess?
a) Needle aspiration, Antibiotics, and ENT consult

2210) What life-threatening infectious complication can develop from the extension of a peritonsillar infection?
a) Septic thrombophlebitis (Lemierre's syndrome)

2211) What findings on a lateral cervical X-ray are consistent with a retropharyngeal abscess caused by Streptococcus or Staphylococcus?
a) Prevertebral space > 6 mm at C2
b) Prevertebral space > ½ the vertebral diameter or > 22 mm in adults or > 14 mm in children at C6

2212) What is the treatment for a retropharyngeal abscess?
a) IV antibiotics and ENT consult with I&D

2213) What bacteria causes a pharyngeal pseudomembrane as a result of an exotoxin, myocarditis, and can lead to an airway obstruction?
a) Diphtheria

2214) What is the treatment of diphtheria?
a) Diphtheria antitoxin and Erythromycin or Penicillin

2215) What type of infection presents with white oral curd-like plaques on an erythematous base that can be scraped off in patients using antibiotics, steroids or are immunocompromised?
a) Candidiasis (thrush)

2216) What is the treatment of oral thrush?
a) Clotrimazole or Nystatin

2217) What are the white plaques on the mucosal surfaces of the mouth that cannot be scraped off, are precancerous, and are seen in tobacco users?
a) Leukoplakia

2218) What type of ulcers can be caused by a virus and are typically diffuse throughout the mouth?
a) Aphthous ulcers

2219) What is the difference of vesicle location between herpetic gingivostomatitis and herpangina?
   a) Gingivostomatitis: anterior vesicles
   b) Herpangina: roof of mouth and posterior vesicles
2220) What virus causes herpangina?
   a) Coxsackie A
2221) What is the most common technique for reducing a dislocated mandible?
   a) Downward posterior force on the mandible under sedation
2222) What bones are involved in a facial tripod fracture?
   a) Zygomatic arch, Zygomatic frontal suture, and Inferior orbital floor fracture
2223) List the three types of LeFort facial fractures.
   a) Type 1: Horizontal maxillary fracture (separates the teeth from the upper face) - fracture passes through the alveolar ridge, lateral nose, and inferior wall of the maxillary sinus
   b) Type 2: Pyramid fracture (maxilla, nose, and infraorbital rim) - fracture passes through the posterior alveolar ridge, lateral wall of the maxillary sinus, inferior orbital rim, and nasal bones
   c) Type 3: Ethmoid, nose, vomer, and zygoma (craniofacial dysjunction) - fracture line passes through nasofrontal suture, maxillo-frontal suture, orbital wall, and zygomatic arch
2224) Where in the mouth do you start with labeling the teeth?
   a) Top right to left (1-16), then bottom left to right (17-32)
2225) What is the treatment for dental caries/pulpitis?
   a) Penicillins and Dental referral
2226) What is the treatment of a periapical or periodontal abscess?
   a) Antibiotics, Possible needle drainage, and Dental referral
2227) What type of Ellis tooth fracture involves just the enamel layer?
   a) Type 1
2228) What type of Ellis tooth fracture involves the enamel and dentin layers?
   a) Type 2
2229) What type of Ellis tooth fracture involves the enamel, dentin, and pulp?
   a) Type 3

2230) What is the treatment used for type 2 and type 3 Ellis fractures?
   a) Cover fracture site with calcium hydroxide composition
2231) What is the recommended treatment for a permanent tooth avulsion?
   a) Re-implant quickly and Splinting
2232) What type of solution is used for tooth fracture transport and storage?
   a) Saliva, Milk, and Hank solution
2233) What emergency oral dental infection involves the destruction of the gums, causing pain and fever, and is treated with antibiotics and dental referral?
   a) Acute necrotizing ulcerative gingivitis
2234) What is the treatment of an impacted permanent tooth?
   a) Surgical reduction by a dentist
2235) What is the treatment for a subluxated tooth?
   a) Bridging to surrounding teeth and Dental referral
2236) What diagnosis is a rapidly spreading facial cellulitis of the submandibular space, usually from dental infections, and can cause airway compromise?
   a) Ludwig's Angina
2237) What is the treatment plan for Ludwig's angina?
   a) Airway protection (intubation), IV Antibiotics and Surgery
2238) What is the treatment for alveolar osteitis (dry socket)?
   a) Pack with iodoform gauze and Pain control
2239) What type of gum infection is seen in a gingival flap over a partially ruptured tooth in pediatric patients?
   a) Pericoronitis
2240) What type of congenital cystic neck mass in a child is laterally located?
   a) Brachial cleft cyst
2241) What type of congenital cystic neck mass in a child is centrally located and connected to the posterior tongue?
   a) Thyroglossal duct cyst
2242) What is the most common site of foreign body obstruction in pediatrics airway?
   a) Cricoid cartilage

2243) What is the most common site of an airway foreign body obstruction in adults?

a) Vocal cords

Ophthalmology

2244) What cranial nerve innervates the superior oblique muscle?
   a) Cranial nerve 4 (trochlear nerve)
2245) What cranial nerve innervates the lateral rectus muscle?
   a) Cranial nerve 6
2246) What cranial nerve innervates the medial rectus muscle?
   a) Cranial nerve 3
2247) What cranial nerve injury causes a weak eyelid and a dilated pupil with a lateral deviated eye?
   a) Cranial nerve 3
2248) What syndrome causes ptosis (droopy eyelid), constricted pupil, and dry skin with unopposed parasympathetics?
   a) Horner's syndrome
2249) Trauma to what area of the body can lead to injury of the sympathetic system and lead to Horner's Syndrome?
   a) Neck and upper spinal cord
2250) What pathologies can cause a cranial nerve 6 palsy?
   a) Cavernous sinus thrombosis, Wernicke Korsakoff, and Idiopathic intracranial hypertension (pseudotumor cerebri)
2251) Do the lateral visual field tract cross midline?
   a) Yes
2252) What type of visual field defect occurs with a left side cerebellar stroke in the vision center?
   a) Right side hemianopsia
2253) What conditions should be considered with bitemporal hemianopsia?
   a) Cavernous sinus thrombosis and Pituitary tumor
2254) What is the eye condition that occurs from an embolic event in the optic artery causing a transient monocular vision loss?
   a) Amaurosis fugax
2255) What artery condition can lead to vision loss in a 55-year-old patient with severe unilateral headaches, and tenderness over the temporal artery?
   a) Temporal arteritis
2256) What lab can be elevated with temporal arteritis?

a) ESR

2257) What is the treatment of temporal arteritis?

a) Steroids

2258) What condition causes inflammation of the eyelid from chronic irritation or a bacterial infection?

a) Blepharitis

2259) What condition causes an infected red swollen lacrimal sac on the medial part of the eye due to a blocked duct?

a) Dacryocystitis

2260) What is the treatment for dacryocystitis?

a) Systemic antibiotics, Warm soaks, and Ophthalmology referral for possible duct stent

2261) What is the treatment for dacryoadenitis (lacrimal gland inflammation or infection)?

a) Warm soaks +/- Systemic antibiotics

2262) What is the term for an internal non-tender, non-inflamed granulomatous reaction of the Meibomian gland?

a) Chalazion

2263) What are the treatments for a chalazion?

a) Warm compresses or Antibiotics

2264) What condition is an abscess of the lid margin that causes pain erythema and can be internal or external on the eyelid?

a) Hordeolum (stye)

2265) What type of conjunctivitis is self-limited with thin watery discharge, lymph node enlargement and is associated with a respiratory infection?

a) Viral (adenovirus)

2266) What is the treatment for viral conjunctivitis?

a) Supportive and Warm compresses

2267) What type of viral conjunctivitis develops chemosis, corneal stippling, and decreased visual acuity?

a) Epidemic keratoconjunctivitis

2268) What type of conjunctivitis presents with unilateral purulent discharge and can be bilateral?

a) Bacterial

2269) What is the treatment of bacterial conjunctivitis?

a) Topical antibiotics (Erythromycin ointment or drops)

2270) What bacteria can be in lens wearers with conjunctivitis?

a) Pseudomonas

2271) What type of neonatal conjunctivitis presents within the first 24-48 hours?

a) Chemical (from the Erythromycin)

2272) What bacterium leads to neonatal conjunctivitis within the first 3-5 days postpartum?

a) Gonorrhea

2273) What is the treatment of gonococcal conjunctivitis?

a) Penicillin or Ceftriaxone

2274) What is the most common bacterium that leads to neonatal conjunctivitis and presents between 5-14 days postpartum?

a) Chlamydia

2275) What is the treatment for conjunctivitis from chlamydia?

a) Topical Erythromycin

2276) What type of bacteria are the leading cause of conjunctivitis after the first month?

a) Staphylococcus and Streptococcus

2277) What are the treatments for allergic conjunctivitis?

a) Antihistamine, Warm compresses, or Vasoconstrictors

2278) What condition caused by trauma and infections leads to decreased visual acuity, aching pain, injected sclera, and miosis?

a) Uveitis and Iritis

2279) What finding on the slit-lamp exam helps diagnosis uveitis and iritis?

a) Cells and Flare in the anterior chamber

2280) What eye finding seen with iritis and uveitis is characterized by white cell accumulation in the anterior chamber?

a) Hypopyon

2281) What are the treatments for iritis and uveitis?

a) Ophthalmology referral, Topical steroids, and Analgesics

2282) What corneal condition commonly in welders not using masks and skiers, presents with painful punctate lesions on the cornea seen on the slit-lamp exam with perilimbal flushing?

a) Keratitis

2283) List the treatment for keratitis.
   a) Topical anesthetics, Eye patch, and Antibiotics
2284) What type of corneal injury and pattern is seen on fluorescein staining with an HSV infection of the eye?
   a) Dendritic ulcer
2285) What is the treatment for a dendritic ulcer from an HSV infection?
   a) Topical antiviral + Oral antiviral and Ophthalmology referral
2286) What physical exam finding consists of vesicles on the tip of the nose and suggests herpes zoster ophthalmicus?
   a) Hutchinson's sign
2287) What is the treatment for a corneal HSV infection?
   a) Referral and Antivirals
2288) What type of glaucoma presents suddenly with a red painful eye, headache, hazy cornea and fixed mid-dilated pupil?
   a) Acute angle glaucoma (AAG)
2289) What corneal pressures suggest AAG?
   a) > 20 mmHg
2290) What is the normal cornea pressure range?
   a) 5-21 mmHg
2291) What class of eye medications can precipitate AAG?
   a) Mydriatics (atropine)
2292) What medications can be used to treat AAG?
   a) Topical Beta-blockers, Alpha agonists, Acetazolamide, Mannitol and Topical Miotic (pilocarpine)
2293) How do beta-blockers, alpha agonist, and Acetazolamide work?
   a) Decreases aqueous humor production
2294) What is the definitive treatment for AAG?
   a) Ophthalmology surgery and decompression
2295) What is the treatment for a subconjunctival hemorrhage?
   a) No treatment needed
2296) What eye emergency presents with decreased vision, pain with eye movements, afferent pupillary defect, and optic disc swelling on the funduscopic exam?
   a) Optic neuritis
2297) What is the diagnostic test used for optic neuritis?
   a) Red desaturation test

2298) What imaging modalities can be used to measure the optic nerve and evaluate for increased intracranial pressure?
   a) Ocular US and CT orbits

2299) What eye emergency presents with complaints of flashes of light, decreased peripheral vision, seeing floaters and is described as a "lowering of a curtain" over their vision?
   a) Retinal detachment

2300) What is the pathognomonic funduscopic exam finding seen with a retinal detachment?
   a) Retinal tear or Elevated retina that appears gray with dark blood vessels

2301) What other eye condition can present similarly to a retinal detachment?
   a) Vitreous hemorrhage

2302) What bedside imaging modality can help diagnose and confirm a retinal detachment or vitreous hemorrhage?
   a) Ocular ultrasound

2303) What is the treatment for retinal detachment and vitreous hemorrhage?
   a) Ophthalmology consult for surgery and reattachment

2304) What eye condition is caused by increased intracranial pressure, and leads to headaches, diplopia, and has bilateral optic disc swelling on a funduscopic exam?
   a) Papilledema

2305) What eye condition causes sudden painless vision loss, afferent pupillary defect, dilated pupil, and a pale retina on the fundoscopic exam?
   a) Central retinal artery occlusion

2306) What finding on a funduscopic exam is pathognomonic for a central retinal artery occlusion?
   a) Cherry red spot in the macula

2307) What are the physical treatments for a central retinal artery occlusion?
   a) Globe massage, Beta-blockers, Carbonic anhydrase inhibitors, ↑pCO_2 (breathing in a bag), and Surgery

2308) What medications can be used for a central retinal artery occlusion?
a) Topical Beta-blockers and Acetazolamide

2309) What vascular eye emergency develops gradual painless vision loss, and has cotton wool spots, macular edema, and retinal hemorrhages on the fundoscopic exam?
a) Central retinal vein occlusion

2310) What is the pathognomonic funduscopic exam seen with dilated retinal veins in central retinal vein occlusion?
a) "Blood and Thunder"

2311) Which type of facial cellulitis around the eye is less emergent with minimal pain, fever, lid edema, and erythema?
a) Periorbital cellulitis

2312) What is the treatment for periorbital cellulitis?
a) Oral antibiotics (Cephalexin or Amoxicillin-Clavulanate)

2313) At what age is it recommended to perform a full septic workup if periorbital cellulitis is diagnosed?
a) < 5 years old

2314) What type of facial cellulitis causes pain with extraocular movement testing limiting extraocular motion, and has surrounding erythema, lid edema, and proptosis?
a) Orbital cellulitis

2315) What are the most common origins of infection leading to orbital cellulitis?
a) Dental and sinus (ethmoid) infection

2316) What is the recommended imaging modality to aid in diagnosing orbital cellulitis?
a) CT orbital scan with IV contrast

2317) What is the recommended plan of care for orbital cellulitis?
a) Admission with IV antibiotics

2318) What emergency eye complication can occur from inflammation of the intraocular cavities and presents with purulent drainage, pain edema, vision loss, and chemosis?
a) Purulent endophthalmitis

2319) What is the treatment of purulent endophthalmitis?
a) Ophthalmology referral and IV antibiotics

2320) What eye condition causes tearing, injection, photophobia, and is due to a foreign body or eye trauma?
   a) Corneal abrasion
2321) What test is used to diagnose a corneal abrasion?
   a) Fluorescein staining
2322) What eye complication occurs with untreated corneal abrasions?
   a) Corneal ulcer
2323) What are the treatments for corneal ulcers and abrasions?
   a) Antibiotics (ofloxacin, erythromycin), Analgesics, and Ophthalmology referral
2324) What vitamin deficiency can lead to a corneal ulcer and night blindness?
   a) Vitamin A deficiency
2325) What should you do to the upper eyelid when you see multiple corneal scratches?
   a) Inverted the eyelid for a foreign body
2326) Does a rust ring on the cornea after foreign body removal need to be removed?
   a) Yes within 24 hours
2327) What test is used to rule out corneal perforation?
   a) Seidel test
2328) What physical exam findings can be seen with a corneal laceration?
   a) Flat anterior chamber and Teardrop shaped pupil
2329) What is the treatment for a corneal laceration?
   a) Ophthalmology referral for surgery
2330) What type of traumatic eye emergency presents with vision loss, and a teardrop pupil, hyphema, and a flat irregular globe on the exam?
   a) Globe rupture
2331) What is the treatment for chemical inoculation of the eyes?
   a) Irrigation
2332) What type of chemical burn of the eye is the worst, and causes liquefaction necrosis?
   a) Alkali

2333) What is the treatment for an alkali burn?
   a) Prolonger eye irrigation
2334) What is the target pH level of the eye that should be used in treatment and irrigation?
   a) 6.8-7.4
2335) What chemical burn causes coagulation necrosis of the eye?
   a) Acid
2336) List the different lid lacerations you need to refer to ophthalmology.
   a) Lid margin, Canalicular system, Tarsal plate, Orbital septum, or Significant de-marginalization
2337) What type of eyelid lacerations are recommended to be repaired in the ED?
   a) Partial-thickness lacerations
2338) What eye emergency can be due to trauma or a spontaneous bleed, and present with blood in the anterior chamber of the eye?
   a) Hyphema
2339) List the four types of hyphema and the percentage of the anterior chamber involved that has blood present with each type.
   a) Type 1: < 33 %
   b) Type 2: 33-50%
   c) Type 3: >50%
   d) Type 4: 100%
2340) What is the most common complication of a hyphema?
   a) Re-bleeding
2341) What medication can be used for a hyphema?
   a) Atropine
2342) What are you supposed to do with a hyphema and ↑ IOP?
   a) Treat it like glaucoma
2343) Which type of hyphema always requires surgical correction?
   a) 100% ("8 ball" hyphema)
2344) Can the lens become dislocated with trauma?
   a) Yes
2345) What imaging modalities can diagnose a lens detachment?
   a) Ocular US and CT orbits

2346) What eye emergency from trauma leads to diplopia, eye pain, and an inhibited upward gaze on extraocular muscle exam?
   a) Orbital blowout fracture

2347) What ophthalmic nerve is the most commonly involved in an orbital blow out fracture?
   a) Infraorbital nerve

2348) What clinical signs can be seen with an orbital blowout fracture with an inferior rectus muscle entrapment?
   a) Decreased vertical ocular mobility, Diplopia, and Infraorbital paresthesia

2349) What is the X-ray view to help diagnose an orbital blow out fracture?
   a) Water's view

2350) What is the positive sign on water's view X-ray seen with an orbital blow out fracture?
   a) Teardrop sign

2351) What is the most common site of fracture in the orbital cavity associated with an orbital blowout fracture?
   a) Medial wall

2352) What traumatic eye injury leads to exophthalmos, acute ↑ IOP, pain, and proptosis?
   a) Retrobulbar hemorrhage

2353) What procedure should immediately be performed to prevent retinal ischemia if a retrobulbar hemorrhage is suspected?
   a) Lateral canthotomy

2354) What imaging modality is used to diagnose a retrobulbar hemorrhage?
   a) CT orbits

2355) What limbal lesion starts to grow over the cornea with time and is seen in areas with high UV light exposure?
   a) Pterygium

2356) What type of visual field loss is seen with an eclipse burn (sungazer's retinopathy)?
   a) Central visual field defect

2357) What is the treatment for scleritis?
   a) Steroids, NSAIDs, or Methotrexate

2358) List the retinal changes seen with diabetic retinopathy.
   a) Microaneurysms, Flame hemorrhages, and Cotton wool spots
2359) List the changes seen in a funduscopic exam with hypertensive retinopathy.
   a) A-V nicking, Arterial narrowing, Flame hemorrhages, and Cotton wool spots
2360) What medications can be used to help remove superglue in the eye or over the eyelid?
   a) Erythromycin or Bacitracin ointment
2361) List two anesthetics used for the eye.
   a) Tetracaine and Proparacaine
2362) List some cycloplegics.
   a) Cyclopentolate, Tropicamide, and Homatropine

Infectious Diseases

2363) Define endemic, epidemic, and pandemic, and the difference between the three terms.
   a) Endemic: Disease affecting many in a population in a localized area
   b) Epidemic: Disease outbreak affecting many people that spread through multiple communities in an area larger than an endemic
   c) Pandemic: Disease affecting many all over the world and is larger than an epidemic

2364) List the different causes of postoperative fever and their associated windows of time they may present.
   a) Atelectasis: 24 hours
   b) Pneumonia: > 2 days
   c) UTI: 3-5 days
   d) DVT: 5 days
   e) Wound infection: 7-10 days

2365) Give the SIRS criteria to help diagnose sepsis.
   a) Temperature > 38°C or < 36°C
   b) Heart rate > 90
   c) Respiratory rate > 20 or $PaCO_2$ less than 32 mmHg
   d) WBC > 12,000 or < 4,000 or bands > 10%

2366) What is the definition of sepsis?
   a) 2 SIRS criteria + source of infection

2367) What are the new criteria to help diagnose sepsis using the quick sequential organ failure assessment tool (qSOFA)?
   a) Altered mental status
   b) Systolic BP ≤ 100 mm Hg
   c) Respiratory rate ≥ 22

2368) What medical condition is the most common condition associated with acute lung injury and acute respiratory distress syndrome (ARDS)?
   a) Sepsis

2369) What specific labs have high sensitivity and predictive power for sepsis?

a) Procalcitonin and CRP

2370) What level of lactate is associated with increased mortality in sepsis?

a) Lactate > 4

2371) What is the definition of septic shock?

a) Sepsis with persistent hypotension despite fluid resuscitation requiring vasopresors to maintain MAP > 65 mmHg or higher, and a lactate level > 2 mmol/L despite adequate volume resuscitation

2372) What labs consist of a full septic workup?

a) CBC, BMP, LFT, Lipase, U/A, Blood cultures x2, Lactate and +/- CSF cultures

2373) Is it recommended to give antibiotics before obtaining blood cultures?

a) No

2374) What is the target fluid resuscitation amount for severe sepsis?

a) 30 mL/kg

2375) What is the target central venous pressure (CVP) during fluid resuscitation in sepsis?

a) CVP 8-12 mm Hg

2376) What is the recommended vasopressor agent used in sepsis?

a) Norepinephrine

2377) What medications can be given to improve hypotension from suspected adrenal insufficiency in sepsis?

a) Hydrocortisone 100 mg or Dexamethasone 10 mg

2378) What diagnosis is suspected in a diabetic patient who presents with a local soft tissue inflammatory response with redness, warmth, and pain?

a) Cellulitis

2379) List risk factors for soft tissue skin infections (cellulitis).

a) Lymphedema, Skin breakdown, Diabetes, Peripheral vascular disease, Immunocompromised, and Obesity

2380) Which risk factor is the most common cause leading to lower extremity cellulitis?

a) Lymphedema

2381) What bacterium has the greatest risk for a poor outcome with treatment for cellulitis?
   a) Methicillin-resistant Staphylococcus aureus (MRSA)
2382) What are the two types of MRSA that can present?
   a) Hospital and Community-acquired
2383) What is the recommended treatment for simple cellulitis not from MRSA?
   a) Cephalexin, Dicloxacillin, Clindamycin, or TMP/SMX
2384) What is the recommended treatment for a patient with cellulitis and who failed outpatient oral antibiotics?
   a) Admit for IV antibiotics
2385) What antibiotics are recommended for the treatment of MRSA skin infections?
   a) Clindamycin, TMP-SMX, Vancomycin, and Linezolid
2386) What superficial skin infection presents with a fever, followed by erythema with sharply demarcated borders on the face?
   a) Erysipelas
2387) What is the treatment for erysipelas?
   a) Clindamycin, Ceftriaxone, Erythromycin, or Vancomycin
2388) What untreated skin infection presents as a hot, red, raised, painful, fluctuant area and can develop in a patient with a history of MRSA?
   a) Abscess
2389) What type of abscess presents with unilateral painful swelling of the labia at 6 or 8 o'clock position?
   a) Bartholin gland abscess
2390) How do you treat a Bartholin abscess?
   a) I & D mucosal surface of abscess followed by Word catheter insertion
2391) What type of chronic skin infection involves reoccurring abscesses of the apocrine sweat glands in both the groin and axilla?
   a) Hidradenitis suppurativa abscesses
2392) What type of abscess involves a gland that is red and tender and contains a capsule that needs surgical removal?
   a) Sebaceous cyst

2393) What is the infection called with pustules or papules in the hair follicles?
   a) Folliculitis
2394) What bacteria commonly leads to folliculitis in a patient recently in a hot tub?
   a) Pseudomonas
2395) What is a collection of infected follicles that can form sinus tracts and an abscess?
   a) Carbuncle
2396) What is the treatment for folliculitis and a carbuncle?
   a) Wound care, Antibiotics, and +/- I & D
2397) What fungal hand infection presents with painless nodules or ulcers and is associated with someone working in a rose garden?
   a) Sporotrichosis
2398) What is the treatment of Sporotrichosis?
   a) Itraconazole or Potassium Iodine
2399) What life-threatening skin infection develops from untreated cellulitis in the immunocompromised patient, and presents with fever, tachycardia, pain out of proportion to a physical exam, necrotic tissue with crepitus?
   a) Necrotizing fasciitis
2400) What bacteria causes necrotizing fasciitis?
   a) Clostridium myonecrosis
2401) What is the most common infection seen with necrotizing fasciitis?
   a) Polymicrobial
2402) Give the plan of care for necrotizing fasciitis.
   a) Broad-spectrum IV antibiotics and Surgery consult for debridement
2403) What infectious syndrome causes a high fever, diffuse desquamating rash, hypotension, and organ failure from a foreign body infection?
   a) Toxic shock syndrome
2404) What bacteria are most associated with toxic shock syndrome from a foreign body?
   a) Staphylococcus aureus

2405) What bacteria is most associated with toxic shock syndrome due to a soft tissue infection?
  a) Streptococcus
2406) What medications are recommended for toxic shock syndrome?
  a) Penicillins, Cephalosporins, Clindamycin, Intravenous immunoglobulin, Methylprednisolone
2407) What are the two main types of influenza?
  a) A & B
2408) What patient populations have the highest risk of mortality with influenza?
  a) < 2 years old, > 65 years old, Immunocompromised, and Pregnant (2nd 3rd trimester), patients, and Patients with chronic illness
2409) What are the antiviral medications used to treat influenza?
  a) Zanamivir and Oseltamivir
2410) What is the most common side effect of the influenza medications Zanamivir?
  a) Bronchospasm
2411) What is the time frame from symptoms onset that it is recommended to initiate antiviral agents for influenza?
  a) Within 48 hrs of symptoms onset
2412) What is the most common bacterium that causes post-viral pneumonia?
  a) Staphylococcus aureus
2413) What bioterrorism bacterial agent can be an infection from handling animals and affects the skin and causes a fever, malaise, and lesions in the lungs?
  a) Anthrax
2414) List the three forms of an anthrax infection.
  a) Cutaneous (eschar), Inhalational, and GI
2415) What type of anthrax infection is the most common?
  a) Cutaneous
2416) What are the pathognomonic skin changes seen with cutaneous anthrax?
  a) Black eschars

2417) What life-threatening lung condition can develop from inhaled anthrax poisoning?
a) Hemorrhagic mediastinitis

2418) What chest X-ray findings suggest anthrax poisoning?
a) Mediastinal widening, Pleural effusions, and Infiltrates

2419) What antibiotics are used to treat anthrax?
a) Ciprofloxacin, Doxycycline, and Penicillins

2420) What medications can be used for prophylaxis against anthrax?
a) Ciprofloxacin, Doxycycline, or Anthrax vaccine

2421) What type of infectious bioterrorism agent is spread by inhalation, and causes fever, headache, cough, vomiting, and raised maculopapular lesions all over the body in the same stage?
a) Smallpox

2422) What type of smallpox is the most common?
a) Variola major (90%)

2423) What stage is smallpox most infectious?
a) Prodromal stage (when in the mucus)

2424) Give the plan of care for a patient with smallpox.
a) Isolation, Cidofovir, and Smallpox vaccine

2425) What is the recommended treatment for those exposed to a smallpox patient?
a) Smallpox vaccine and VIG 0.3 mg/kg injection

2426) What bioterrorism agent leads to a descending paralysis, diplopia, and dysphagia due to neurotoxins, and can be seen in contaminated food or improperly home-canned products?
a) Botulism

2427) What proteins are disrupted by the botulism toxin?
a) SNARE proteins

2428) What food product is not recommend in infants until age 1 to prevent botulism toxin ingestion?
a) Honey

2429) What is the most common symptom in pediatrics with botulism?
a) Constipation

2430) Give the plan of care for a patient with botulism.
a) Botulism antitoxin, Botulism IG, and Supportive care

2431) What bacteria toxin causes muscle rigidity, pain, stiffness, dysphagia, and trismus?
a) Tetanus

2432) What is the term for spasms of the muscles causing backward arching of the head, neck, and spine from severe tetanus?
a) Opisthotonos

2433) What chemical drug poisoning can also lead to opisthotonos?
a) Strychnine

2434) What is the most common symptom seen in a tetanus infection?
a) Stiff painful jaw or "Lockjaw"

2435) What are the criteria for giving a tetanus boost in the emergency department in those with dirty and clean wounds, cuts, or skin breaks?
a) Dirty wound and last tetanus boost > 5 years
b) Clean wound and last tetanus booster > 10 years

2436) What are the treatment recommendations for tetanus?
a) Tetanus immune globulin (3,000-5,000), Wound debridement, Muscle relaxants, and Antibiotics

2437) Which antibiotics are recommended for tetanus treatment?
a) Metronidazole

2438) Should the tetanus IG be given before or after wound debridement during tetanus treatment?
a) Before wound debridement

2439) Based on the patient's history of immunization, what treatment regime should be used in a patient with an uncertain tetanus vaccine history and a wound?
a) Tetanus vaccine and Tetanus immune globulin

2440) Based on the patient's history of immunization, what treatment regime should be used in a patient with incomplete tetanus vaccine history < 2 doses and a clean wound?
a) Tetanus vaccine

2441) What are the side effects of IV immunoglobulin (IVIG) administration?
a) Seizures, Vomiting, and Hypotension

2442) What bacterium spreads by secretion droplets, causes a fever, headache, vomiting, stiff neck, altered mental status, and a petechial rash?
   a) Neisseria meningitidis

2443) What are the gram stain and culture findings with neisseria meningitides?
   a) Gram-negative diplococcus

2444) What is the condition caused by Neisseria meningitides leading to hemorrhagic disease and failure of the adrenal glands?
   a) Waterhouse-Friderichsen syndrome

2445) What are the antibiotic options for Neisseria meningitis?
   a) Ceftriaxone or Penicillin G

2446) What are the antibiotic options for prophylaxis in those exposed to a patient with Neisseria meningitis?
   a) Ciprofloxacin, Ceftriaxone, or Rifampin

2447) What bacterial infection presents with fevers, night sweats, weight loss, cough, hemoptysis, and a parenchymal infiltrate on chest X-ray in an immigrant?
   a) Mycobacterium tuberculosis (TB)

2448) What type of TB infection is initially asymptomatic and occurs in the middle-lower lung fields?
   a) Primary

2449) What type of TB infection is the most common clinical form in the U.S. and involves the apical and upper lobes?
   a) Reactivation

2450) Which form of TB causes multiple diffuse tiny infiltrates bilaterally on chest X-ray and can affect other organs and bone marrow?
   a) Miliary TB

2451) List the different classes of patients at risk for TB.
   a) Homeless, Alcoholics, HIV, IV Drug users, Elderly, Nursing home residents, and Prisoners

2452) What bacteria is the number one infectious cause of death worldwide?
   a) TB

2453) List the tests used to diagnose TB.

a) PPD (Mantoux), Chest radiograph, Cultures, Acid-fast stain, Quantiferon Gold TB test

2454) When do you check a PPD test after the 0.1 mL PPD injection?
a) 48-72 hours

2455) What size of induration after a PPD test is a positive test in the different patient populations?
a) > 15 mm in Healthy patients
b) > 10 mm in Immigrants, High-risk employees or residents, IV Drug abusers, and Children < 4 years old
c) > 5 mm in patients with a suppressed immune system, HIV patients, Recent TB contacts, Patients with previous chest X-ray findings suggesting TB

2456) What is the next step after a positive PPD finding?
a) Chest X-ray

2457) What drugs are used in combination to treat TB?
a) Rifampin, Isoniazid (INH), Pyrazinamide, and Ethambutol (RIPE)

2458) What two medications cannot be used in multidrug-resistant TB?
a) Isoniazid (INH) and Rifampin

2459) What is the treatment for a patient with a + PPD without an active TB infection?
a) Isoniazid (INH)

2460) What TB medication can cause hepatitis, peripheral neuropathy, and seizures as a side effect?
a) Isoniazid (INH)

2461) What TB medication can cause optic neuritis as a side effect?
a) Ethambutol

2462) What TB medication can cause gout as a side effect?
a) Pyrazinamide

2463) What TB medication can cause orange urine and lacrimations as a side effect?
a) Rifampin

2464) Are universal precautions necessary for a suspected TB case?
a) Yes with isolation (negative pressure room)

2465) What is the diagnostic finding for TB on a gram stain and culture?

a) Aerobic acid-fast rods

2466) Is TB an AIDS-defining illness in HIV patients?

a) Yes

2467) What is the main vector of rabies worldwide?

a) Dogs

2468) What is the main vector of rabies in the US?

a) Bats

2469) List the symptoms of rabies.

a) Excitation, Agitation, Opisthotonus, Hydrophobia, Salivation, Paralysis, and Lacrimation

2470) What are the pathognomonic pathological bodies found on brain biopsy in rabies patients?

a) Negri bodies

2471) How does the rabies virus spread to the central nervous system?

a) Via retrograde spread up peripheral nerves

2472) On what days is the post-exposure rabies vaccine supposed to be administered.

a) Day 0-3-7-14

2473) In what situation do you give rabies immunoglobulin and vaccine?

a) When the source animal cannot be tested or observed, or bat exposure

2474) How long are animals with an unknown vaccination history monitored for rabies symptoms and quarantined after biting a human?

a) 10 days

2475) What protozoal disease causes repetitive cyclical fevers, headache, and malaise in a patient with a recent travel history?

a) Malaria

2476) What specific type of mosquito transmits malaria?

a) Anopheles

2477) What are the four species of Plasmodium malariae?

a) Falciparum

b) Vivax

c) Malariae

d) Ovale

2478) What species is the most common, has the highest mortality, and is Chloroquine-resistant?
   a) Falciparum

2479) What labs help confirm malaria?
   a) Thick and thin blood smears and Giemsa stain

2480) What is the recommended oral treatment for malaria?
   a) Chloroquine, Quinine, Atovaquone-Proguanil, Mefloquine-primaquine, or Doxycycline

2481) What oral medications can be used for malaria prophylaxis?
   a) Chloroquine, Quinine, Atovaquone-Proguanil, Mefloquine-primaquine, or Doxycycline

2482) Which Malaria medication causes abdominal cramping and neuro symptoms?
   a) Mefloquine

2483) What type of Malaria infection from P. Falciparum causes jaundice, fever, and massive hemolysis?
   a) Blackwater fever

2484) What mosquito-borne illness more commonly seen in warm humid climates causes headache flu-like symptoms, and can progress to encephalitis and paralysis?
   a) West Nile virus

2485) What is the most common sexually transmitted disease (STD), and presents with urethritis, epididymitis, and urethral discharge?
   a) Chlamydia trachomatis

2486) What are the medications used for chlamydia treatment?
   a) Azithromycin or Doxycycline

2487) What STD presents with shallow painless genital ulcer and painful inguinal lymph nodes (Groove sign), fever, and arthralgias?
   a) Lymphogranuloma venereum

2488) What bacteria causes lymphogranuloma venereum?
   a) Chlamydia trachomatis

2489) What is the treatment for lymphogranuloma venereum?
   a) Doxycycline or Erythromycin for 3 weeks

2490) What STD is caused by the bacteria Klebsiella granulomatis and presents with a painless ulcer and Donovan bodies on tissue biopsy?

a) Granuloma inguinale

2491) Which STD causes urethritis, cervicitis, epididymitis, urethral discharge, and can lead to a disseminated disease with joint pains and a diffuse rash?
a) Nisseria gonorrhea

2492) What is the microscopic finding for gonorrhea on the gram stain and culture?
a) Gram-negative diplococci

2493) List the signs of disseminated gonorrhea.
a) Tender pustules on an erythematous base, Arthritis, and Conjunctivitis

2494) What is the treatment for gonorrhea?
a) Ceftriaxone 250mg IM or Cefixime 400mg PO

2495) What are the symptoms with 1° Syphilis?
a) Painless genital ulcers (Chancre)

2496) What bacteria causes syphilis?
a) Treponema pallidum

2497) What labs are ordered to diagnose syphilis?
a) Serology (VDRL/RPR), FTA-ABS, and Dark field microscopy

2498) What are the symptoms with 2° syphilis?
a) Maculopapular rash on palms and soles 2-10 weeks after ulcer

2499) What are the smooth flat warts in the genital region called in 2° syphilis?
a) Condyloma lata

2500) List the other organ involvement seen with 3° syphilis.
a) Neurosyphilis, Cardiovascular syphilis (aneurysm), Skin lesions (Gummas), and Bone changes (Charcot joint)

2501) What is the treatment for syphilis?
a) Penicillin 2.4 million units intramuscular

2502) What is recommended for treatment for syphilis in a Penicillin allergic?
a) Desensitization of Penicillin for treatment

2503) What is the reaction of fever, arthralgias, headache, and myalgias that occurs after treatment of syphilis?
a) Jarisch-Herxheimer reaction

2504) What medication can be given 2 hours before treating syphilis with antibiotics to prevent symptoms from Jarisch-Herxheimer reaction?
a) Tylenol

2505) What STD causes painful genital ulcers and unilateral adenopathy with drainage?
a) Chancroid

2506) What is the bacteria that causes chancroid?
a) Haemophilus ducreyi

2507) Give the treatments for chancroid.
a) Ceftriaxone, Azithromycin, or Ciprofloxacin

2508) What STD causes painful clustered vesicular lesions, ulcers, and prodrome of fever, myalgias, and a headache?
a) Herpes simplex virus (HSV)

2509) What type of herpes is the most common type found in genital herpes?
a) HSV 2

2510) What type of herpes is the most commone type found with head and neck herpes?
a) HSV 1

2511) What lab testing can be done to confirm HSV?
a) Tzanck smear

2512) What is the treatment for HSV?
a) Antivirals (Acyclovir or Famciclovir)

2513) What neurological complication can occur with HSV and is typically in the temporal region?
a) HSV meningitis

2514) What STD is from a flagellated protozoan and causes green-yellow malodorous penile or vaginal discharge?
a) Trichomoniasis

2515) What is cervical finding suggests trichomonas?
a) Strawberry cervix

2516) What is the treatment of trichomonas?
a) 2 grams metronidazole or (500mg Bid 7 days in OB)

2517) What STD causes condyloma accuminata, flat painless flesh-colored skin lesions in the rectal penile and perineal areas?

a) Human papilloma virus (HPV)

2518) List the treatment for HPV.

a) Podofilox topical or Cryotherapy

2519) What is the period called for seroconversion to occur with HIV over 3 months?

a) Window period

2520) What are the initial presenting symptoms for HIV patients which leads to a misdiagnosis?

a) Viral syndrome (fever, malaise, adenopathy, and rash)

2521) Give the different body fluids which HIV can be transferred by.

a) Blood, Saliva, Semen, Vaginal secretions, Breast milk, CSF, Tears, and Alveolar fluid

2522) What is the most common population with the highest transmission rates?

a) Men who have sex with men

2523) What lab tests diagnose HIV?

a) HIV-1 antibody, ELISA, Western blot, Single-use diagnostic system, or HIV plasma RNA

2524) During what period can HIV can the lab tests give a false negative?

a) Window period

2525) What CD4 count delineates AIDS?

a) Less than 200 cells/mm3

2526) List some AIDS-defining illnesses in HIV patients.

a) Pneumocystis, Kaposi sarcoma, TB, Cryptococcus, Esophagitis, Cytomegalovirus, or Cryptosporidium

2527) What is the most common eye condition leading to blindness seen in AIDS with CD4 count < 50 cells/mm3?

a) Cytomegalovirus (CMV) retinitis

2528) What are the funduscopic findings with CMV retinitis?

a) Cotton wool spots, and tallow patches

2529) What viral infection is the most common in patients with a history of a liver transplant?

a) CMV hepatitis

2530) What is the treatment for CMV retinitis and CMV hepatitis?

a) Ganciclovir or Foscarnet

2531) What is the most common type of pneumonia that can develop in HIV/AIDS patients?
a) Pneumocystis jiroveci pneumonia (PCP)

2532) What infection is the most common identifiable cause of death in AIDS patients?
a) PCP

2533) What are the indications for steroid use in PCP pneumonia?
a) PaO_2 < 70 or A-a gradient >35

2534) What antibiotics are used for the treatment of PCP in HIV patients?
a) TMP-SMX

2535) What bacteria from cats and undercooked meat, commonly affects the immunocompromised and can cause ring-enhancing lesions on brain CT?
a) Toxoplasmosis

2536) What medications treat toxoplasmosis?
a) Pyrimethamine + Sulfadiazine + Folinic acid

2537) What is the most common cause of meningitis in HIV/AIDS patients?
a) Cryptococcosis

2538) What is the treatment of cryptococcosis meningitis?
a) Amphotericin B + Flucytosine

2539) What skin condition in HIV patients presents with painless purple areas?
a) Kaposi's sarcoma

2540) What is the treatment for candida esophagitis in immunocompromised patients?
a) Fluconazole

2541) What is the most common serious opportunistic viral disease in HIV?
a) CMV

2542) What is the most common occurring neoplasm in HIV?
a) Non-Hodgkin's lymphoma

2543) What are the combinations of highly active antiretroviral therapy (HAART) used to treat HIV?

a) 2 nucleoside analog reverse transcriptase inhibitors (NRTI) + 1 protease inhibitor (PI), or non-nucleoside reverse transcriptase inhibitors (NNRTI), or Integrase strand transfer inhibitors

2544) List the NRTI medications.
a) Zidovudine, Stravudine, Emtricitabine, and Tenofovir

2545) List the NNRTI medications.
a) Efavirenz and Nevirapine

2546) List some Protease inhibitors.
a) Indinavir, Rotinavir, and Saquinavir

2547) List an Integrase strand transfer inhibitors.
a) Raltegravir

2548) Which HIV drug can lead to nephrolithiasis?
a) Indinavir

2549) What class of HIV medications can lead to bone marrow suppression and lactic acidosis?
a) Nucleoside analog reverse transcriptase inhibitors (Zidovudine, Stravudine, Emtricitabine, and Tenofovir)

2550) What type of mycobacterium avium complex (MAC) illness can develop in patients after starting HAART for HIV?
a) Immune reconstruction illness to MAC

2551) What are the indications to start HAART therapy in the ED?
a) CD4 < 350, HIV neuropathy, HIV in pregnancy, HIV potential exposure, and HIV with a hepatitis B history

2552) What is the risk of developing HIV after a needle stick?
a) 0.3%

2553) What is the recommendation for HIV post exposure prophylaxis (PEP) for a patient with a needle stick when the source is not able to be tested?
a) Initiate PEP within 72 hours

2554) What is the preferred HIV PEP regimen?
a) Raltegravir + Tenofovir, and Emtricitabine

2555) What type of bacteria from uncooked fish causes flushing, headache, and vomiting?
a) Scombroid

2556) What is the treatment for scombroid poisoning?
a) Antihistamines

2557) List the typical fish that can contain scombroidae bacteria.
a) Mackerel, Albacore tuna, Mahi-mahi, and Kingfish

2558) What type of bacteria from uncooked fish presents with headache, muscle aches, paresthesias, burning sensation on contact with cold and sodium channel abnormalities?
a) Ciguatera

2559) What electrolyte abnormality can be seen with ciguatera poisoning?
a) Hyponatremia

2560) What is the treatment of ciguatera poisoning?
a) IV Mannitol

2561) What type of bacterial infection from water leads to chronic painful cutaneous granulomas after swimming in the ocean?
a) Mycobacterium marinum

2562) What type of bacteria is usually seen in cellulitis with hemorrhagic bulla from a saltwater skin injury?
a) Vibrio vulnificus

2563) What is the antibiotic treatment for Vibrio induced cellulitis?
a) Doxycycline

2564) What bacteria is typically seen with freshwater infections of the skin?
a) Aeromonas hydrophila

2565) What is the antibiotic treatment for Aeromonas?
a) Ciprofloxacin or Piperacillin-Tazobactam

2566) What is the vector of transfer for Lyme, Q fever, and RMSF?
a) Ticks

2567) What tick-borne disease has a triad of symptoms including fever, followed by a petechial rash that first appears on extremities and spreads to the trunk?
a) Rocky Mountain Spotted Fever (RMSF)

2568) What lab findings can be seen with RMSF?
a) Thrombocytopenia, Hyponatremia, and Elevated liver enzymes

2569) What organism causes RMSF?
a) Rickettsia

2570) What type of tick vector carries rickettsia?
a) Dermacentor ticks

2571) What is the drug of choice for RMSF?

a) Doxycycline

2572) What is the preferred treatment of choice for RMSF in pediatric patients?

a) Doxycycline

2573) What is the most common tick-born vector infection in the US?

a) Lyme disease

2574) What is the treatment of acute Lyme disease?

a) Doxycycline 21-day course

2575) What is the spirochete organism transmitted by the Ixodes tick that leads to Lyme disease?

a) Borrelia burgdorferi

2576) What is the pathognomonic rash seen with Lyme disease?

a) Erythema migrans

2577) How many stages of Lyme disease can develop?

a) Three

2578) What cardiovascular and neurologic complications can occur from Lyme disease?

a) Myocarditis, AV block, and Bilateral bell's palsy

2579) What lab diagnoses Lyme disease?

a) Serology ELISA test

2580) What is the time frame that a tick is attached to the skin that increases the risk of a Lyme infection transmission?

a) 72 hours or more

2581) What is the prophylactic dose of Doxycycline used for tick bites in endemic Lyme areas?

a) Doxycycline 200 mg x1

2582) What muscle condition from a tick bite can develop with reversible ascending paralysis?

a) Tick paralysis

2583) Which infection is transmitted by ticks and rabbits, can lead to ulceroglandular pulmonary disease, and is treated with Streptomycin?

a) Tularemia

2584) What is the treatment for tularemia?

a) Gentamycin or Streptomycin

2585) Which tick-borne disease causes a malaria-like illness, and can cause hemolysis and elevated LFT's?
a) Babesiosis

2586) What is the treatment of Babesiosis?
a) Quinine + Clindamycin or Atovaquone + Azithromycin

2587) Which tick-borne disease causes a fever, rash, thrombocytopenia, leucopenia, and liver dysfunction?
a) Ehrlichiosis

2588) What are the two types of ticks that carry Ehrlichiosis?
a) Dermacentor and Amblyomma (lone star tick)

2589) What antibiotic is recommended for Ehrlichiosis?
a) Doxycycline

2590) What tick-borne infection causes an acute viral illness, fever, chills, and photophobia and is seen in the western U.S.?
a) Colorado tick fever

2591) What type of tick bites cause Colorado tick fever?
a) Dermacentor andersoni (wood tick)

2592) What is the treatment for Colorado tick fever?
a) Supportive

2593) What type of bacteria causes the plague from flea bites?
a) Yersinia pestis

2594) What is the most common form of the plague?
a) Bubonic

2595) What are the significant findings with the Bubonic plague?
a) Swollen tender lymph nodes, Fever, Headache, and Chills

2596) Which type of the plague can cause a rapid spreading blood infection and ischemia of end arteries leading to gangrene?
a) Septicemic plague

2597) List the antibiotics used to treat the plague.
a) Gentamicin, Streptomycin, or Doxycycline

2598) What infection caused by the Aedes aegypti mosquito leads to fever, abdominal pain, and hemorrhagic shock?
a) Dengue fever

2599) What lab tests are used to diagnose Dengue fever?
a) PCR and IgM ELISA

2600) Which arbovirus from a mosquito presents with fever, headache nausea, and generalized arthralgias in patients who recently traveled to Africa or Asia?
   a) Chikungunya
2601) What lab test is used to diagnose Chikungunya?
   a) ELISA for IgM and IgG anti-chikungunya antibodies
2602) What bacteria causes fever, headache, bloody diarrhea, and bradycardia, from ingesting contaminated food or water with the infected feces of a symptomatic carrier?
   a) Salmonella typhi (Typhoid fever)
2603) How is typhoid diagnosed?
   a) Stool culture
2604) What bacterial infection comes from contact with cattle and goats, and leads to relapsing fever, abdominal pain, joint pains, lymphadenopathy, and hepatosplenomegaly?
   a) Brucellosis
2605) What is the treatment for Brucellosis?
   a) Doxycycline, Rifampin, or Gentamycin
2606) Give the names of the two infections caused by bites of the ixodid ticks in travelers to the African and Asia areas, and leads to fever, eschars, and splenomegaly.
   a) African tick typhus and Scrub typhus
2607) What regions of the world have the epidemic louse-borne typhus from Rickettsia prowazekii, causing fevers, headaches, and rash?
   a) Mexico, Guatemala, Ethiopia, and the Himalayas
2608) What is the medical treatment for typhus?
   a) Doxycycline
2609) What spirochete infection is due to skin contact with contaminated water with infect animal urine and leads to hepatitis, nephritis, and jaundice?
   a) Leptospirosis
2610) What is the severe condition of leptospirosis called that causes jaundice, conjunctival hemorrhages, hepatitis, and DIC?
   a) Weil's disease
2611) What is the treatment for leptospirosis?

a) Penicillin or Doxycycline

2612) What medical condition in agricultural workers in the African, Asian, and Middle East regions, leads to fever, thrombocytopenia, liver and renal injury, hemoptysis, and GI bleeding?

a) Crimean-Congo Hemorrhagic fever (CCH)

2613) What is the treatment for CCH?

a) Ribavirin

2614) What mosquito-borne illness seen in equator countries causes a flulike illness, hemorrhagic fever, black emesis, albuminuria, and shock?

a) Yellow fever

2615) What is the treatment of yellow fever?

a) Supportive

2616) What worm infection from undercook pork leads to a CNS infection and causes seizures?

a) Cysticercosis (pork tapeworm)

2617) What type of worm infection from street vendor foods contaminated with feces causes dry cough consisting of expectorated worms?

a) Ascariasis

2618) What type of worm infection from fecal-oral contact of contaminated objects leads to intense perianal itching and is diagnosed with cellophane tape over the anus at night?

a) Enterobiasis (pinworm)

2619) What type of worm infects its host by the larvae penetrating the skin leading to a red cutaneous larva migrans skin burrow and can migrate to the lung and GI tract?

a) Ancylostoma duodenale and Nector Americanos (hookworm)

2620) Give the treatment for Ascariasis, pork tapeworm, pinworm, and hookworm.

a) Mebendazole, Albendazole, or Pyrantel pamoate

2621) What worm infection is from eating contaminated fish and leads to B12 deficiency?

a) Diphyllobothrium latum

2622) What worm infection is from eating contaminated beef and causes abdominal pain, bowel obstruction, and diarrhea?

a) Taenia saginata

2623) What worm infection if from eating contaminated pork?

a) Taenia solium

2624) Give the treatment for Taenia solium, Taenia saginata, and Diphyllobothrium latum.

a) Praziquantel

2625) What infection is transmitted by the tsetse fly and causes a chancre, fevers, neurologic changes, and hemolysis?

a) African trypanosomiasis (African sleeping sickness)

2626) What is the treatment of African sleeping sickness?

a) Suramin

2627) What infection from trypanosoma cruzi from a reduviid "kissing bug" bite causes unilateral periorbital edema, painful cutaneous edema at the bite, and a heart murmur?

a) Chagas disease

2628) What is the treatment for Chagas disease?

a) Nifurtimox or Benznidazole

2629) How are Chagas disease and African sleeping sickness diagnosed?

a) On peripheral blood smear

2630) What protozoan infection from a sand-fly bite in the jungle, causes fever, weight loss, hepatosplenomegaly, pancytopenia, and hypergammaglobulinemia?

a) Leishmaniasis (visceral)

2631) What is the treatment for leishmaniasis?

a) Sodium stibogluconate or Meglumine antimonate

2632) What infection comes from exposer to snail larvae in freshwater causing GI symptoms, and a macular papular pruritic dermatitis?

a) Schistosomiasis (snail fever)

2633) What organ does schistosomiasis commonly deposit in causing eosinophilia and eggs in mid-day urines?

a) Bladder

2634) What is the treatment of schistosomiasis?

a) Praziquantel

2635) What infectious organism from the Asia and Africa areas, causes colitis, fever, and abdominal pain, and can lead to a liver abscess?

a) Entamoeba histolytica (Amebiasis)

2636) What parasite is from drinking contaminated river water with animal (beaver) urine and leads to greasy diarrhea, and stomach aches?

a) Giardia

2637) How are Amebiasis and Giardia diagnosed?

a) Stool culture for ova and parasites

2638) What is the treatment for Amebiasis and Giardia?

a) Metronidazole

2639) List the TORCH infections.

a) Toxoplasmosis, Rubella, Cytomegalovirus, Herpes, Epstein-Barr, and Syphilis

2640) What condition presents with a sudden onset flaccid limb weakness in a patient with a recent viral URI, and has grey matter lesions on the spinal cord found on an MRI?

a) Acute flaccid myelitis

2641) What is the most common infectious cause of acute flaccid myelitis?

a) Enterococcus

Neurology

2642)   List the muscle reflex nerves for biceps, brachioradialis, triceps, knee, and plantar.
   a)   1) Bicep: C5-C6
   b)   2) Brachioradialis: C6
   c)   3) Triceps: C7
   d)   4) Patellar: L4
   e)   5) Plantar: S1

2643)   List the dermatome nerve innervation for the thumb & index, middle, and little fingers.
   a)   Thumb & index: C6
   b)   Middle finger: C7
   c)   Little finger: C8

2644)   List the dermatome nerve innervation at the nipple line.
   a)   T4

2645)   List the dermatome nerve innervation at the umbilicus.
   a)   T10

2646)   List the scoring for the Glasgow coma scale (GCS) for the eyes.
   a)   4: Spontaneously
   b)   3: To verbal
   c)   2: To pain
   d)   1: None

2647)   List the scoring for the Glasgow coma scale for the motor response.
   a)   6: Follows commands
   b)   5: Localizes pain
   c)   4: Withdraws
   d)   3: Decorticate (abnormal flexion)
   e)   2: Decerebrate (extension posturing)
   f)   1: None

2648)   List the scoring for the Glasgow coma scale for the verbal category.
   a)   5: Oriented
   b)   4: Confused
   c)   3: Inappropriate words

d) 2: Incomprehensible speech

e) 1: None

2649) List common causes of altered mental status or coma.

a) Alcohol, Dehydration, Drugs, Electrolytes, Fever, Glucose levels, Hypercapnia, Hypoxia, Infections, Psychiatric, Poisons, Seizure, Stroke, Thyroid levels, and Uremia

2650) What cranial nerve lesion causes anisocoria?

a) CN 3

2651) Describe nystagmus.

a) Rapid, uncontrollable movement of the eyes described by the direction of the fast component

2652) What neurological reflex checking brain function is test by holding the eye open and rotating the head from side to side and indicates intact brainstem if the eyes move the opposite direction of the head movements?

a) Oculocephalic reflex (dolls eyes)

2653) What neurological reflex is tested by instilling hot or cold water into the ear canal and is normal if the eyes nystagmus away from the cold water?

a) Oculovestibular reflex (caloric)

2654) With an intact oculovestibular reflex, what direction do the eyes deviate after instilling warm water into the ear canal?

a) Same side the warm water was instilled on

2655) What type of brainstem reflex is testing the CN V and CN VII and indicates an intact brainstem with blinking?

a) Corneal reflex

2656) What neurological abnormality can lead to a unilateral dilated pupil (blown pupil)?

a) Ipsilateral bleed or Uncal herniation

2657) What eye finding on funduscopic exam indicates increased intracranial pressure?

a) Papilledema

2658) List the medications commonly used for a coma cocktail in the ED.

a) Dextrose, Oxygen, Naloxone, Normal saline, and Thiamine

2659) What is the most common cause of a breakthrough seizure?

a) Medication non-compliance

2660) What type of seizure is characterized by diffuse body part movements and shaking with loss of consciousness?

a) Generalized tonic-clonic (Grand mal)

2661) What type of seizure is characterized by sudden staring with loss of consciousness?

a) Absence seizure(Petit mal)

2662) What type of seizure presents with a sudden collapse and flaccid period of muscles?

a) Atonic seizure

2663) What type of seizure is characterized by a focal tonic muscle spasms with consciousness maintained?

a) Simple partial siezure

2664) What is the term for a simple partial seizure progressing to a generalized seizure?

a) Jacksonian march

2665) What type of seizure is characterized by mild impairment, lips smacking, picking, hallucinations, and confusion?

a) Complex partial seizure

2666) What type of seizures present with movements of the extremities, intact consciousness, is commonly seen in psychiatric patients and is not followed by postictal phase?

a) Pseudoseizure or Psychogenic non-epileptic seizures

2667) What type of seizure is the most common cause in pediatrics, and is associated with a recent respiratory infection and fever?

a) Febrile seizure

2668) What is the suspected cause of a new-onset seizure in an alcoholic patient?

a) Alcohol withdrawal seizure

2669) What is the recommended treatment of an alcohol withdrawal seizure?

a) Benzodiazepine

2670) What type of seizure presents in a patient with an anxiety history who recent stopped taking their antianxiety medications?

a) Benzodiazepine withdrawal seizure

2671) Can the lactate level increase due to seizures?

a) yes

2672) What blood lab can help decipher between a seizure versus a syncope episode? (Clinical pearl)
   a) Prolactin

2673) What metabolic/electrolyte abnormalities can lead to intractable seizures?
   a) Hyponatremia and Hypoglycemia

2674) What is the suspected cause of a new-onset seizure in a 30-week pregnant patient?
   a) Eclampsia

2675) What is the definition of status epilepticus?
   a) Persistent seizure activity > 5 mins or two or more seizures without full recovery of consciousness

2676) What is the term for a postictal paralysis seen after a seizure that can last up to 24 hours?
   a) Todd's paralysis

2677) What bacteria is associated with gastroenteritis in a pediatric patient and seizures?
   a) Shigella

2678) What is the first-line medication treatment used for seizures?
   a) Benzodiazepines

2679) What are the 2nd, 3rd, and 4th line agents used for seizures after benzodiazepines fail to break the seizure?
   a) Phenytoin/Fosphenytoin
   b) Phenobarbital
   c) Levetiracetam

2680) What is the loading dose for Phenytoin and Fosphenytoin?
   a) 18 mg/kg

2681) What is the loading dose for Phenobarbital?
   a) 20 mg/kg

2682) What is the loading dose for Levetiracetam?
   a) 30-50 mg/kg

2683) What sedation medication also has an antiepileptic component?
   a) Propofol

2684) What medication should be administered in a patient with a seizure who is receiving INH for TB treatment?
a) Pyridoxine

2685) What neurological condition presents with severe intermittent attacks of facial pain from a compressed nerve?
a) Trigeminal neuralgia (Tic douloureux)

2686) What is the treatment for trigeminal neuralgia?
a) Carbamazepine

2687) What is the most common type of headache, characterized by bilateral frontal aching pain with neck tightness?
a) Tension headache

2688) What type of headache presents with an aura followed by severe throbbing unilateral headache with nausea and vomiting?
a) Migraine

2689) What are the three types of migraine headaches?
a) Classic
b) Non-classic
c) Complex

2690) What type of migraine is the most common?
a) Non-classic 80% (migraine without aura)

2691) Which type of migraine present with auras?
a) Classic

2692) What type of migraine presents with headache, vomiting, photophobia, numbness, tingling, and weakness?
a) Complex migraine

2693) List the medications used for abortive migraine therapy.
a) Ergotamine, Sumatriptan, Opioids, Metoclopramide, Promethazine, Magnesium, and Steroids

2694) List the medications used to prevent chronic migraines.
a) Tricyclic antidepressants, Beta-blockers, and Calcium channel blockers

2695) What type of headache presents more commonly in middle age males with unilateral pain, conjunctival injection, lacrimation, and rhinorrhea?
a) Cluster headache

2696) What is the treatment for a cluster headache?

a) Oxygen and Analgesics

2697) What medication can be used to prevent cluster headaches?

a) Verapamil

2698) What neurological condition presents as chronic headaches in young obese females, with nausea, vomiting, and visual changes?

a) Idiopathic intracranial hypertension (Pseudotumor Cerebri)

2699) What is the cause of the headaches in pseudotumor cerebri?

a) Elevated CSF pressure

2700) How is pseudotumor cerebri diagnosed?

a) Lumbar puncture (LP) opening pressure

2701) Give the treatments for idiopathic intracranial hypertension.

a) Repeat lumbar punctures, Acetazolamide, or ventricular shunt

2702) What level of opening pressure on LP is considered abnormal in adults?

a) > 25 cm H_2O

2703) What type of headache presents in a patient that is pulsatile, worse with upright posture in a patient who received a recent lumbar puncture?

a) Spinal headache

2704) What is the definitive treatment for a spinal headache after a lumbar puncture?

a) Blood patch

2705) What neurological emergency needs ruled out in a patient with sudden onset severe headache that is the worst of their life?

a) Subarachnoid hemorrhage (SAH)

2706) What procedure can be done to rule out meningitis or subarachnoid hemorrhage?

a) Lumbar puncture

2707) How many hours after the onset of a posterior headache does a CT head have a sensitivity of 99% for detecting a subarachnoid hemorrhage?

a) 6 hours or less

2708) What is the most common cause of a subarachnoid hemorrhage?

a) Secondary to aneurysm

2709) What RBC finding in the CSF fluid obtained on lumbar puncture is suggestive of a brain bleed?

a) A RBC count in the spinal fluid that does not decrease or resolve from tubes 1-4

2710) What is the term used to describe the yellowish appearance of CSF that occurs several hours after bleeding into the subarachnoid space and is caused by presence of bilirubin in the CSF?

a) Xanthochromia

2711) What medication is used to prevent arterial spasms and worsening bleeding in SAH?

a) Nimodipine

2712) What neurological condition presents with a headache, nausea, vomiting, altered mental status, papilledema, and has dilated ventricles on head CT?

a) Hydrocephalus

2713) What neurological condition presents with dilated ventricles on a brain CT, progressive altered mental status changes, shuffling or ataxic gait, and urinary incontinence?

a) Normal-pressure hydrocephalus

2714) What are the treatment options for symptomatic normal-pressure hydrocephalus in the ED?

a) Elevated the head of the bed, Mannitol, Hyperventilate, and Neurology consult for shunt

2715) What are the most common causes of a ventricular shunt headache?

a) Malfunction or Infection

2716) What imaging is used to diagnose a shunt malfunction?

a) Shunt series (X-ray: head, neck, chest, and abdomen) or Brain CT

2717) What type of brain bleed is the most common following head trauma?

a) Traumatic SAH

2718) What neurological emergency is suspected in an elderly patient complaining of a headache after a fall with altered mental status?

a) Subdural hematoma

2719) Injury to what vessels lead to a subdural hematoma?

a) Torn bridging veins

2720) What is the finding of a subdural hematoma on a brain CT?
   a) Concave/crescent shaped hyperdense area that crosses suture lines
2721) What neurological bleed is characterized by head trauma with loss of consciousness followed by a lucid interval, headache, and progression to decreased mental status?
   a) Epidural hematoma
2722) What is the pathognomonic finding of an epidural hematoma on brain CT?
   a) Lens shape hematoma (hyperdense area)
2723) What vessel injury leads to an epidural hematoma?
   a) Middle Meningeal artery
2724) What is the treatment of increased intracranial pressure?
   a) Mannitol
   b) Hypertonic saline 3%
   c) Hyperventilation
   d) Neurosurgery consult
   e) +/- Anticonvulsants
2725) What is the targeted PaCO2 range for the treatment of increased intracranial pressure (ICP) with hyperventilation?
   a) 25-30 mmHg
2726) What is the targeted ICP in the treatment of patients with increased intracranial pressure?
   a) < 20 mmHg
2727) Name the two types of stroke.
   a) Ischemic and Hemorrhagic
2728) What is the most common type of stroke?
   a) Ischemic
2729) List some causes of hemorrhagic stroke.
   a) Arteriovenous malformation, Aneurysm, SAH, Subdural or epidural hematoma, and Head trauma
2730) What is the term for stroke-like symptoms that resolve within 24 hours?
   a) Transient ischemic attack (TIA)

2731) What cerebral artery is most commonly associated with an ischemic stroke and causes aphasia and contralateral motor and sensory loss greater in the upper extremities?
a) Middle cerebral artery

2732) What area of the brain is affected in a patient who cannot understand directions with stroke symptoms?
a) Wernicke's

2733) What area of the brain is affected in a patient who cannot speak appropriately with stroke symptoms?
a) Broca's

2734) What side of the brain is the most common dominant side containing Broca's and Wernicke's areas?
a) Left

2735) What cerebral artery is affected causing a stroke with contralateral motor and sensory loss greater in the lower extremities?
a) Anterior cerebral artery

2736) What cerebral artery is affected with contralateral homonymous hemianopsia and a cranial nerve 3 palsy?
a) Posterior cerebral artery

2737) What brain artery is affected in a patient with vertigo, nystagmus, diplopia, dysarthria, and dysphagia?
a) Vertebrobasilar artery

2738) What brain artery is effected that causes a "locked-in syndrome" of quadriplegia with a reserved pupil function?
a) Basilar artery

2739) What syndrome occurs with a lateral brainstem infarct of the proximal vertebral artery, causing vertigo, ipsilateral facial numbness, and contralateral loss of pain and temperature of the trunk and limbs?
a) Wallenberg's syndrome (Lateral medullary syndrome)

2740) What is the time window in which most ischemic strokes do not show up on brain CT?
a) < 24 hours

2741) What is the most sensitive brain imaging for acute stroke?
a) MRI

2742) What medication can be given to reverse CVA symptoms?
   a) Alteplase (TPA)
2743) What is the dosing of TPA for a CVA?
   a) 0.9mg/kg max 90mg (10% bolus and the remainder infused over 1 hour)
2744) What is the risk of intracranial hemorrhagic bleed after TPA administration?
   a) 6 %
2745) Give the absolute contraindications for TPA administration.
   a) CVA < 3 months
   b) Hemorrhagic CVA history
   c) Intracranial surgery or trauma < 3 months
   d) Intracranial mass or AVM
   e) Aortic dissection suspected
   f) Active internal bleeding
   g) Uncontrolled hypertension > 185/110
   h) Major surgery < 14 days
   i) Thrombocytopenia < 100,000
   j) Pregnancy
   k) Current anticoagulant therapy
2746) What is the target blood pressure that is needed to give TPA in a stroke patient?
   a) < 180/110 mmHg
2747) What is the onset of stroke symptoms window for TPA administration?
   a) < 3-4.5 hours
2748) Is it typical to see an elevated blood pressure in an ischemic stroke?
   a) Yes
2749) Why is it not recommended to decrease the blood pressure in an ischemic stroke if the BP is less than 220/110 mmHg in patients who do not meet criteria for TPA treatment?
   a) Due to worsening ischemia
2750) At what blood pressure range is control of the blood pressure recommended in an ischemic stroke for patients that do not meet criteria for TPA treatment?

a) > 220/110 mmHg

2751) What is the target systolic blood pressure to prevent increased bleeding in a hemorrhagic stroke?
a) < 140 mmHg

2752) What medications can be given to lower blood pressure to target goals for ischemic and hemorrhagic strokes?
a) Nicardipine, Labetalol, and Nitroprusside

2753) What products can be given to reverse anticoagulants in a patient with a hemorrhagic stroke?
a) Prothrombin complex concentrate (PCC), Fresh frozen plasma (FFP), or Cryoprecipitate

2754) List factors that increase mortality and lead to worse prognosis with an acute stroke.
a) Hyperglycemia, Fever, Hypoxia, and Hypotension

2755) What stroke mimic is caused predominantly by malignant hypertension and is characterized by headache, confusion, seizures, and visual loss that improve with blood pressure control?
a) Posterior reversible encephalopathy syndrome (PRES)

2756) What neurologic condition presents with severe posterior headaches in patients on birth control or who are pregnant, and has an empty delta sign on head CT?
a) Cerebral venous thrombosis

2757) What is the treatment for a cerebral venous thrombosis?
a) Heparin and Neurology consult

2758) What vascular emergency presents with sudden onset neck pain, aphasia, paralysis, ptosis, and miosis in a patient with Marfan's syndrome?
a) Carotid/Vertebral artery dissection

2759) What imaging study is required to diagnose a carotid or vertebral artery dissection?
a) MRA or CT angiography

2760) What autoimmune demyelination neurologic condition is seen after a viral infection, and has pathognomonic areflexia and ascending weakness?
a) Guillain-Barré syndrome

2761) What life-threatening condition can occur with a severe untreated Guillain-Barre attack and is defined by an inspiratory force < 30 and FVC < 20 mL/kg?
a) Respiratory failure

2762) What are the treats used for Guillain-Barre disease?
a) Plasmapheresis or IV Immunoglobulin

2763) What is the finding on CSF labs in a patient with Guillain-Barre'?
a) Increased protein

2764) What neurological disorder presents more commonly in females in their 30's and causes multiple episodes of intermittent weakness, numbness and double vision that can be permanent or resolve with time?
a) Multiple sclerosis (MS)

2765) What is the pathognomonic finding on the ocular physical exam with MS?
a) Bilateral internuclear ophthalmoplegia

2766) What are the lab findings on CSF with MS?
a) Increased proteins and Oligoclonal bands

2767) What are the treatments used for a MS flare?
a) Steroids, Interferon, or ACTH

2768) What imaging studies are used to help diagnose MS?
a) MRI Brain and Spine

2769) What autoimmune neurologic muscle condition is caused by antibodies against acetylcholine receptors and presents with ptosis, diplopia, and proximal limb weakness with repetitive use?
a) Myasthenia Gravis (MG)

2770) List the precipitants of MG.
a) Infections, Dehydration, Fever, and Stress

2771) What tumor is related to MG?
a) Thymoma

2772) What test is used to diagnose MG?
a) Tensilon (Edrophonium) test

2773) What is the side effect that can occur with Edrophonium administration and can be prevented with atropine administration first?
a) AV block

2774) Give the different treatment options for a MG flare.
   a) Physostigmine, Neostigmine, Steroids (mild to moderate), and Plasmapheresis (severe)
2775) What neurological condition similar to MG is due to antibodies against the calcium channels preventing the release of acetylcholine from axons leading to proximal weakness?
   a) Lambert-Eaton syndrome
2776) What is the recommended treatment for Lambert-Eaton?
   a) Plasmapheresis
2777) What mosquito-borne illness can lead to flaccid paralysis and has CSF findings of increased protein and antibodies?
   a) West Nile virus
2778) What medical condition presents as a stroke with unilateral upper and lower facial weakness, inability to close the eyelid and is usually seen after a viral infection?
   a) Bell's palsy
2779) How do you tell the difference between Bell's palsy facial paralysis and facial paralysis from a stroke?
   a) Bell's involves both upper and lower cranial nerve 7 whereas CVA facial weakness is in the lower face only
2780) What congenital brain condition can lead to chronic headaches and increased intracranial pressure from non-communicating hydrocephalus?
   a) Arnold-Chiari malformation
2781) What pain medication, when given to patients with a seizure history increases the seizure potential?
   a) Tramadol
2782) What type of dementia typically presents in patients > 70 years old and is due to protein deposits in the brain causing symptoms to wax and wane with visual hallucinations and REM disturbance?
   a) Lewy body dementia
2783) What type of dementia can occur in a patient less than 65 years old and leads to disinhibited action and yelling out?
   a) Frontotemporal dementia
2784) What life-threatening complication of Parkinson's disease has a clinical picture similar to neuroleptic malignant syndrome and

causes severe akinesis, dysphagia, hyperthermia, dysautonomia, and +/- increased CK levels?

    a)   Akinetic crisis in Parkinson's disease

2785)   List the common indications for a brain CT before performing a LP.

    a)   Altered mental status, Focal neurologic deficits, Seizures, Papilledema, Age > 60, Immunodeficiency, and Suspicion for a SAH

2786)   What spinal emergency condition follows a recent viral infection and presents with back pain that radiates around to the front of the body in a dermatomal pattern?

    a)   Transverse myelitis

2787)   What treatments are available for transverse myelitis?

    a)   IV Steroids, Neurology consult, and +/- Plasmapheresis

Obstetrics and Gynecology

2788)   List the vital sign changes that occur with pregnancy.
   a)   Elevated Heart rate 15-20 bpm, Decreased systolic BP 5-10 mmHg and decreased diastolic BP 10-15 mmHg, and Increased respiratory rate

2789)   List the physiological changes seen in pregnancy.
   a)   Increased cardiac output, Cardiac murmur, Increase tidal volume and minute ventilation, Decreased gastric motility, and Increased renal filtration

2790)   What basal metabolic change occurs indicating ovulation?
   a)   Increased basal temperature

2791)   What vascular structure is compressed in late-term obstetric patients > 20 weeks when lying flat?
   a)   Vena cava

2792)   What position is recommended for late-term obstetric patients when lying flat?
   a)   Left lateral decubitus (30 degrees)

2793)   What is the anatomic location of the uterine fundus at 12 weeks?
   a)   Pubic symphysis

2794)   What is the anatomic location of the uterine fundus at 20 weeks?
   a)   Umbilicus

2795)   At what β-hCG level can pregnancy be seen on a transvaginal (pelvic) ultrasound?
   a)   1,500-2,000

2796)   At what β-hCG level can pregnancy be seen on a transabdominal ultrasound?
   a)   5,000-6,000

2797)   At what range of β-hCG does the appearance of the fetal pole occur on transvaginal US?
   a)   10,000-20,000

2798)   Over what time period is the β-hCG supposed to double in pregnancy?
   a)   Every 48 hours

2799) Give a list of the drugs to avoid in pregnancy.
  a) Sulfas, Fluoroquinolones, Tetracycline's, Amiodarone, Antipsychotic medications, ACE inhibitors, NSAIDs, and Seizure mediations
2800) What is a major side effect of Amiodarone if given in pregnancy?
  a) Fetal neurotoxicity
2801) Are the insulin requirements in pregnancy increased or decreased when treating diabetes?
  a) Increased
2802) Exposure to how many rads of radiation is teratogenicity associated with during pregnancy?
  a) > 10 rads
2803) What diagnosis should be suspected with unilateral pelvic pain, cramping, vaginal bleeding, and a positive pregnancy test?
  a) Ectopic pregnancy
2804) What is the most common location for implantation of an ectopic pregnancy in the fallopian tubes?
  a) Ampulla
2805) What is the most deadly site of the insertion of an ectopic pregnancy?
  a) Cornual
2806) List the risk factors for ectopic pregnancy.
  a) PID, IUD, Tubal sterilizations, Older age, Infertility treatment, Previous ectopic, and Race.
2807) What is the number one risk factor for ectopic pregnancy?
  a) Previous ectopic pregnancy
2808) What is the study of choice for diagnosing an ectopic pregnancy?
  a) Ultrasound
2809) What is the pathognomonic US Doppler finding seen with an ectopic when looking at an adnexal mass that shows an increased vascularity?
  a) Ring of fire
2810) What are the US findings that suggest an ectopic pregnancy?
  a) Extrauterine gestational sac and yolk sac, Free pelvic fluid with a mass, Tubal ring, Ring of fire, and Hepatorenal free fluid

2811) What is the most common cause of an empty uterus with a + β-hCG?
   a) Ectopic pregnancy
2812) What intrauterine structure (in the setting of an ectopic pregnancy) can be seen on an obstetric US and give a false-positive finding of an IUP?
   a) Pseudogestational sac
2813) Give the criteria followed for methotrexate drug treatment of ectopic pregnancies.
   a) Unruptured ectopic < 4 cm, No fetal heart tones, and β-hCG < 5000 (due to higher failure rate)
2814) What complication can fertility drug-assisted pregnancy lead to?
   a) Heterotopic pregnancy (IUP & ectopic)
2815) Does the level of the β-hCG determine whether you can perform an US to rule out an ectopic if it is suspected?
   a) No (ectopic may be present even under 1,000)
2816) What is the treatment plan for a patient with an indeterminate or low β-hCG and abdominal pain?
   a) Repeat β-hCG in 48 hours, OB consult, +/- US if high suspicion
2817) What is the risk of pregnancy after tubal ligation?
   a) 1-2:1000
2818) List the five different types of miscarriage.
   a) Threatened, Inevitable, Incomplete, Complete and Missed
2819) What are the findings with a threatened miscarriage?
   a) Bleeding with a normal exam and Closed cervical OS
2820) What are the findings with an inevitable miscarriage?
   a) Excessive bleeding and Dilated cervical OS
2821) What are the findings with an incomplete miscarriage?
   a) Bleeding with partial expelled fetal parts and Open cervical OS
2822) What are the findings with a complete miscarriage?
   a) Bleeding with complete expulsion of fetal parts, Closed cervical OS, and Empty uterus on ultrasound
2823) What are the findings with a missed miscarriage?
   a) Intrauterine fetal death with a normal exam
2824) What medication is given in an Rh-negative pregnant patient > 12 weeks with vaginal bleeding?

a) 300 mcg Rhogam (Rho D immunoglobulin)

2825) What is the Rhogam dose for a pregnant patient < 12 weeks?
   a) 50 mcg

2826) What is the blood test used to measure the amount of fetal Hb transferred from a fetus to a mother's bloodstream with bleeding?
   a) Kleihauer-Betke test

2827) What test differentiates maternal hemoglobin from fetal hemoglobin?
   a) Alkali denaturation test (APT)

2828) What complication can be seen from an infection of fetal parts or the endometrium following a miscarriage and present with a fever, vomiting, and purulent discharge?
   a) Septic abortion

2829) What is the treatment for a septic abortion?
   a) Dilation and Curettage, and Antibiotics (Gentamycin + Ampicillin)

2830) What uterine complication can occur entering the second trimester, presents with severe rectal pressure, cervical prolapse, and urinary obstruction?
   a) Uterine incarceration

2831) What is the term given for excessive vomiting in pregnancy?
   a) Hyperemesis gravidarum

2832) What is the typical length of morning sickness?
   a) 13 weeks or First trimester

2833) List the antiemetic's used in pregnancy.
   a) Doxylamine, Pyridoxine, Metoclopramide, Prochlorperazine, and Zofran

2834) What is the best ED treatment for abdominal cramping during pregnancy?
   a) IV Hydration

2835) What is the hypertensive emergency seen in pregnant patients > 20 weeks, with blood pressures > 140/90, headache, edema, and proteinuria?
   a) Preeclampsia

2836) What is the blood pressure criteria for severe preeclampsia?
   a) > 160/110 mmHg

2837)   What hypertensive emergency in pregnant patients > 20 weeks is seen with preeclampsia plus a seizure?
   a)   Eclampsia
2838)   What antihypertensive medications are used to treat preeclampsia and eclampsia?
   a)   Labetalol, Hydralazine, and Sodium Nitroprusside
2839)   What is the treatment for seizures in eclampsia?
   a)   IV Magnesium (4-6 grams)
2840)   What are the signs of magnesium toxicity?
   a)   Loss of deep tendon reflexes, Decreased respiratory rate, Decreased blood pressure, and Decreased fetal heart tones
2841)   What other medications can be used for seizures with eclampsia after magnesium administration?
   a)   Benzodiazepines and Phenobarbital
2842)   What syndrome consists of hemolysis, elevated liver enzymes, and low platelets and is associated with preeclampsia?
   a)   HELLP syndrome
2843)   What placental complication is defined by painless bright vaginal bleeding and placental insertion over the cervix?
   a)   Placenta previa
2844)   Is it recommended to do a vaginal exam with placenta previa?
   a)   No
2845)   What placental emergency is seen with painful bright vaginal bleeding and is a separation of the placenta from the uterus?
   a)   Abruptio placenta
2846)   List the risk factors that can lead to an abruptio placenta.
   a)   Cocaine use, Trauma, Gestational hypertension, and Smoking
2847)   What pregnancy complication can occur spontaneously or with trauma and present with sudden severe abdominal pain, vaginal bleeding, and uterine tenderness with irregular contour?
   a)   Uterine rupture
2848)   What obstetric disease is caused by a hydatidiform mole and presents with severe hyperemesis gravidarum, with preeclampsia symptoms < 20 weeks and can lead to cancer?
   a)   Gestational trophoblastic disease (GTD)

2849) What lab finding should raise your suspicion of a molar pregnancy?

    a) Abnormally elevated β-hCG for gestational age

2850) Give the two types of a hydatidiform (molar) pregnancy.

    a) Complete and Partial molar pregnancy

2851) What type of uterine cancer does GTD increase the risk for?

    a) Choriocarcinoma

2852) What is the pathognomonic ultrasound finding seen with GTD?

    a) Grapelike appearance / Snowstorm pattern

2853) Is it recommended to treat bacteria found on urinalysis without symptoms in a pregnant patient?

    a) Yes (asymptomatic bacteria)

2854) What is the most common bacterial infection in pregnancy?

    a) UTI

2855) List the safe antibiotics used for UTI and pyelonephritis in OB patients.

    a) Cephalosporins, Nitrofurantoin (not in 1st trimester), Penicillins, Macrolides, and Clindamycin

2856) Is it recommended to admit OB patient >24 weeks for IV antibiotics with pyelonephritis?

    a) Yes (due to preterm labor risks)

2857) What abdominal pathology is the most common cause of surgery in pregnancy?

    a) Appendicitis

2858) What is the 1st recommended imaging modality to diagnose appendicitis in a pregnant patient?

    a) Ultrasound

2859) What are the indications for a postmortem C-section after trauma?

    a) Gestational age > 28 weeks and Fetal heart tones on the US

2860) What is the time frame to do a postmortem C-section after maternal death?

    a) Within 5 minutes of maternal death

2861) What is the technique used for a postmortem C-section versus a normal planned C-section?

    a) Vertical incision above the umbilicus

2862) If conservative antibiotic treatment for cholecystitis fails, in what trimester is a cholecystectomy recommended?
   a) Second trimester
2863) Does pregnancy increase the risk of blood clots?
   a) Yes
2864) What trimester is the risk for pulmonary emboli (PE) highest during pregnancy?
   a) During 1st trimester
2865) What types of imaging are used to rule out a PE in pregnancy?
   a) CT chest with contrast or Ventilation-perfusion scan (VQ)
2866) What imaging modality is preferred to rule out PE during pregnancy to decrease radiation risk?
   a) V/Q scan
2867) What blood-thinning medication is recommended for DVT or PE treatment in OB patients?
   a) Enoxaparin
2868) What is the most common cause of nonsurgical maternal death during pregnancy?
   a) PE
2869) Is it recommended to use a D-Dimer to rule out blood clots in a pregnant patient?
   a) No due to false positives
2870) What imaging study is suggested to be performed before considering a CT chest or VQ scan in a pregnant patient being worked up for PE?
   a) Venous Doppler to rule DVT
2871) What type of uterine contractions occur irregularly, have no cervical changes, and are deemed to be false contractions?
   a) Braxton-Hicks
2872) What week gestation is considered full term?
   a) > 37 weeks
2873) What obstetric complication is the leading cause of neonatal death?
   a) Preterm labor
2874) List the risk factors for preterm labor.

    a)   Premature rupture of membranes, Urinary infections, Vaginal infections, and Cervical incompetence

2875)   What criteria determines preterm labor?

    a)   Ruptured membranes, Cervical dilation or progression, < 37 weeks

2876)   What is the treatment of preterm labor?

    a)   Give Magnesium and beta-agonists to arrest labor, and OB consult

2877)   What tests are used to determine ruptured membranes?

    a)   Nitrazine paper and Ferning on microscopy

2878)   What two maneuvers can be used to help with the delivery of shoulder dystocia?

    a)   McRobert's, Rubin's, Woods corkscrew, Delivery of the posterior arm, or Intentional clavicle fracture

2879)   Give the body position of McRobert's maneuver.

    a)   Hyperflexion of maternal legs with abduction while supine

2880)   Describe the procedure of the Wood corkscrew?

    a)   Apply pressure to the anterior part of posterior shoulder with a 180-degree counterclockwise rotation

2881)   Why is it necessary to palpate the infant neck after delivery of the head?

    a)   To check for a nuchal cord

2882)   What is the treatment for cord prolapse with delivery?

    a)   Elevate the cord and Slow delivery

2883)   What is the treatment for a nuchal cord present during delivery?

    a)   Reduce or clamp and cut the cord

2884)   What is the most common cause of postpartum hemorrhage?

    a)   Uterine atony

2885)   What volume of blood loss in the first 24 hours after a vaginal delivery meets the criteria for postpartum hemorrhage?

    a)   > 500 ml

2886)   What volume of blood loss in the first 24 hours after a C-section birth meets the criteria for postpartum hemorrhage?

    a)   > 1000 ml

2887)   What are the treatments used for postpartum hemorrhage?

a) Uterine massage + Oxytocin or Methylergometrine

2888) What uterine complication presents with symptoms of foul-smelling lochia, fever, and abdominal pain and commonly occurs after C-section or a D&C?

a) Endometritis

2889) What is the treatment for endometritis?

a) Broad-spectrum antibiotics

2890) What complication can develop post vaginal delivery and presents with a fever, tachycardia, and unilateral pelvic pain and is treated with heparin and antibiotics?

a) Septic pelvic thrombophlebitis

2891) What breast infection occurs in breastfeeding moms complaining of hot, red, tender, and swollen breasts?

a) Mastitis

2892) What is the treatment of mastitis?

a) Continue breastfeeding and Antibiotics (Penicillin)

2893) What location of the vagina is an episiotomy made if needed?

a) Posterior lateral

2894) What obstetric complication involving amniotic fluid in the 2nd-3rd trimester can lead to anaphylaxis, dyspnea, cardiovascular collapse, and mortality?

a) Amniotic fluid embolism

2895) What disease occurs from the extension of an untreated STD into the abdomen leading to fever and RUQ pain?

a) Pelvic inflammatory disease (PID)

2896) What vaginal exam finding suggests the diagnosis of PID?

a) Cervical motion tenderness (Chandelier's sign)

2897) What syndrome develops with PID involving perihepatic inflammation of the liver?

a) Fitz-Hugh-Curtis syndrome

2898) What is the outpatient treatment for PID?

a) 250mg IM Ceftriaxone and Doxycycline 14 days PO

2899) What do you do with an IUD in a patient with PID?

a) Remove it

2900) List the admission criteria for PID.

a) Pregnancy, Sepsis, Failed outpatient treatments, Peritoneal signs, HIV, Uncontrolled pain, or a Tubal ovarian abscess

2901) List the medication regimens used for the inpatient treatment of PID.
a) Cefoxitin plus Doxycycline
b) Clindamycin plus Gentamycin
c) Ampicillin-Sulbactam plus Doxycycline

2902) What complication of PID presents with unilateral pelvic pain, adnexal mass on vaginal exam, fever, and an elevated WBC?
a) Tubo-ovarian abscess

2903) What imaging modalities are used to diagnose a tubo-ovarian abscess from an untreated STD?
a) Ultrasound

2904) What bacteria causes thin white vaginal discharge, a PH > 4.5, a fishy odor, and is the most common cause of vulvovaginitis?
a) Gardnerella (bacterial vaginosis or BV)

2905) What are the 4 Amsel criteria to diagnose BV?
a) pH > 4.5, Fish odor, > 20% clue cells, and Thin discharge

2906) What are the findings on the wet mount exam for bacterial vaginosis?
a) Clue cells

2907) What is the treatment for bacterial vaginosis?
a) Metronidazole (500 mg BID x 7 days) or Clindamycin (oral or cream)

2908) What is the treatment of BV during pregnancy?
a) Clindamycin (intravaginal cream or oral), Metronidazole vaginal cream, or Metronidazole (250 or 500 mg BID x 7 days)

2909) What is the recommended route of administration for Clindamycin and Metronidazole for the treatment of BV in pregnancy?
a) Intravaginal cream

2910) What vaginal infection causes thick white cottage cheese discharge vaginal itching, with a normal pH?
a) Candidal vaginitis (yeast infection)

2911) What is the finding for a yeast infection on the wet mount exam?

a) Pseudohyphae

2912) What is the treatment for candida vaginitis?

a) Fluconazole 150 mg 1x

2913) What is the treatment for candida vaginitis in a pregnant female?

a) Intravaginal (topical) Clotrimazole

2914) What is the treatment for a Bartholin gland abscess?

a) I &D with the placement of a Word catheter

2915) What type of ovarian cyst occurs in the first 2 weeks of the menstrual cycle and can cause sudden severe unilateral pelvic pain with rupture?

a) Follicular cyst

2916) What type of ovarian cyst can be complex or simple and cause resting pain and pain with sudden rupture leading to free fluid in the pelvis on the US?

a) Corpus luteal cyst

2917) What type of ovarian cyst is loculated, asymmetric in shape, and has septations that require further workup and evaluation by OB due to an increased risk of malignancy?

a) Complex cyst

2918) What size of ovarian cyst increases the risk of developing an ovarian torsion and may need surgical removal?

a) Cysts > 5 cm

2919) What is the term for mid menstrual cycle pain with light vaginal spotting?

a) Mittelschmerz

2920) What medication can be used for mittelschmerz?

a) NSAIDs

2921) What is the term for crampy abdominal pain with menstrual cycles?

a) Dysmenorrhea

2922) What is the first and second-line treatment for dysmenorrhea?

a) 1st line: NSAIDs

b) 2nd line: Oral contraceptives

2923) What is the average time frame between menstrual cycles?

a) 21-35 days

2924) What condition is the most common cause of prepubertal vaginal bleeding?
  a) Non-specific vulvovaginitis
2925) What type of abnormal vaginal bleeding in a non-pregnant female is defined as prolonged amenorrhea with intermittent vaginal bleeding?
  a) Dysfunctional uterine bleeding (DUB)
2926) What is the most common cause of dysfunctional uterine bleeding?
  a) Anovulation
2927) What medication can be given in severe DUB?
  a) IV Estrogen
2928) What is the outpatient treatment for DUB?
  a) Oral contraceptives
2929) How much blood loss during menses qualifies for abnormal bleeding and menorrhagia?
  a) > 70 mL
2930) What are the top three causes of post-menopausal bleeding?
  a) 1st: Atrophy
  b) 2nd: Cancer
  c) 3rd: Endometrial hyperplasia
2931) What is the most common cause of postmenopausal bleeding?
  a) Atrophic vaginitis
2932) What is the workup for post-menopausal bleeding?
  a) US, OB referral, Endometrial biopsy, and then Hysterectomy
2933) What is the treatment of lichen sclerosis?
  a) Topical steroids (Clobetasol)
2934) What ovarian emergency is due to a lack of blood flow, and presents with sudden severe unilateral pain and rebound tenderness in a patient with history of ovarian cysts?
  a) Ovarian torsion
2935) What is the imaging modality of choice to rule out ovarian torsion?
  a) Transvaginal Doppler ultrasound
2936) What is the treatment for ovarian torsion?
  a) OB consult with surgical reduction < 6 hours

2937) What gynecological disease causes pelvic pain associated with menses, hypermenorrhea, and chocolate cysts?
a) Endometriosis

2938) How is endometriosis diagnosed?
a) Laparoscopy

2939) List the treatments for endometriosis.
a) NSAIDs, Birth control, +/- Surgery

2940) What are the most common benign tumors of the uterus?
a) Leiomyomas

2941) What is the most common gynecologic cancer?
a) Adenocarcinoma of the uterus

2942) What diagnosis needs to be considered with postmenopausal painless vaginal bleeding?
a) Uterine cancer

2943) What type of gynecological cancer is seen with abdominal bloating, pain, ascites, and a unilateral mass on the pelvic exam?
a) Ovarian cancer

2944) What is the most common virus that leads to cervical cancer?
a) Human papillomavirus

2945) What is the most common type of cervical cancer?
a) Squamous cell (from HPV 16,18 & 21)

2946) What gynecological syndrome from excess gonadotropin release, leads to bloating, ascites, nausea, and weight gain?
a) Ovarian hyperstimulation syndrome

2947) What gynecological conditions can lead to increased testosterone levels in females?
a) PCOS, Hyperthecosis, and Sertoli-Leydig ovarian cell tumors

2948) Name the three types of uterine fibroids based on the growth in the uterus that can cause heavy painless vaginal bleeding.
a) Intramural, Submucosal, and Subserosal

2949) What complication can occur 2-10 days post embolization of uterine fibroids and presents with fever, nausea, pelvic pain, and leukocytosis?
a) Post embolization syndrome

2950) What complication from a hysterectomy develops 10-14 days post-op, and presents with watery vaginal discharge?
a) Vesicovaginal fistula

2951) What is the antibiotic treatment for cuff cellulitis post hysterectomy?
   a) Ampicillin + Gentamycin + Clindamycin
2952) What bacteria is the most common cause of infection with a retained foreign body in the vagina?
   a) E. coli
2953) What are the effects of hormone replacement therapy on cholesterol levels?
   a) ↑ HDL and ↓ LDL
2954) List the risk factors for developing osteoporosis.
   a) Steroid use, Caucasian, BMI < 18.5, and Smoking
2955) What are the treatment options for osteoporosis?
   a) Calcium and Bisphosphonates
2956) What is the definition of active labor?
   a) 3-5 contractions per 10 mins, or as frequent as every 2-5 min
2957) What type of deceleration during labor is a symmetric fall in the fetal heart rate beginning at or after the peak of the uterine contraction that returns back to baseline after the contraction has ended?
   a) Late deceleration
2958) What type of deceleration during labor is caused by fetal head compression during uterine contraction and causes slowing of the fetal heart rate that begins at the onset of contraction and returns with the end of the contraction?
   a) Early deceleration
2959) What is the average fetal heart rate during pregnancy?
   a) 120-160
2960) Are variable decelerations considered concerning for fetal distress?
   a) No
2961) How do you tell the difference between variable early decelerations and early decelerations with contractions?
   a) Early deceleration from contractions are > 30 secs
2962) What is the main cause of late deceleration during labor?
   a) Uteroplacental insufficiency
2963) What are the treatment options for late decelerations during labor?
   a) Turn the mother onto her left side, Stop Pitocin, Start Oxygen, Fluid bolus, +/- Terbutaline (for increased contractions)

Psychiatry

2964) What behavior disorder causes a gradual disturbance in cognition, impaired memory, and has a normal level of consciousness?
   a) Dementia
2965) What behavioral disorder causes an acute global impairment in cognitive functioning with fluctuating symptoms of inattention and hallucinations?
   a) Delirium
2966) List the causes of delirium.
   a) Infection, Electrolyte abnormalities, Toxins, Hypercapnia, and Head injuries
2967) What type of psychiatric disorder has a gradual onset, with clear sensorium, and can have associated auditory hallucinations?
   a) Functional disorders
2968) What type of psychiatric disorder is from a medical pathology and is typically acute in onset with disorientation and visual hallucinations?
   a) Organic disorders
2969) What disorder is an impairment of memory, or loss of memory, that is brief, long term, or global in nature, and is due to a thiamine deficiency or brain trauma?
   a) Amnesia
2970) What type of amnesia causes an inability to form new memories and typically resolves within 24 hours with a good prognosis?
   a) Transient global amnesia
2971) What dissociative disorder is from a loss of memory and assumption of a new identity when traveling?
   a) Dissociative fugue
2972) What psychiatric disorder causes an acute or chronic disturbed perception of reality with delusion, hallucinations, and disorganized speech?
   a) Psychosis
2973) List the positive symptoms with schizophrenia.

a) Auditory hallucinations, Delusions, Disorganized speech, or Catatonic behavior

2974) List the negative symptoms with schizophrenia.
a) Blunted affect, Emotional withdrawal, Anhedonia, and Impaired attention

2975) What is the length of time symptoms must be present to diagnose schizophrenia?
a) > 6 months

2976) What behavior has muscle rigidity, mutism, and grimacing with schizophrenia?
a) Catatonia

2977) What type of schizophrenic disorder has symptoms < 6 months?
a) Schizophreniform

2978) What type of schizophrenic disorder has symptoms < 4 weeks?
a) Brief psychotic disorder

2979) What type of personality disorder associated with schizophrenia has symptoms of voluntary social withdrawal?
a) Schizoid personality disorder

2980) What type of personality disorder associated with schizophrenia has odd eccentric magical thinking?
a) Schizotypal personality disorder

2981) What condition is associated with psychosis with non-bizarre delusions?
a) Delusional disorder

2982) Which personality disorder has a history of conduct issues, impulsive behavior, and disrespecting others?
a) Antisocial

2983) Which personality disorder is seen in emotionally unstable patients, that have multiple relationships, splitting behavior, and are frequently suicidal?
a) Borderline

2984) Which personality disorder has emotional dramatic attention seeking and seductive behavior?
a) Histrionic

2985) Which personality disorder has an exaggerated sense of self-importance and abilities and unrealistic ambitions?

a) Narcissistic

2986) What personality disorder is characterized by an obsession with repetitive acts and ritualistic behavior to relieve anxiety?

a) Obsessive-compulsive

2987) What type of personality disorder do the patients rely on others, and are typically in abusive relationships?

a) Dependent

2988) In what condition do patients have a distorted self-body image, poor oral intake, weight loss, and amenorrhea > 3 months?

a) Anorexia nervosa

2989) List the symptoms seen with anorexia nervosa.

a) Orthostatic hypotension, Bradycardia, Hypothermia, Dry brittle hair, and Downy body hair.

2990) What psychiatric condition is associated with binging and purging cycles after eating, and have body weights that can be normal?

a) Bulimia nervosa

2991) What physical exam findings suggest anorexia or bulimia?

a) Dental enamel erosion and Pharyngeal abrasions or calluses over the dorsal aspect of the fingers

2992) List the criteria for admitting eating disorder patients.

a) Bradycardia, Hypotensive, < 75% ideal body weight, Suicidal, or Electrolyte disturbances.

2993) What methods can be used for the agitated patient?

a) Verbal de-escalation, Comforting items, Quiet room, and Physical restraints

2994) List common medications used for the agitated patient in the ED.

a) Antipsychotics, Benadryl, and Benzodiazepines

2995) What mood disorder is a loss of interest, with feelings of worthlessness, hopelessness, loss of appetite, fatigue, and sleep disturbances all lasting > 2 weeks?

a) Major depression

2996) Is it recommended to start an antidepressant in the ED?

a) No (increased risk of suicide)

2997) What mood disorder has recurrent cyclic episodes of mania and depression, grandiose ideas, racing thoughts, insomnia, and pressured speech?
   a) Bipolar disorder
2998) What type of bipolar disorder involves mania?
   a) Bipolar type 1
2999) What mood disorder has chronic fluctuating low-grade depression lasting 2 years or more?
   a) Dysthymic disorder
3000) What length of time of anxiety symptoms is used to diagnose generalized anxiety disorder?
   a) > 6 months
3001) What anxiety disorder presents with chest pain, nausea, hyperventilation, and paresthesias from recurrent episodes of fear?
   a) Panic attack
3002) What anxiety disorder is from a past traumatic event and leads to a severe anxiety reaction to repetitive psychosocial stressors that they perceive as life threatening?
   a) Post-traumatic stress disorder (PTSD)
3003) What anxiety disorder is from unfounded fears of specific objects or things that arouse a state of panic?
   a) Phobias
3004) What medication class is used to treat anxiety disorders?
   a) Benzodiazepines (i.e. Alprazolam or Lorazepam)
3005) What psychiatric disorder has unexplained physical symptoms consisting of 2 GI symptoms, 1 sexual symptom, and 1 neurologic symptom?
   a) Somatization disorder
3006) In what somatoform disorder does a patient unconsciously and voluntarily produce symptoms of a physical disorder that leads to a loss of physical functioning as a response to a stressor?
   a) Conversion disorder (Functional neurological symptom disorder)
3007) What is the term used for individuals who are preoccupied with the fear of a serious illness and frequent the ED?
   a) Hypochondriasis

3008) Are you as a physician able to hold a suicidal or homicidal patient against their will?
   a) Yes (by state authority)
3009) Who can write a pink slip for suicidal or homicidal patients?
   a) Law officer, Licensed practitioner, Health officer, or Psychologist
3010) What is the term for a patient who voluntary simulates a disease with exaggerated symptoms, is motivated by external incentives, and often have a coinciding antisocial personality disorder?
   a) Malingering
3011) What is the main difference between malingering and conversion disorder?
   a) Malingering is voluntary
3012) What do you have to be suspicious of in a drug-seeking patient with hematuria complaining of flank pain, who refuses to have an abdominal CT scan?
   a) Fictitious hematuria
3013) What psychiatric condition is a voluntary fabrication of disease symptoms to gain medical attention and are willing to undergo procedures and admissions?
   a) Munchausen syndrome
3014) What is the term used when a parent induces a medical complaint in their child to seek attention?
   a) Munchausen by proxy
3015) List the side effects that occur with antipsychotic medications.
   a) Extrapyramidal symptoms, Anticholinergic, QT prolongation, Neuroleptic malignant syndrome, and Hypotension
3016) List the different antipsychotic medications that cause extrapyramidal effects.
   a) Aripiprazole, Clozapine, Olanzapine, Quetiapine, Risperidone, Lurasidone, and Ziprasidone
3017) What medication side effect is caused by dopamine antagonism from antipsychotic medications and causes acute muscle spasms?
   a) Dystonic reaction
3018) What is the treatment for dystonia?

a) Diphenhydramine or Benztropine, and Stop the inciting drug

3019) What medication side effect from antipsychotic medications causes facial muscle twitching and can be permanent?

a) Tardive dyskinesia

3020) What extrapyramidal side effect from neuroleptics is defined by motor restlessness involving the legs?

a) Akathisia

3021) What extrapyramidal side effect from neuroleptics, is defined by a triad of tremor, muscular rigidity, and loss of the power of movement (akinesia)?

a) Parkinsonism or Pseudoparkinsonism

3022) What antipsychotic medication side effect manifests with fever, encephalopathy, muscle rigidity, unstable vitals, and a ↑CPK level?

a) Neuroleptic malignant syndrome (NMS)

3023) What are the medications used to treat NMS?

a) Dantrolene or Bromocriptine

3024) What medication classes are used to treat depression?

a) Selective serotonin reuptake inhibitors (SSRI), Tricyclic antidepressants (TCA), and Monoamine oxidase inhibitors (MAOI)

3025) What syndrome can occur from a SSRI overdose that presents with acute onset of confusion, muscle rigidity, fever, tachycardia, diaphoresis, and hyperreflexia?

a) Serotonin syndrome

3026) What drugs combined with SSRI's can lead to serotonin syndrome?

a) MAOI, Sympathomimetics, Tramadol, St. John's Wort, and Lithium

3027) What is the treatment of serotonin syndrome?

a) Cyproheptadine and Stop the inciting drug

3028) What physical exam finding is pathognomonic for serotonin syndrome?

a) Clonus

3029) What type of reaction presents with agitation, diaphoresis, tachycardia and AMS, and occurs in patients on MAOIs who ingest certain wines or cheeses containing tyramine?

a) MAOI reaction

3030) Linezolid + Pseudoephedrine or an MAOI can lead to what type of reaction?

a) MAOI reaction

3031) List the complications of a MAOI's toxicity.

a) Intracranial hemorrhage, Hypertensive urgency, Myocardial infarction, and Serotonin syndrome

3032) What antihypertensive medication should be avoided when treating a catecholamine hypertensive crisis due to a MAOI toxicity?

a) Beta-blockers (due to unopposed alpha activity)

3033) Alcohol metabolized at a constant rate of 15-20mg/dL/hr is described by what type of drug elimination?

a) Zero-order kinetics

3034) List the high-risk factors for suicide completion.

a) Single

b) Drug abuse

c) Alcoholic

d) Unemployed

e) Previous attempts

f) Mental disorder

g) Access to weapons

h) Chronic disease

3035) Which psychiatric condition has hyper-energetic patients with inattention to detail, and is seen in adults and children?

a) Attention deficit hyperactivity disorder (ADHD)

3036) What is it called when someone has uncontrolled random bouts of vocal or motor tics?

a) Tourette syndrome

3037) What is the condition called when a patient continuously ingests non-nutritional substances like ice and dirt due to the lack of iron intake?

a) PICA

3038) What substance withdrawal can lead to sudden death and causes agitation, anxiety, tremors, psychosis, seizures, and tachycardia?

a) Alcohol withdrawal

3039) At what time range does the risk of delirium tremens increase with alcohol withdrawal?
   a) > 48 hours
3040) What medications are used to treat alcohol withdrawal?
   a) Benzodiazepines
3041) What are the most common vitamin deficiencies seen with chronic alcohol abuse?
   a) Thiamine (B1), Folic acid, and Vitamin B12
3042) What is the most common electrolyte deficiency seen in alcohol abuse and can lead to torsades?
   a) Magnesium
3043) What guidelines are used to treat alcohol withdrawal?
   a) The Clinical Institute Withdrawal Assessment for Alcohol-Revised (CIWA)
3044) What medical condition from chronic alcohol abuse has a CN 6 palsy, nystagmus, confusion, ataxia, amnesia, and confabulation?
   a) Wernicke Korsakoff's syndrome
3045) What drug can be used to help with alcohol abuse and can cause nausea and vomiting if alcohol is ingested with it?
   a) Antabuse (Disulfiram)
3046) What metabolic disorder can be caused by alcohol abuse, and is due to impaired gluconeogenesis?
   a) Hypoglycemia
3047) What drug withdrawal causes dilated pupils, nausea, vomiting, diarrhea, and myalgias?
   a) Opioid withdrawal
3048) What pain medication can induce opioid withdrawal in a chronic opioid user?
   a) Buprenorphine (partial agonist and antagonist)
3049) What medication is used to reverse the symptoms of an opioid overdose?
   a) Naloxone
3050) What medications can help with opioid withdrawal symptoms?
   a) Clonidine
3051) What drug withdrawal causes anxiety, insomnia, confusion, tachycardia, hypertension, and withdrawal seizures?

a) Benzodiazepine withdrawal

3052) Withdrawal from which drugs lead to depression, fatigue, loss of sleep, and increased appetite?

a) Cocaine or Methamphetamine withdrawal

3053) Can you have marijuana withdrawal?

a) Yes

3054) What addiction term for substance use, is associated with social and medical problems that result from the repetitive use of a substance?

a) Abuse

3055) What addiction term for substance use, refers to a patient that continues to require larger dosages of a substance, has cravings, and can have withdrawal symptoms?

a) Tolerance

Musculoskeletal / Orthopedics

Upper extremity

3056)　What type of distal radius fracture has volar angulation?

a)　Smith's fracture

3057)　What type of distal radius fracture has dorsal angulation?

a)　Colles' fracture

3058)　What type of splint is used to treat a stable Colles' fracture?

a)　Volar wrist splint

3059)　What type of splint is used to treat an unstable Colles' fracture?

a)　Sugar tong

3060)　What is the most common fall that causes a Colles' fracture?

a)　Fall on an outstretched hand (FOOSH)

3061)　What is a Barton's fracture?

a)　Dorsal or volar rim fracture of the distal radius

3062)　What is the most common carpal bone fracture?

a)　Scaphoid fracture

3063)　What fracture should you be concerned about with snuffbox tenderness?

a)　Scaphoid fracture

3064)　What is the most common complication of a scaphoid fracture?

a)　Avascular necrosis

3065)　What is the most common type of fall that causes a scaphoid fracture?

a)　Fall on an outstretched hand (FOOSH)

3066)　What splint is recommended for a nondisplaced scaphoid fracture?

a)　Thumb spica splint

3067)　How do you test for median nerve compression or carpal tunnel syndrome?

a) Phalen's test, Compression test, or Tinel's test

3068) What are the symptoms of carpal tunnel syndrome?

a) Pain at the wrist, Tingling, Numbness, and Weakness of the first 3 digits

3069) What are the treatment options for carpal tunnel syndrome?

a) Night splinting, Steroid injections, or Surgery

3070) What is cubital tunnel syndrome?

a) Ulnar nerve entrapment at the elbow

3071) What are the symptoms of cubital tunnel syndrome?

a) Pain at the elbow, Tingling, Numbness, and Weakness of the 4th and 5th digits

3072) What is the treatment of a subungual hematoma > 50% of the nail bed?

a) Trephination

3073) Where do most lacerations occur in a "fight bite"?

a) Over the MCP

3074) What is the most common anaerobic bacteria seen in a human bite?

a) Bacteroides

3075) What are the most common aerobes in a human bite?

a) Streptococcus and Staphylococcus

3076) What antibiotics are recommended for human bites?

a) Amoxicillin-Clavulanate or Clindamycin

3077) Which bone is fractured in a boxer's fracture?

a) Fracture of the 5th metacarpal neck

3078) What is the accepted angulation of the metacarpal head at the 4th and 5th digits in a boxer's fracture?

a) 40°

3079) What is the most sensitive test in the assessment of sensation in the hand?

a) Two-point discrimination < 6 mm

3080) What is the definitive treatment of a hand flexor laceration?

a) Orthopedic referral and Splint

3081) What ligament is torn in a Gamekeeper's thumb injury?
a) Ulnar collateral ligament

3082) What is the treatment of a Gamekeepers' thumb injury?
a) Thumb spica cast

3083) What type of abscess in the palmer aponeurosis presents with extension of the fingers, and can be caused by a splinter?
a) Collar button abscess

3084) What type of fracture is described by a fracture of the ulnar base of the thumb at the metacarpal joint, displaced by the abductor pollicis longus?
a) Bennett's fracture

3085) What type of thumb fracture is a comminuted intra-articular fracture through the base of the metacarpal?
a) Rolando fracture

3086) What is the most common location of a clavicle fracture?
a) Middle third (80%)

3087) Give the Neer classification for operative verse nonoperative treatment of clavicle fractures.
a) Nonoperative: < 100% displacement
b) Operative: > 100% displacement

3088) What are the criteria that suggest the need for surgical correction for a clavicle fracture?
a) > 2 cm displacement or shortening or > 1 cm superior displacement/100% displacement

3089) What is the ED treatment for an uncomplicated clavicle fracture?
a) Arm sling and Orthopedic follow up

3090) What is the most commonly dislocated carpal bone?
a) Lunate

3091) What carpal dislocation has X-ray findings of the lunate in line with the radius and dorsal displacement of the capitate and the rest of the carpal bones?
a) Perilunate dislocation

3092)	What is a Terry Thomas sign?
a)	A scapholunate ligament dissociation, commonly a result of a fall on the outstretched hand. A gap of more than 3mm is pathognomonic.

3093)	What type of finger injury is diagnosed by flexion of the DIP and extensor tendon avulsion?
a)	Mallet finger

3094)	What type of finger abnormality is diagnosed by hyperextension of the PIP and flexion of the DIP?
a)	Swan neck deformity

3095)	What type of finger abnormality is diagnosed by the flexion of the PIP with hyperextension of the DIP?
a)	Boutonniere deformity

3096)	What diagnosis is seen with an inflamed MCP pulley with flexor tendon swelling that catches with bending?
a)	Trigger finger

3097)	What hand complication is seen with hyperextension of the MCP with flexion of the PIP from ulnar nerve palsy?
a)	Claw hand

3098)	What nerve is involved in Guyon's canal syndrome, often seen in cyclists, presenting with numbness and tingling in the 4th and 5th digits?
a)	Ulnar nerve

3099)	What hand abnormality develops due to the contracture of the longitudinal bands of the palmer aponeurosis?
a)	Dupuytren's contracture

3100)	What is a painless, cystic lesion, fixed to deep tissue and a nerve called?
a)	Ganglion cyst

3101)	What is the treatment for a ganglion cyst?
a)	Orthopedic referral for removal

3102)	What is the definitive treatment for a high-pressure injection hand injury?
a)	Orthopedic referral for surgery and Antibiotics

3103) What thumb injury is diagnosed with Finkelstein's test?
   a) DeQuervain's tenosynovitis
3104) What tendons are involved in DeQuervain's tenosynovitis?
   a) Abductor pollicis longus and Extensor pollicis brevis
3105) What is the treatment of DeQuervain's tenosynovitis?
   a) Thumb spica
3106) What is a paronychia?
   a) Infection of the soft tissue around a fingernail
3107) What is the treatment of a paronychia?
   a) I&D and Antibiotics
3108) What finger infection is associated with a vesicular bullous viral infection?
   a) Herpetic whitlow
3109) What type of finger infection is a deep infection of the pulp space of the fingertip?
   a) Felon
3110) What I&D approach is used for felon drainage?
   a) Unilateral longitudinal incision 5mm distal to DIP
3111) What areas do you avoid performing the I&D for a felon in the 2nd, 3rd, 4th, and 5th fingers due to complications?
   a) Radial aspect of 2nd and 3rd
   b) Ulnar aspect of 4th and 5th
3112) List the four Kanavel signs used to diagnose tenosynovitis of the finger.
   a) Slightly flexed finger
   b) Tenderness over the tendon
   c) Pain with passive extension
   d) Symmetrical swelling
3113) What is the 1st and earliest Kanavel sign to appear on the exam with tenosynovitis?
   a) Pain with passive extension
3114) List the indications for reimplantation.
   a) Injury to multiple digits with digits still attached
   b) Most amputations of the thumb

c) Amputations in children

d) Clean amputations of the wrist, hand, or forearm

3115) How do you care/preserve an amputated part?

a) Clean with lactated ringer's, wrap in moistened saline gauze, place in a sterile iced container

3116) What type of hand burns should be referred to a burn center?

a) Circumferential digit burns and Third-degree burns

3117) What is the pathophysiology of compartment syndrome?

a) Increased compartment pressure leading to compromised circulation

3118) What is the earliest symptom seen with compartment syndrome?

a) Pain

3119) What are the 6 Ps of compartment syndrome, seen after a fracture, injury or infection?

a) Pain out of proportion to exam

b) Pain with passive range of motion

c) Paresthesia

d) Paralysis

e) Pallor

f) Pulselessness

3120) What intracompartment pressure is concerning for compartment syndrome?

a) Pressure > 30 mmHg

3121) What is normal intercompartmental pressure?

a) 0-8 mmHg

3122) How is the delta pressure measured?

a) Diastolic pressure - Measured compartment pressure

3123) What delta pressure in compartment syndrome indicates a need for a fasciotomy?

a) 30 mmHg or less

3124) What are the treatments for compartment syndrome?

a) Remove cast or dressing and Fasciotomy for pressures > 30 mmHg

3125) What type of forearm fracture involves a fracture of the radius with a distal ulna dislocation?
a) Galeazzi fracture

3126) What type of forearm fracture involves a fracture of the proximal ulna with a radial head dislocation?
a) Monteggia fracture

3127) What deformity can occur as a complication of a forearm fracture and inadequate circulation?
a) Volkmann's contracture

3128) What bone is commonly fractured in the forearm with a nightstick injury?
a) Ulna shaft

3129) What injury involves a radial head fracture, interosseous membrane disruption, and a dislocated distal radial ulnar joint?
a) Essex-Lopresti injury

3130) What specific X-ray finding is seen with a radial head fracture without a bone abnormality?
a) Posterior fad pad

3131) What are the four types of radial head fracture?
a) Type 1: Nondisplaced
b) Type 2: Displaced and Angulated
c) Type 3: Comminuted
d) Type 4: All above plus dislocation

3132) What is the treatment for type 1 and 2 radial head fractures?
a) Sling

3133) What artery and nerve are frequently injured in a supracondylar fracture?
a) Brachial artery and Median nerve

3134) What is the most common injury pattern seen with supracondylar fractures?
a) Fall on out stretched hand (FOOSH)

3135) What is the specific X-ray finding seen with a supracondylar fracture?
a) Posterior fat pad sign

3136) What bone on a lateral elbow X-ray is the anterior humeral line supposed to transect the anterior 1/3 of when evaluating for a supracondylar fracture?
   a) Capitellum
3137) List the three types of supracondylar fractures.
   a) Type 1: Nondisplaced
   b) Type 2: Posterior cortex affected
   c) Type 3: Cortex disrupted
3138) Name the four muscles that make up the rotator cuff.
   a) Supraspinatus, Subscapularis, Teres Minor, and Infraspinatus
3139) What is the most commonly injured rotator cuff muscle?
   a) Supraspinatus
3140) List the physical exam tests used to diagnose a rotator cuff injury.
   a) Neer's test
   b) Hawkin's test
   c) Empty can test
   d) Drop arm test
   e) Lift off test
   f) Apley scratch test
3141) Name the two types of sternoclavicular (SC) joint dislocations.
   a) 1st degree-partial tear, 2nd degree-complete tear
3142) What type of SC dislocation, anterior or posterior, is the most common?
   a) Anterior dislocation
3143) What is the ED treatment for an anterior SC joint dislocation?
   a) Reduction with conscious sedation, Sling and swathe, and Orthopedic referral
3144) What is the treatment for a posterior SC joint dislocation?
   a) Orthopedic surgery for closed reduction
3145) How many types of acromioclavicular (AC) joint dislocations are there?
   a) 6

3146) What is the management of type 1 and 2 AC joint dislocations?
   a) Arm sling and Orthopedic follow up
3147) Which joint is the most commonly dislocated?
   a) Shoulder
3148) What is the most common type of shoulder dislocation?
   a) Anterior dislocation
3149) What two fractures can occur with a shoulder dislocation?
   a) Hill-Sachs deformity and Bankart lesion
3150) What type of deformity is seen with a compression fracture of the posterolateral humeral head after a shoulder dislocation?
   a) Hill-Sachs lesion
3151) What type of deformity is seen with a fracture of the anterior inferior aspect of the glenoid after a shoulder dislocation?
   a) Bankart Lesion
3152) What is the most common nerve injury associated with anterior shoulder dislocation?
   a) Axillary nerve
3153) What X-ray finding is seen with posterior shoulder dislocation?
   a) Light bulb sign
3154) Which shoulder dislocation is associated with seizures?
   a) Posterior shoulder dislocation
3155) "Luxatio erecta" is another name for which type of shoulder dislocation?
   a) Inferior shoulder dislocation
3156) What type of injury most commonly leads to scapular fractures?
   a) High-velocity injury
3157) What is the classification used to type humeral head fractures?
   a) Neer's classification

3158) What is the most common nerve injury associated with a midshaft distal humeral fracture?
  a) Radial nerve

3159) What is the most common nerve injury associated with a proximal humeral fracture?
  a) Axillary nerve

3160) What is the most common physical exam finding seen with a radial nerve palsy?
  a) Wrist drop

3161) What is the most common complication from a proximal humeral head fracture?
  a) Adhesive capsulitis

3162) What anatomical part of the bicep is typically associated with bicep rupture?
  a) Long head

3163) What type of tendonitis is associated with pain in the anterior shoulder with abduction and rotation of the shoulder and a positive Speed's test?
  a) Bicep tendonitis

3164) Name the three types of thoracic outlet syndrome.
  a) Neurologic, Venous, and Arterial

3165) What type of thoracic outlet syndrome is the most common?
  a) Neurologic

3166) What tests are used to diagnose thoracic outlet syndrome?
  a) Adson's and Roos test

3167) What is another name for pain over the lateral epicondyle that occurs from repetitive use and tendonitis?
  a) Tennis elbow

3168) What is the treatment of tennis elbow or lateral epicondylitis?
  a) Immobilization of the arm in flexion and supination with the wrist extended

3169) What is the treatment of olecranon bursitis?
  a) Anti-inflammatory +/- Aspiration

3170) What is a contraindication to aspirating an infected bursa?
   a) Cellulitis overlying the site
3171) What type of orthopedic injury is seen in a 3-year-old child who comes in holding the arm in flexion and pronation after abrupt traction on an arm with wrist pronation?
   a) Radial head subluxation (nursemaid's elbow)
3172) What ligament is torn in a nursemaid's elbow?
   a) Annular ligament
3173) What are the two techniques for the reduction of a radial head subluxation (nurse maid's elbow)?
   a) Hyperpronation of the wrist and forearm
   b) Supination of the forearm and flex the elbow
3174) What is another name for medial epicondylitis?
   a) Golfers elbow
3175) What is the most common elbow dislocation after a fall on an outstretched hand?
   a) Posterior
3176) What is the treatment of a posterior elbow dislocation?
   a) Reduction and Posterior splint
3177) What nerve and artery are commonly injured in elbow dislocations?
   a) Brachial artery and Ulnar nerve
3178) What sign occurs while testing thumb adduction and is due to the weakness of the adductor pollicis muscle from an ulnar nerve palsy?
   a) Froment's sign (thumb flexes when gripping paper)
3179) What ligament flexes the DIP joint of the finger?
   a) Flexor digitorum profundus
3180) What ligament flexes the PIP joint of the finger?
   a) Flexor digitorum superficialis
3181) What type of pediatric extremity fracture is defined as an incomplete or buckling fracture that shows a bulging of the cortex on an X-ray?

a) Torus fracture

3182) What type of pediatric extremity fracture is due to the bone bending under pressure, leading to a break of only one side of the cortex and periosteum?
   a) Greenstick fracture

Pelvis and lower extremity

3183) How do you stabilize an open book pelvic fracture?
   a) Pelvic binder

3184) What are the two most common sites of pelvic dislocation?
   a) Pubic symphysis or Sacroiliac joint (SI)

3185) What is the most common visceral injury seen in pelvic fractures?
   a) Lower urinary tract

3186) What specific sign is consistent with a rectal hematoma as a complication of a pelvic fracture?
   a) Earle sign

3187) What type of pelvic fracture consists of a widened pubic symphysis and SI joint?
   a) Anterior-posterior compression fracture

3188) What type of pelvic fracture consists of internal rotation of the hemipelvis?
   a) Lateral compression fracture

3189) What type of pelvic fracture consists of a cephalad-displaced hemipelvis?
   a) Vertical shear fracture

3190) What type of pelvic fractures is seen in skeletally immature patients, ages 14-17, and typically involves the ASIS or ischial tuberosity?
   a) Avulsion fracture

3191) What is the most common type of pelvic fracture?
   a) Compression fracture

3192) What type of hip injury is seen with a shortened, flexed, adducted, and internally rotated hip?
   a) Posterior hip dislocation

3193) What is the most common type of hip dislocations?

a) Posterior hip dislocation

3194) What type of injury occurs with a posterior hip dislocation?
a) Nerve injury

3195) What type of injury occurs with an anterior hip dislocation?
a) Vascular injury

3196) What complication is seen with hip dislocations?
a) Avascular necrosis

3197) What percentage of elderly patients die within one year of a hip fracture?
a) 15-20%

3198) What are the two most common types of hip fractures?
a) Femoral neck and Intertrochanteric fractures

3199) Can hemorrhagic shock develop due to hip or femoral fractures?
a) Yes

3200) What blood volume loss can be associated with a hip and femur fractures?
a) Up to 1,500 mL

3201) What imaging modality would you consider if suspicion is high for an occult hip fracture with a negative hip X-ray?
a) CT scan

3202) What type of splint is used for immobilization of a midshaft femoral fracture?
a) Traction splint

3203) What is the most common type of femur fracture?
a) Transverse with displacement

3204) What artery is commonly injured from a knee dislocation?
a) Popliteal artery

3205) Which type of knee dislocation is the most common and is more associated with a lower extremity vascular injury?
a) Anterior

3206) Which test should be done to rule out arterial injury?
a) Ankle-brachial index (ABI)

3207) What ABI percentage indicates a potential artery injury?
   a) < 0.9
3208) What is the treatment of a posterior knee dislocation with decreased pulses?
   a) Immediate reduction and Splinting in 15°-20° flexion
3209) What test should you order to rule out artery injury with a knee dislocation?
   a) Angiogram
3210) List the Ottawa knee rules for ordering radiography.
   a) Patient > 55 years old
   b) Fibular head tenderness
   c) Patellar tenderness
   d) Inability to flex 90°
   e) Inability to transfer after injury
3211) What is the treatment of a patellar dislocation?
   a) Closed reduction (flex hip with knee extension and medial pressure)
3212) What muscle tear is seen with an inability to extend the knee after trauma?
   a) Quadriceps tear
3213) What tendon is ruptured with a physical exam finding of a high riding patella on knee extension?
   a) Inferior patella tendon
3214) What test is used to diagnose patellofemoral syndrome?
   a) Patellar grind test
3215) What specific symptom with a patella fracture is an orthopedic emergency?
   a) If the patient is unable to extend the knee
3216) What ligament is injured with a positive anterior drawer test of the knee?
   a) ACL
3217) What pathognomonic fracture is seen with an ACL injury?
   a) Segond fracture
3218) What is a Segond Fracture?

a) Lateral proximal tibia fracture

3219) What is the most common ligament injury of the knee?

a) ACL

3220) What is the most sensitive test to diagnose an ACL tear?

a) Lachman's test

3221) Which knee ligament tear is most associated with acute hemarthrosis?

a) ACL

3222) Injury to which ligament presents with a positive posterior drawer test?

a) PCL

3223) What tests are used to diagnose meniscal tears?

a) Apley's test and McMurray test

3224) What is the most common meniscal tear?

a) Medial

3225) Define the three ligaments involved in the "Terrible triad" injury?

a) MCL, Medial meniscus, and ACL

3226) What type of knee fracture is most commonly seen with valgus/varus stress?

a) Lateral plateau fracture

3227) What is lipohemarthosis on a strait leg lateral knee X-ray associated with?

a) Tibial plateau fracture

3228) What disease is associated with active adolescents and tibial tuberosity tenderness?

a) Osgood-Schlatter's

3229) What type of cyst involves inflammation of the gastrocnemius bursa, with a painful swollen popliteal fossa, and can be diagnosed with ultrasound?

a) Bakers cyst

3230) Which nerve is commonly injured from a proximal fibula fracture?

a) Peroneal nerve

3231) What type of fibula head fracture is seen with ankle injuries and is caused by an interosseous membrane tear?
   a) Maisonneuve fracture

3232) List the criteria for Ottawa ankle rules.
   a) Bone tenderness distal 6cm distal tibia or fibula
   b) Tenderness base of 5th metatarsal
   c) Inability to bear weight after injury or in ED for four steps.

3233) What type of ankle dislocation is the most common?
   a) Posterior

3234) What is the most common injury pattern leading to an ankle ligament injury?
   a) Inversion and rotation (85%)

3235) Name the three lateral ankle ligaments.
   a) Anterior talofibular, Calcaneofibular, and Posterior talofibular

3236) What ankle ligament is the most commonly injured?
   a) Anterior talofibular

3237) How many types of ankle sprains are there?
   a) 3

3238) Which degree of an ankle sprain is associated with a complete ligament tear and a significant functional loss?
   a) 3rd degree

3239) What test is used to help diagnose an Achilles tendon rupture?
   a) Thompson's test

3240) What age range is most common for Achilles tendon rupture?
   a) 30-40's

3241) What imaging modalities are the best to diagnose an Achilles tendon rupture?
   a) Ultrasound and MRI

3242) What type of splint is used to treat an Achilles tendon rupture?
   a) Plantar-flexed posterior short leg splint

3243) What type of foot fracture involves a transverse fracture of the diaphysis of the 5th metatarsal?
a) Jones fracture

3244) What is the management of a Jones fracture?
a) Posterior splint and Surgery (open reduction and internal fixation)

3245) What type of foot fracture involves an avulsion fracture of the proximal 5th metatarsal?
a) Pseudo-jones (Dancer's) fracture

3246) What is the management of a Pseudo-Jones fracture?
a) Hard sole shoes or Cast shoe

3247) What foot fracture has the highest rate of nonunion and risk for infection?
a) Calcaneus fracture

3248) What angle measured on a calcaneal X-ray is normally 20°- 40° and is used to diagnose a calcaneal fracture?
a) Boehler's angle

3249) What is a common complication of a talus fracture?
a) Avascular necrosis

3250) What unstable foot fracture has a widened space between the 1st and 2nd metatarsal heads, a small fracture of the 1st metatarsal head, and malalignment of the medial edge of 2nd metatarsal and the 2nd cuneiform on foot X-ray?
a) Lisfranc fracture

3251) What is the treatment for a Lisfranc fracture?
a) Posterior short leg splint and Orthopedic consult for surgery

Bone and joint

3252) What is the most common bacteria associated with septic arthritis?
a) Staphylococcus

3253) What bacteria is most commonly associated with septic arthritis in a sickle cell patient?
a) Salmonella

3254)　What bacteria is the most common cause of prosthetic joint infection in the early post-op period?
　a)　MRSA

3255)　List the synovial fluid lab orders needed to diagnose septic arthritis.
　a)　Cell count, Gram stain, Culture, and Crystals

3256)　What synovial fluid WBC count indicates the diagnosis of septic arthritis?
　a)　> 50,000

3257)　Elevation of which two inflammatory markers indicate septic arthritis in the setting of a hot, swollen, painful joint?
　a)　ESR and CRP

3258)　What are the best imaging modalities to diagnose septic arthritis in pediatric patients?
　a)　MRI and Ultrasound

3259)　What is the most common cause of a painful hip in a child with a limp, with a history of a recent viral infection or trauma, and needs to have septic arthritis ruled out?
　a)　Transient (toxic) synovitis

3260)　What type of bacteria is commonly seen in IV drug abusers with bone and joint infections?
　a)　Pseudomonas

3261)　What is the best study for diagnosing osteomyelitis?
　a)　Bone scan

3262)　What type of injury is due to trauma to the bone and is a painful osteonecrotic local lesion seen on an X-ray?
　a)　Osteochondritis dissecans

3263)　What is diagnosed when calcification and bone develop in the muscle after a traumatic injury?
　a)　Traumatic myositis ossificans

3264)　Exposure to and toxicity of what metal leads to bands of increased density at the metaphysis of tubular bones, possibly seen on X-ray of an inner-city child living in an old home?
　a)　Lead (i.e. lead lines)

3265) What type of Salter-Harris fracture involves a fracture through the physis/growth plate and a slipped/displaced epiphysis?
   a) Type 1
3266) What type of Salter-Harris fracture involves a fracture through metaphysis and physis?
   a) Type 2
3267) What type of Salter-Harris fracture is the most common?
   a) Type 2
3268) What type of Salter-Harris fracture is through the epiphysis and physis?
   a) Type 3
3269) What type of Salter-Harris fracture is a fracture through the metaphysis, physis, and epiphysis?
   a) Type 4
3270) What type of Salter-Harris fracture is a crush injury involving part or all of the physis?
   a) Type 5
3271) Orthopedic consult in the ED should be done for which types of Salter-Harris fractures?
   a) Slipped, angulated, or displaced Types 1,2,3
   b) All Type 4 and 5 fractures
3272) What is the most common cause of monoarticular arthritis in a young adult?
   a) Gonococcal arthritis
3273) What bone disease is defined by rapid inflammatory bone resorption with chaotic weak bone formation, normal calcium levels, and increased alkaline phosphatase?
   a) Paget's disease

Spine
3274) List the back pain high-risk factors (red flags) requiring imaging.
   a) Recent trauma, Progressive, HIV, Cancer, Steroid use, IV drug abuse, Fever, Urinary retention, Bowel

incontinence, Widespread neurological deficits, and Structural deformity.

3275) What spinal emergency presents with worsening sensory loss, saddle anesthesia, overflow incontinence, bilateral sciatica, leg weakness, and is caused by a tumor or central disc herniation?
a) Cauda equina syndrome

3276) What is the most consistent symptom seen in cauda equina syndrome?
a) Urinary retention (90%)

3277) What are the symptoms seen with conus medularis syndrome?
a) Cord compression with non-dermatomal sensory loss

3278) What test is more specific for disc herniation than the regular straight leg test?
a) Crossed straight leg test

3279) What bacteria is the leading cause of spinal epidural abscesses?
a) Staphylococcus aureus

3280) Elevation of what specific labs help with the diagnosis of a spinal epidural abscess?
a) ESR and CRP

3281) What are the classic symptoms associated with a spinal epidural abscess?
a) Midline spine pain, Fever, and Neurological deficits

3282) What is the preferred test for diagnosing a spinal epidural abscess?
a) MRI with and without contrast.

3283) What antibiotics are recommended for spinal epidural abscesses?
a) Vancomycin + Metronidazole + Ceftriaxone

3284) What is the definitive treatment for a spinal epidural abscess?
a) Surgical decompression and drainage

3285) What spinal emergency should be considered in a patient on anticoagulants with back pain, numbness, and tingling, with a history of a recent spinal injection?
a) Epidural hematoma

3286) What medical conditions are unstable C 1/2 Atlantoaxial dislocations associated with?
   a) Rheumatoid arthritis and Ankylosing spondylitis
3287) What part of the pediatric cervical spine has a natural pseudosubluxation and is seen on cervical imaging?
   a) C2-C3
3288) What spinal line on cervical imaging should be intact in the presence of a C2-C3 pseudosubluxation?
   a) Spinolaminar line
3289) Name the difference between spondylosis and spondylolisthesis.
   a) Spondylolisthesis is a pars defect with anterior vertebral displacement
   b) Spondylosis is degenerative changes to the spine
3290) What condition presents with burning pain down the lateral thigh, is commonly seen in pregnant women and men with work belts, and is caused by a lateral femoral nerve impingement?
   a) Meralgia parasthetica
3291) What type of crystal is found in the synovial fluid in gout?
   a) Negative birefringent needle crystals
3292) What is the most common site for gout?
   a) Great toe (podagra)
3293) What type of crystal is seen in the synovial fluid with pseudogout?
   a) Calcium pyrophosphate rhomboid crystals
3294) What is the treatment of acute gout and pseudogout?
   a) NSAIDs, Colchicine, or Steroids
3295) What medication is used to prevent uric acid crystal production and gout?
   a) Allopurinol
3296) What complication of rheumatoid arthritis presents with joint pain, edema, motility dysfunction, and includes neutropenia and splenomegaly?
   a) Felty Syndrome

Nephrology / Urology

3297) What is the definition of oliguria in adults and pediatrics?
   a) Adults: < 500 mL of urine in 24 hours
   b) Pediatrics: < 300 mL of urine in 24 hours
3298) What is the definition of anuria?
   a) < 100 mL/day
3299) What is the normal expected urine production rate per mL/kg/hr in a healthy patient?
   a) 0.5-1.5 mL/kg/hr
3300) What classification system is used for staging acute kidney injury (AKI)-previous known as acute renal failure?
   a) RIFLE classification (risk, injury, failure, loss of function, ESRD)
3301) What lab is the most useful to an ED physician in the diagnosis of AKI?
   a) Creatinine level
3302) What Cr increase from baseline defines AKI?
   a) ↑ 1.5-3x baseline Cr
3303) What amount of Cr increase and GFR decrease from baseline is defined by the RIFLE classification for each of the following: risk, injury, and failure?
   a) Risk: ↑ 1.5x baseline or ↓ GFR > 25%
   b) Injury: ↑ 2x baseline or ↓ GFR > 50%
   c) Failure: ↑ 3x baseline or ↓ GFR > 75%
3304) What two medications commonly lead to renal injury?
   a) NSAIDs and ACE inhibitors
3305) Name the three types of acute kidney injury (AKI).
   a) Prerenal, Renal, and Postrenal
3306) Which type of AKI is the most common?
   a) Prerenal
3307) Which type of AKI is caused by dehydration and hypovolemia, and can be corrected with IV fluids?
   a) Prerenal
3308) What is the BUN to creatinine ratio in prerenal AKI?
   a) 20:1
3309) What is the urine Na^+ secretion amount in prerenal AKI?

a) Low < 20

3310) Give the calculation to find the fractional excretion of Na^+.

    a) Na^+ $(FeNa^+) = (UNa^+/PNa^+) \div (UCr/PCr) \times 100$

3311) What is the factional excretion of Na^+ in prerenal AKI?

    a) < 1

3312) What is the most common cause of hospital-acquired AKI?

    a) Acute tubular necrosis (Intrinsic renal failure)

3313) What is the most common cause of community-acquired AKI?

    a) Prerenal acute renal failure

3314) What is the imaging study of choice for most ARF patients?

    a) Renal US

3315) What type of renal failure is most commonly caused by acute tubular necrosis (ATN) or acute interstitial nephritis due to ischemia and neprotoxic agents?

    a) Intrinsic renal failure

3316) What type of glomerulonephritis is caused by immune complexes attacking the glomeruli, leading to oliguria, edema, proteinuria, and RBC casts on urinalysis?

    a) Acute nephritic syndrome

3317) What are some causes of acute nephritic syndrome?

    a) Post-streptococcal GN, IgA nephropathy, HSP, HUS, HELLP, TTP, Wegener's, and Goodpasture's

3318) What is the treatment for acute nephritic syndrome?

    a) Steroids

3319) What type of glomerulonephritis has edema, hematuria, and hypertension and is seen 1-2 weeks after a throat infection?

    a) Post-streptococcal glomerulonephritis

3320) What medication can be used to treat edema from post-streptococcal glomerulonephritis and which medication should be avoided?

    a) Treat: Hydrochlorothiazide

    b) Avoid: Furosemide

3321) What autoimmune disease involves the sinuses, lungs, and kidney causing epistaxis, hemoptysis, and hematuria and is due to the ANCA antibody?

    a) Wegener's granulomatosis

3322) What autoimmune disease affects the kidneys and lungs causing hematuria and hemoptysis and is due antibodies that attack type 4 collagen and the glomerular basement membrane?

a) Goodpasture's syndrome

3323) What is the recommended treatment for Wegener's and Goodpasture's disease?

a) Steroids

3324) What type of chronic renal failure is associated with hypoalbuminemia, proteinuria, edema, and hyperlipidemia?

a) Nephrotic syndrome

3325) List some diseases that cause nephrotic syndrome.

a) Minimal changes disease, Membranous glomerulonephritis, Focal segmental glomerular sclerosis, and Amyloidosis

3326) What is the most common cause of nephrotic syndrome?

a) Minimal change disease

3327) What vascular complication can be seen with nephrotic syndrome?

a) Renal vein thrombosis

3328) What are the treatment options for nephrotic syndrome?

a) Furosemide and Steroids

3329) List the drugs that can cause acute interstitial nephritis (AIN).

a) Penicillins, Sulpha, Diuretics, and NSAIDs

3330) What are the typical findings seen with AIN?

a) Fever, Rash, Eosinophiluria, and WBC casts

3331) What type of casts are seen in the urine with AIN?

a) WBC casts

3332) What is the leading cause of renal failure?

a) Acute tubular necrosis (ATN)

3333) What type of casts are seen in the urine with ATN?

a) Muddy brown (granular) casts

3334) What type of urinary casts is benign?

a) Hyaline casts

3335) What are the most common causes of postrenal AKI?

a) Obstruction from stones, Prostate hypertrophy, or Ureteral or Urethral abnormalities

3336) What are the management options for postrenal AKI due to prostate hypertrophy and ureteral obstructions?

a) Catheter placement (prostatic hypertrophy) or percutaneous nephrostomy (ureteral obstructions)

3337) What is the most common cause of AKI in children?
a) Hemolytic uremic syndrome (HUS)

3338) What is the leading cause of chronic kidney disease?
a) Diabetes

3339) List the medical conditions for emergent dialysis for patients.
a) Uremic encephalopathy, Uremic pericarditis, Cardiac tamponade/effusion, Pulmonary edema, or Refractory hyperkalemia, Overdoses, Hyponatremia (< 115), Hypernatremia (> 165), and Severe acid-base disturbances

3340) What Cr and BUN levels indicate the need for emergent dialysis treatment in renal failure?
a) Cr > 10 mg/dL or BUN > 100 mg/dL

3341) What complication from end stage renal disease (ESRD), presents with chest pain, diffuse ST-segment elevation and PR depression ECG changes +/- altered mental status and elevated BUN level?
a) Uremic pericarditis

3342) What is the most common electrolyte problem found in renal failure or patients that miss dialysis?
a) Hyperkalemia

3343) What ECG changes are seen with hyperkalemia?
a) Bradycardia, Peaked T- waves, and a Widened QRS

3344) List the treatments used for hyperkalemia.
a) Calcium gluconate, Bicarbonate, Insulin with Dextrose, Albuterol, and Sodium polystyrene

3345) Does Calcium chloride need to be administered through a central line?
a) Yes

3346) What electrolyte changes can be seen in ESRD?
a) Hypocalcemia. Hypokalemia, Hyperkalemia, and Hypomagnesemia

3347) What cell changes normally occur with ESRD?
a) Anemia, Decreased WBC, and Dysfunctional platelets (increased bleeding)

3348)   What medication is given during dialysis that can increase the risk of bleeding, subdural hematomas, and can be reversed with protamine?
   a)   Heparin
3349)   What is the most common dialysis complication?
   a)   Hypotension
3350)   Are patients with ESRD classified as immunocompromised?
   a)   Yes
3351)   Why should a regular dose of insulin not be given to treat hyperglycemia in the ED for patients with ESRD?
   a)   Due to the increased half-life in ESRD, it can induce hypoglycemia
3352)   What is the most common cause of ESRD?
   a)   Diabetes
3353)   What syndrome can occur with dialysis due to increased intracranial pressure from the osmotic shift, and causes a headache, nausea, muscle cramps, and confusion?
   a)   Disequilibrium syndrome
3354)   What complication can occur in a patient receiving peritoneal dialysis that presents with abdominal pain, fever, and abdominal distention?
   a)   Peritonitis
3355)   What are the lab changes used to diagnose peritonitis?
   a)   WBC's > 100 and PMN's > 50%
3356)   What bacteria is the most common cause of peritonitis in a patient receiving peritoneal dialysis?
   a)   Staph. epidermidis
3357)   What is the treatment for peritonitis?
   a)   Intraperitoneal antibiotics (Vancomycin & Aminoglycoside)
3358)   What type of bacterias cause infections around peritoneal catheters?
   a)   Staph and Pseudomonas
3359)   What antibiotics can be used for peritoneal catheter infections?
   a)   Ciprofloxacin or Cephalosporins
3360)   What clinical finding is consistent with a clotted fistula?
   a)   Loss of the thrill

3361) What sign indicates high output cardiac failure in an ESRD patient and is defined by a drop in the heart rate when a fistula is pressed on?
   a) Branham's sign
3362) What autosomal dominant kidney disease presents with flank pain, hematuria, and has renal cysts on imaging?
   a) Polycystic kidney disease
3363) What neurovascular condition is associated with polycystic kidney disease?
   a) Cerebral aneurysms
3364) Are nitrites or leukocytes more specific for a urinary tract infection (UTI)?
   a) Nitrites (87%)
3365) What amount of bacteria seen on urine culture meets the criteria for a UTI?
   a) > 10^5 CFU's
3366) How much bacteria on a dipstick urinalysis is consistent with 10^5 bacteria CFU's?
   a) 2+
3367) How many WBC's found on urinalysis microscopy should be considered low-level pyuria?
   a) 2-5 WBC on HPF
3368) Does the use of Phenazopyridine (Pyridium) skew the urinalysis results?
   a) Yes
3369) What is the most common bacteria accounting for UTIs?
   a) E. Coli (80%)
3370) What bacteria are associated with negative nitrite UTIs?
   a) Enterococcus, Pseudomonas, and Acinetobacter
3371) What is the most common infection in the elderly?
   a) UTI
3372) List the antibiotic choices to treat a UTI.
   a) Fluoroquinolones, TMP-SMX, Doxycycline, Cephalosporins, or Penicillins
3373) In what patient population do you treat asymptomatic bacteriuria?
   a) Pregnant

3374) List the antibiotics that are safe for UTI treatment during pregnancy.

a) Penicillins, Cephalosporins, and Nitrofurantoin (2nd-3rd trimester only)

3375) What renal complication can occur with an untreated UTI and usually presents with flank pain, nausea, fever, and dysuria?

a) Pyelonephritis

3376) What type of urinary casts are seen with pyelonephritis?

a) WBC casts

3377) What renal complications can occur with untreated pyelonephritis?

a) Perinephric abscess and AKI

3378) What antibiotics are recommended for the treatment of pyelonephritis?

a) Fluoroquinolones,TMP-SMX (Bactrim), Amoxicillin/Clavulanate, or Cephalosporins

3379) What is the treatment length for pyelonephritis for each of the following antibiotics: Fluoroquinolones, TMP-SMX, Amoxicillin/Clavulanate, and Cephalosporins?

a) Fluoroquinolones: 10 days

b) TMP-SMX (Bactrim): 14 days

c) Amoxicillin/Clavulanate: 10-14 days

d) Cephalosporins: 10-14 days

3380) List the criteria used to define a complicated UTI to determine a patient's risk of a treatment failure.

a) Pregnant patients, Newborns, UTI's resistant to multiple all oral antibiotics, Immunodeficiency, UTI with ureteral stone, UTI with a ureteral stent, or UTI with a Foley catheter

3381) Can you rely on the urinalysis to diagnose a UTI that is taken from a chronic indwelling catheter?

a) No (asymptomatic colonization is common)

3382) What other medical conditions excluding a UTI can also present with dysuria?

a) Sexually transmitted diseases (urethritis), Prostatitis, and Epididymitis

3383) Where is the most likely location of urinary tract bleeding when hematuria is present at the onset of urination?
a) Urethral

3384) Where is the most likely location of urinary tract bleeding when hematuria is present late after starting urination?
a) Bladder, Prostate, or Kidney

3385) List the causes of hematuria.
a) Kidney stones, Trauma, Prostatitis, Pyelonephritis, UTI, AVM, Nephritis, Prior pelvic radiation, Cancers: Prostate, Bladder, Kidney, or Urethral

3386) What is the most common cause of hematuria?
a) UTI

3387) What is the workup for uncomplicated hematuria?
a) U/A and Culture, CT Urogram, or Renal US, and Urology referral

3388) What molecule can cause a positive blood result on a urine dipstick test but be negative for RBCs on the urinalysis?
a) Myoglobin

3389) What is it called when a malingering drug-seeking patient presents with flank pain and RBCs are only seen on initial unwitnessed urinalysis and not a witnessed urinalysis?
a) Pseudohematuria

3390) What urologic condition presents with sudden onset waxing and waning flank pain, urinary frequency, blood in the urine, nausea, and vomiting?
a) Ureteral stone (passing kidney stone)

3391) What type of stone is the most common cause of nephrolithiasis?
a) Calcium

3392) What type of stone typically leads to a struvite stone or staghorn calculus?
a) Magnesium-ammonium-phosphate

3393) What is the treatment of struvite stones?
a) Surgical removal

3394) What type of kidney stone can develop in patients with history of gastric bypass and is due to fat binding and saponification from the increased fat in the bowel?
a) Calcium/oxalate stones

3395) What type of renal stone is radiolucent on imaging?
   a) Uric acid
3396) What size renal stones have a high spontaneous passage rate?
   a) 4-5 mm
3397) What is the most common location in the urinary tract for nephrolithiasis obstruction?
   a) Ureterovesical junction (UVJ)
3398) What is the second most common location in the urinary tract for stone obstruction?
   a) Ureteropelvic junction (UPJ)
3399) What HIV drug commonly leads to nephrolithiasis?
   a) Indinavir
3400) Does hematuria or RBC's on urinalysis mean there is a kidney stone?
   a) No (absent in 15-20% of cases)
3401) What is the most common imaging study used in the ED to diagnose a passing kidney stone and its size?
   a) CT abdomen and pelvis without contrast
3402) What quick bedside imaging study can be performed to rule out hydronephrosis with obstructive uropathy?
   a) Renal ultrasound
3403) A dilated renal pelvis on an abdominal CT or renal ultrasound suggests what complication from passing a kidney stone?
   a) Hydronephrosis
3404) What are the typical medications used to treat nephrolithiasis?
   a) Pain medications, Antiemetic's, Tamsulosin, and +/- Antibiotics (for UTI)
3405) List the admission criteria for nephrolithiasis.
   a) Single kidney with obstruction, Uncontrolled pain, Intractable vomiting, Renal insufficiency (↑ Cr), Infected stent, or Coexisting UTI (questionable-urology consult)
3406) What are the treatment options for a very large stone or an obstructed ureteral stone?
   a) Lithotripsy, Open surgery, or Ureteral stenting
3407) What is the recommended therapy for an infected ureteral stent?
   a) Urology consult and Antibiotics +/- Removal

3408) What two lab tests are "required" for kidney stones?
   a) Basic metabolic profile (kidney function check) and Urinalysis (U/A)
3409) What is the medical term for post-lithotripsy urinary obstruction from stone fragments?
   a) Steinstrasse
3410) What complication should be suspected in a patient with a ureteral stent who presents with severe gross hematuria, syncope, and hypotension?
   a) Ureteral arterial fistula
3411) What life-threatening vascular condition can also present with a sudden onset of flank pain and is commonly misdiagnosed as renal colic?
   a) Abdominal aortic aneurysm (AAA)
3412) What urological infection presents with dysuria, low back and perineal pain, fever, pain with defecation, and positive bacteria on urinalysis?
   a) Prostatitis
3413) Why is it not recommended to perform a prostate exam with prostatitis?
   a) It can induce bacteremia
3414) What is the recommended antibiotic treatment length for acute prostatitis?
   a) 4-6 weeks
3415) What are the recommended antibiotics for acute prostatitis?
   a) Fluoroquinolones or TMP-SMX
3416) What polymicrobial skin infection of the groin spreads rapidly due to necrotizing fasciitis and usually seen in the immunocompromised?
   a) Fournier's scrotal gangrene
3417) What is the management for Fournier's gangrene?
   a) IV broad spectrum antibiotics, Surgical debridement, and Oxygen
3418) What condition presents with discharge, itching, redness, and pain around the glands and is more commonly in uncircumcised patients?
   a) Balanoposthitis

3419) What is the most common infectious cause of balanitis?
   a) Candidal
3420) What is the condition called when an uncircumcised patient is unable to retract the foreskin of the penis proximally, causing pain and possibly urinary retention?
   a) Phimosis
3421) What is the treatment for phimosis?
   a) Dorsal slit of the foreskin
3422) What penile emergency presents with a proximally retracted foreskin that is unable to be reduced manually, causing pain and swelling to the glans?
   a) Paraphimosis
3423) Give the treatment options in order for paraphimosis.
   a) 1st: Compression with reduction
   b) 2nd: Dorsal slit of the foreskin
   c) 3rd: Needle puncture of the gland to relieve edema
3424) Injury to what part of the penis leads to ecchymosis and swelling in a fractured penis?
   a) Tunica albuginea
3425) Give the plan of care for a fractured penis.
   a) Urology consult and Hematoma evacuation
3426) What are the two types of priapism that can occur?
   a) Low flow (ischemic) and High flow (arterial)
3427) What lab test can be used to determine low flow verse high flow priapism and is taken from a blood aspirate from the penis?
   a) Blood gas
3428) What blood gas results suggest low flow priapism?
   a) $pO_2 < 60$ kPa, $pCO_2 > 70$ kPa, or a pH < 7.0
3429) List the conditions that can lead to low-flow priapism.
   a) Sickle cell, Spinal cord injury, Leukemia, Prostate cancer, Groin trauma, and Medications (Sildenafil or Antidepressants)
3430) List the treatment options for low flow priapism.
   a) Corporeal aspiration, Phenylephrine penile injection, or Terbutaline subcutaneous injection
3431) What locations do you perform a penile block at the base of the penis?
   a) 10 o'clock and 2 o'clock, or 12 o'clock

3432) What anatomical location of the penis do you perform drainage or flushing of the blood in low flow priapism to avoid a vascular infiltration or injury?
a) Corpus cavernosum at the 10 and 2 o'clock positions

3433) What is the treatment for high flow priapism?
a) Embolization or Surgery

3434) What emergency renal condition needs to be worked up in a post-renal transplant patient 1-2 weeks out with tenderness over the graft, decreased urine output, low-grade fever, and malaise?
a) Acute graft rejection

3435) What is the time frame to diagnose hyperacute rejection?
a) 1-2 days post-transplant

3436) What are the treatments for acute and hyperacute rejections?
a) Glucocorticoids and OKT3

3437) Rise of what specific test from baseline can indicate renal transplant rejection?
a) Creatinine

3438) What is the most common infectious cause of life-threatening infections in transplant patients?
a) Cytomegalovirus (CMV)

3439) What is the most important side effect to know about Cyclosporine that is commonly used in transplant patients?
a) Renal insufficiency

3440) What bacteria commonly cause infections immediately following an organ transplant?
a) Staph, Strep, and E.coli

3441) What scrotal emergency presents with an acute onset of a hard, painful, elevated, swollen, erythematous testicle?
a) Testicular torsion

3442) What direction is the most common in testicular torsion?
a) Medially

3443) What method of de-torsion may be used in the emergency department before surgical reduction for testicular torsion?
a) Open book reduction (medial-lateral)

3444) Presence of what specific clinical test on the physical exam can be used to rule out testicular torsion?
a) Cremaster reflex (stroke inner thigh)

3445) What congenital deformity leads to an increased risk of testicular torsion?
   a) Bell-clapper (improper anchoring of the testicle)
3446) Can a patient have recurrent or intermittent episodes of testicular torsion with spontaneous resolution?
   a) Yes
3447) What is the recommendation for intermittent testicular torsion?
   a) Urology consult for elective orchiopexy
3448) What imaging modality is used to help diagnose a testicular torsion and is suggested with the absence of arterial flow?
   a) Color Doppler ultrasound
3449) What is the treatment for testicular torsion?
   a) Surgical bilateral orchiopexy
3450) What is the time frame for surgical reduction for testicular torsion?
   a) < 6 hours
3451) Torsion of what testicular structure can mimic testicular torsion and is recognized by the pathognomonic "blue dot" sign on trans-illumination?
   a) Testicular appendage torsion
3452) How is a torsed testis appendix treated?
   a) Analgesics and Bedrest
3453) What scrotal infection can mimic testicular torsion and presents with gradual scrotal swelling, pain, dysuria, and has relief of pain with testicle elevation?
   a) Epididymitis
3454) What is the finding on scrotal Doppler ultrasound with epididymitis?
   a) Increased flow in the epididymis
3455) What clinical exam sign helps relieve pain by elevating the testicle in epididymitis?
   a) Prehn's sign
3456) What is the most common cause of epididymitis in patients < 35 years old?
   a) STDs (Gonorrhea & Chlamydia)
3457) What bacteria typically cause epididymitis in > 35 years old?

a) E. coli, Pseudomonas, and Gram-positive bacteria

3458) What scrotal infection can mimic testicular torsion and presents with a hard testicle, scrotal swelling, pain, dysuria, and mild relief of pain with testicle elevation?

a) Orchitis

3459) What is the finding on scrotal Doppler ultrasound with orchitis?

a) Increased blood flow in the testicle

3460) What is the management for epididymitis and orchitis?

a) Scrotal elevation, Analgesics, and Antibiotics (cover for STDs and E. coli)

3461) What is the recommended way to remove a zipper with groin anatomy stuck in the zipper?

a) Cut the median bar

3462) What scrotal venous abnormality can also mimic testicular torsion and presents with painful swollen scrotal veins like a "bag of worms" and is more commonly on the left side?

a) Varicocele

3463) Why are varicoceles more common on the left?

a) Due to the angle of the testicular vein

3464) What cyst-like structure can develop in the epididymis and causes pain?

a) Spermatocele

3465) What type of scrotal swelling is a non-tender fluid collection around the testicle that develops gradually, and can be transparent on the light illumination exam?

a) Hydrocele

3466) Where does the fluid collect in a hydrocele?

a) In the tunica vaginalis

3467) What anatomical defect leads to a pediatric hydrocele?

a) Patent tunica vaginalis

3468) What post-void residual volume of retained urine seen a bladder scan suggests urinary retention?

a) > 50 – 100 mL

3469) What is the most common cause of urinary retention in an adult male?

a) Benign prostate hypertrophy (BPH)

3470) List drugs that can lead to urinary retention.

a) Anticholinergic, Sympathomimetic, Antihypertensive, and Opioid medications

3471) What is the ED workup for overflow incontinence or urinary retention?
a) Post void residual testing, U/A, BMP, and Medication review

3472) What is the treatment urinary retention in the ED?
a) Place a Foley catheter, Urology referral, and +/- Antibiotics (for UTI)

3473) What medical condition can lead to renal failure from muscle breakdown products like myoglobin, and is diagnosed with elevated creatinine kinase levels > 5x the normal limit?
a) Rhabdomyolysis

3474) List the conditions that lead to rhabdomyolysis.
a) Seizures (status epilepticus), Trauma (crush injury), Drug use (cocaine, meth, MDMA, & heroin), Statins, Dehydration (severe), and Excessive muscle use (i.e. lifting, marathons)

3475) What is the treatment for rhabdomyolysis?
a) IV Hydration, Urine alkalization, and +/- Admission or Nephrology consult

3476) What medication can be given to alkalinize the urine to prevent kidney injury in rhabdomyolysis with renal failure?
a) Bicarbonate

3477) What is the target urine output during treatment for rhabdomyolysis?
a) 3 mL/kg/hr or about 200 mL/hr

3478) What is the number one treatment for IV contrast-induced nephropathies?
a) IV Fluids

3479) What are the treatment options in the ED for urine urgency and frequency?
a) Anticholinergics and Urology referral (bladder stimulation or Botox injections)

3480) What is the treatment for bladder spasms?
a) Oxybutynin

Environmental

3481) In order of anatomical depth name the three zones of a burn?
   a) Hyperemia, Stasis, and Coagulation
3482) What method of calculating the percentage of total body surface area burned is used for a quick estimation?
   a) Wallace rule of nines
3483) Give the rule of nines per body area on the adult body.
   a) Head-9%, Trunk-18%, Back-18%, Arm-9%, Leg-18% , Genitalia-1%
3484) Give the rule of nines per body area on the children's body.
   a) Head-17%, Trunk-13%, Back-13%, Arm-19%, Leg-13% , Genitalia-1%
3485) Give the rule of nines per body area on the infant's body.
   a) Head-18%, Trunk-18%, Back-18%, Arm-9%, Leg-14% , Genitalia-1%
3486) What is the percentage area of the back of a patient's hand generally equivalent to when estimating total body surface area with a burn?
   a) 1%
3487) What burn diagram can give a more precise estimation of the percentage of area burned than the estimated rule of nines?
   a) Lund and Browder diagram
3488) Which degree of burn involves the epidermal layer and red painful skin without blisters?
   a) 1st degree
3489) Which degree of burn involves the epidermis and superficial dermis, has skin blisters, and is painful?
   a) 2nd degree Superficial partial-thickness
3490) Which degree of burn involves the deep dermis, has skin blisters, pale white skin, and is absent of pain?
   a) 2nd degree Deep partial-thickness
3491) Which degree of burn is a full-thickness burn through the epidermal and dermal layers, appears charred, pale, painless, and leathery?
   a) 3rd degree

3492) Which degree of burn is a full-thickness burn extending deep into the fat, muscle and bone and is life-threatening?
   a) 4th degree
3493) List the burn center referral criteria.
   a) 2nd-degree partial thickness > 10%, Burns to (Feet, Hand, Genitalia), Circumferential burns, Burns over large joints, 3rd-degree burns, Electrical, Chemical inhalation burns, and Burns with trauma
3494) Name the adult formula and equation used for fluid resuscitation in 2nd and 3rd-degree burn patients.
   a) Parkland formula: 4ml x wt. (kg) x % BSA
3495) Give the pediatric parkland equation used for fluid resuscitation.
   a) 3ml x wt. (kg) x % BSA + Maintenance
3496) How much fluid from the parkland formula is to be given over the first 8 hours?
   a) Half in the first 8 hours (use "remaining" over the next 16 hours)
3497) Which antibiotics are used for 2nd and 3rd-degree burns?
   a) Silvadene or Bacitracin
3498) What axis do you cut for performing an escharotomy?
   a) Long axis sides
3499) What is the treatment for elemental metal burns?
   a) Cover with Mineral Oil
3500) What are the proper steps of decontamination and removing lime or cement powder on the skin of a patient?
   a) Brush off then irrigate
3501) What is the most common arrhythmia seen in lightning strikes?
   a) Asystole
3502) List common complications from lightning strikes.
   a) TM rupture, Cataracts, and Skin burns (ferning)
3503) What pathognomonic skin burn is seen with lightning strikes?
   a) Lichtenberg ferning/feathering
3504) What type of trauma triage is needed for a lightning mass casualty event?
   a) Reverse triage (sickest patients first i.e. black))

3505) What type of electric current causes more extensive injuries AC or DC?

a) AC

3506) What complication is seen with an electric oral commissure burn?

a) Delayed labial artery bleed

3507) What is the treatment plan for a labial artery bleed from a mouth burn?

a) Stop the bleed, Discharge, and Plastics referral

3508) What degree of hypothermia causes lethargy, confusion, shivering, and ataxia with temperatures 32°-35° C (90°-95° F)?

a) Mild

3509) What degree of hypothermia causes delirium, bradycardia, no shivering, and CNS depression, with temperatures 28°-32° C (82°-90° F)?

a) Moderate

3510) What degree of hypothermia causes coma, dysrhythmias, areflexia, apnea, fixed pupils, and an absent pulse with temperatures < 28° C (< 82° F)?

a) Severe

3511) What is the complication of antidiuretic hormone inhibition (ADH) with severe hypothermia?

a) Cold diuresis

3512) List types of external rewarming for hypothermia treatment.

a) Removing wet clothes, Drying skin, Heat room, Immersion, and a Heating blanket

3513) List the different methods for internal core rewarming.

a) Heated oxygen, Heated IV fluids through Gastric, Bladder or Thoracic lavage, or Cardiopulmonary bypass

3514) At what temperature does V. fibrillation become refractory to electric shock in cardiac arrest?

a) < 30° C (86° F)

3515) What type of frostbite is defined by superficial erythema, numbness, and edema?

a) 1st degree

3516) What type of frostbite is defined by superficial erythema, edema, and clear superficial blisters?

a) 2nd degree

3517) What type of frostbite is defined by erythema with deep hemorrhagic blisters?

a) 3rd degree

3518) What type of frostbite is defined by deep injury to the subcutaneous tissues, muscle, and bone?

a) 4th degree

3519) What is the recommended range water temperature is supposed to be for immersion rewarming with circulating water used for frostbite?

a) 40°-42° C

3520) What cold injury is associated with a pail, mottled, pulseless, wet foot that leads to cold insensitivity, and hyperhidrosis?

a) Trench foot

3521) What cold injury is seen with painful inflamed skin, and is due to chronic exposure to wet or damp environments and cold temperatures?

a) Chilblains

3522) What medical treatments are used for Chilblains?

a) Nifedipine, Steroids, and Pentoxifylline

3523) What is the pathognomonic ECG finding seen with hypothermia < 32° C?

a) J-wave (Osborn Wave)

3524) Which syndrome is from sudden and unexpected immersion in water with temperatures < 15° C, causing syncope from a dysrhythmia and leads to more deaths than hypothermia?

a) Coldwater immersion syndrome (Cold-water shock)

3525) Name the four types of heat loss.

a) Radiation
b) Convection
c) Conduction
d) Evaporation

3526) What type of heat loss is the most efficient in humans?

a) Evaporation

3527) What is the primary mechanism of heat loss in a cold environment?

a) Radiation

3528) What type of heat injury causes painful spasmodic muscle after exercise with dehydration?
   a) Heat cramps
3529) What is the treatment of heat edema?
   a) Self-limited
3530) What is the treatment for heat rash "prickly heat"?
   a) Antihistamine
3531) What type of heat injury is defined by headache, weakness, nausea, syncope, tachycardia, sweating, and hypotension?
   a) Heat exhaustion
3532) What is the recommended treatment for heat exhaustion?
   a) Hydration, Cool environment, Rest, and Fanning
3533) What type of heat injury is associated with temperature > 104° F, tachycardia, hypotension, hyperventilation, coma, sweating that stops, and has a high mortality rate?
   a) Heatstroke
3534) What is the target temperature goal for cooling in a patient with heatstroke?
   a) 39° C (0.2° C/min)
3535) What complications can develop from heatstroke?
   a) Encephalopathy, Rhabdomyolysis, Renal failure, ARDS, Liver failure, Hyperkalemia, and MI
3536) What are the treatments used to decrease the body temperature in heatstroke?
   a) Fanning, Cool water immersion, IV Hydration, and Ice pack application
3537) What is the treatment of pit viper and coral snake bites in a patient with systemic symptoms?
   a) Antivenin (CroFab)
3538) What are the side effects that you need to know about with antivenin use?
   a) Anaphylaxis, Serum sickness, and Fever
3539) List symptoms associated with a pit viper bite.
   a) Pain, Burning, Numbness, Nausea, Vomiting, DIC, Cardiovascular, and Vascular Collapse

3540) What snake is black with red on yellow stripes, is seen in the south, and its toxin causes respiratory failure and weakness through inhibiting acetylcholine receptors at the neuromuscular junction?
   a) Coral snake
3541) Which spider bite is painful, has the latrotoxin, and leads to painful muscle rigidity, abdominal pain, and hypertension?
   a) Black widow spider
3542) What are the treatments for a black widow spider bite?
   a) Benzodiazepines and +/- Antivenom
3543) What spider bite is painless and leads to a delayed skin reaction and large ulcer lesion?
   a) Brown recluse
3544) What treatments can be used for a scorpion sting?
   a) Benzodiazepines and Atropine for bradycardia
3545) What type of scorpion sting causes pathognomonic roving eye movements and muscle jerks?
   a) Bark scorpion centruroides
3546) What is the treatment for a stonefish, lionfish, turkey fish, and zebrafish sting?
   a) Hot water rinse
3547) What is the treatment of a stingray sting?
   a) Hot water rinse
3548) What is the treatment for jellyfish, sea anemones, and coral stings?
   a) Remove nematocysts and Rinse with seawater
3549) Which type of jellyfish is the deadliest in the world and treatment requires antivenin?
   a) Box jellyfish (Chironex)
3550) What syndrome develops after a Carukia jellyfish sting and consists of hypertension, tachycardia, pain, and diaphoresis?
   a) Irukandji syndrome
3551) What type of infection develops painful marginated plaques after handling fish?
   a) Erysipelothrix

3552) What diving complication leads to altered mental status, loss of consciousness, headache, vision changes and sudden death within 10 minutes after rapid ascent?

a) Arterial gas embolus

3553) What is the treatment for an arterial gas embolus?

a) Hyperbaric therapy

3554) Which diving complication is from a blocked Eustachian tube and leads to a ruptured TM, vertigo, and facial nerve palsy while descending?

a) Middle ear barotrauma (middle ear squeeze)

3555) Which type of barotrauma is caused by the squeeze of the facemask on decent?

a) Facial barotrauma

3556) What is the most common type of barotrauma on decent?

a) Middle ear squeeze

3557) Which diving complication is from the development of nitrogen in the blood, and causes muscle and joint pains, cutis marmorata, weakness, and headache?

a) Decompression syndrome (DCS)

3558) How many types of DCS are there?

a) 3

3559) What type of DCS can have air bubbles in the urinary system or spinal cord and causes CNS symptoms and a severe cough "the chokes"?

a) Type 2 DCS

3560) What is the definitive treatment of DCS?

a) Hyperbaric therapy

3561) What are the risk factors for DCS?"

a) Fast ascent, obesity, deep diving, alcohol use, and flying within 24 hours of diving.

3562) What diving condition can present with dives > 100 ft. and altered mental status?

a) Nitrogen narcosis

3563) What is the treatment of nitrogen narcosis?

a) Ascent

3564)   What condition causes nausea, headaches, decreased appetite, and fatigue in a patient who recently traveled to a high altitude for a skiing trip?
   a)   Acute mountain sickness (AMS)
3565)   What is the treatment for mild AMS?
   a)   Hold ascent
3566)   List the treatment options for moderate AMS with nausea, vomiting, headache, fatigue, and insomnia?
   a)   Oxygen
   b)   Acetazolamide
   c)   Dexamethasone
   d)   Descent
3567)   What medications can you give to prevent AMS for someone traveling?
   a)   Acetazolamide or Dexamethasone
3568)   What type of altitude sickness causes confusion, altered mental status, seizures, and vision changes due to retinal hemorrhages?
   a)   High altitude cerebral edema (HACE)
3569)   What is the first-line treatment for HACE?
   a)   Decent
3570)   What are the other treatment options for HACE after decent?
   a)   Diuretics and Oxygen
3571)   Which type of altitude sickness causes severe dyspnea, altered mental status, and possible fever?
   a)   High altitude pulmonary edema (HAPE)
3572)   What is the first-line treatment for HAPE?
   a)   Decent
3573)   What are the other treatments are used for HAPE after decent?
   a)   Diuretics, Nifedipine, and Oxygen
3574)   What is the treatment for a tetanus infection?
   a)   Antibiotics, Tetanus Immune globin, and active immunization
3575)   How do you treat bee and wasp stings?
   a)   Remove the stinger, H-2 blocker, Steroids, and Benadryl
3576)   What is the cold water reflex called with bradycardia, apnea, and shunting of blood to CNS during a cold water immersion?
   a)   Mammalian diving reflex

3577) What is the number one thing to do in a diving/ drowning accident after securing ABC's?
   a) Secure C-spine
3578) List the three types of radiation.
   a) α (alpha), β (beta), and γ (gamma)
3579) What type of radiation is the most lethal?
   a) γ (gamma)
3580) What is the most common source of gamma radiation exposure?
   a) X-rays
3581) What type of particles are alpha (α) and beta (β) radiation types?
   a) Alpha: Neutrons
   b) Beta: Electrons
3582) What is the median lethal dose of radiation exposure?
   a) 4.5 Gy
3583) How many rads are in 1 Gy?
   a) 100 rads
3584) When determining radiation dosing how many Sieverts (Sv) are in a Gray (Gy) and Rems in a Rad?
   a) 1 Sv = 1 Gy
   b) 1 Rem = 1 Rad
3585) What amount of radiation exposure in Grays (Gy) can manifest cutaneous, hematopoietic, gastrointestinal and neurovascular syndromes?
   a) Cutaneous: < 2 Gy
   b) Hematopoietic: > 2 Gy
   c) Gastrointestinal: > 6 Gy
   d) Neurovascular: > 20 Gy
3586) What are the different phases of radiation syndrome?
   a) 1st: Prodromal (nausea, vomiting, diarrhea)
   b) 2nd: Latent (symptoms free)
   c) 3rd: Manifest illness
   d) 4th: Death phase
3587) What are the first symptoms of acute radiation sickness?
   a) Nausea and Vomiting
3588) What is the first cell damaged with radiation exposure?
   a) Lymphocytes

3589) What lab test do we follow for radiation sickness at 48 hours?
   a) Absolute lymphocyte count
3590) What absolute lymphocyte count levels indicate a good and poor prognosis, and an increased risk of death in acute radiation syndrome?
   a) Death: < 300
   b) Poor prognosis: < 500
   c) Good prognosis: >1200
3591) What type of skin condition can develop with acute radiation syndrome from a large dose of radiation exposure?
   a) Radiation cutaneous syndrome
3592) What type of biologic toxin is a cytotoxin from castor beans, and causes cough, fever, and pulmonary hemorrhage?
   a) Ricin
3593) What symptoms can nerve agents such as Sarin, VX, and Soman cause?
   a) Salivation, Lacrimation, Urination, Defecation, Emesis, and Miosis
3594) What are the 1st and 2nd line treatments for the neuromuscular toxicity from Sarin, VX, and Soman?
   a) 1st line: Atropine (initial dosing 2mg)
   b) 2nd line: 2-PAM (initial dosing 600mg)
3595) What is the time period required for antidote administration for Sarin poisoning?
   a) Within 5 hours
3596) What is the time period required for antidote administration for Soman poisoning?
   a) Within 5 min
3597) What type of vesicant gas used in World War I can cause necrotic blisters on the skin and in the lungs?
   a) Mustard gas
3598) What is the treatment of an exposure of the biochemical Benzilate (BZ) causing vision disturbance, dehydration, and AMS?
   a) Physostigmine
3599) What is the treatment for a symptomatic patient with a chlorine exposure?
   a) Supportive

3600) What gas should be suspected in a family presenting with flu-like symptoms, nausea, and headaches during the winter?
a) Carbon monoxide (CO)

3601) Does the pulse oxygenation drop with carbon monoxide poisoning?
a) No

3602) What causes the dysfunction of hemoglobin in CO poisoning?
a) Increased affinity for oxygen by COHgb

3603) What way does the oxygen dissociation curve shift with carbon monoxide poisoning
a) Left

3604) How is carbon monoxide poisoning diagnosed?
a) COHgb level

3605) What is the recommended treatment for mild to moderate carbon monoxide poisoning?
a) 100% oxygen

3606) What chemical exposure can cause delayed carbon monoxide poisoning?
a) Methylene chloride

3607) List the criteria for hyperbaric chamber treatment in carbon monoxide poisoning.
a) Neurological deficits
b) Loss of consciousness
c) Coma
d) Ischemic EKG changes
e) MI
f) CO levels greater than 25%
g) Pregnant patient with CO level > 15%

3608) How long do the symptoms of ophthalmic burning, coughing, and tearing from pepper spray typically last?
a) 15 minutes

3609) What precautions should be taken to treat and clean up exposures to the T2-Mycotoxin fungus that is toxic to humans and animals, and causes, skin burns, coughing, vomiting, and vision changes?
a) Hazmat clean up

Endocrine

3610) Name the anion gap formula.
   a) Anion gap (AG)= Na^+- (Cl + HCO3)
3611) What is the normal range of an anion gap?
   a) 8-12
3612) Name the causes of an anion gap acidosis that make up the pneumonic "MUDPILES".
   a) Methanol, Uremia, DKA, Paraldehyde, (Iron, Isoniazid, Inhalants), Ethanol/Ethylene, and Salicylates
3613) What is the most common cause of metabolic acidosis?
   a) Lactic acidosis
3614) List causes of HCO3 losses that can cause a non-anion gap acidosis.
   a) **HARDUP:** Hypoaldosteronism, Acetazolamide, Addison's disease, Proximal renal tubular acidosis, Diarrhea, Uretosigmoidostomy, and Pancreatic fistula
3615) How do you calculate the osmolar gap (OG)?
   a) OG=2(Na^+) + BUN/2.8 + Glucose/18
3616) What is the normal OG range and gap?
   a) 280-295 (15)
3617) Name some causes of a wide OG.
   a) Isopropyl alcohol, Methanol, Ethanol, Ethylene glycol, Uremia, Mannitol, and Glycerol,
3618) What etiologies can lead to respiratory alkalosis (decreased PaCO2)?
   a) Anxiety, CNS disease, Metabolic acidosis, Pain, and Hypermetabolic state
3619) What etiologies can lead to a metabolic alkalosis?
   a) NG suctioning, Vomiting, and Dehydration (contraction alkalosis)
3620) What electrolyte abnormities can occur from vomiting?
   a) Hypochloremia and Hypokalemia
3621) What are the early and late symptoms of hyponatremia?
   a) Early: Nausea, Headache
   b) Late: Lethargy, Seizures

3622) At what sodium level do symptoms from hyponatremia typically occur?
　　a) < 130 mEq/L (severe < 120 mEq/L)
3623) List the three classifications of hyponatremia.
　　a) Hypovolemic, Hypervolemic, and Euvolemic
3624) List the causes of hypovolemic hyponatremia.
　　a) Na^+ loss > free water loss, Vomiting, Diarrhea, Burns, Pancreatitis, and Renal losses
3625) What is the treatment used for hypovolemic hyponatremia?
　　a) Normal saline
3626) List a differential for the causes of hypervolemic hyponatremia.
　　a) CHF, Liver cirrhosis, Decreased free water losses, Nephrotic syndrome, and Renal failure
3627) What are the treatments used for hypervolemic hyponatremia?
　　a) Salt and water restriction, Diuretics, and Dialysis
3628) List a differential for the causes of euvolemic hyponatremia.
　　a) SIADH, Psychogenic polydipsia, and Hypothyroidism
3629) What is the treatment used for euvolemic hyponatremia?
　　a) Water restriction
3630) What conditions can cause pseudohyponatremia?
　　a) Hyperglycemia, Hyperproteinemia, and Hypertriglyceridemia
3631) What type of fluids are used for the treatment of severe hyponatremia (<120) with seizures?
　　a) 3% NaCl (rate (mL/hr) = weight (kg) / 2)
3632) What is the target goal of Na^+ correction in hyponatremia?
　　a) 0.5-1 mEq/L/hr, max 12 mEq/day
3633) What is a delayed complication caused by rapid correction of hyponatremia?
　　a) Osmotic demyelination syndrome / Central pontine myelinolysis
3634) What is the most common cause of hypernatremia?
　　a) Dehydration
3635) At what sodium level do symptoms from hypernatremia typically occur?
　　a) > 150 mEq/L
3636) What are symptoms of hypernatremia?

a) Spasticity, Vomiting, Lethargy, Coma, and Seizures

3637) What is the maximum amount of sodium reduction in 24 hours when treating hypernatremia?

a) 10 mEq/L

3638) What CNS complication can occur with rapid correction of hypernatremia?

a) Cerebral edema

3639) Give the calculation for determining a free water deficit (FWD).

a) FWD = (measured [Na^+]/desired [Na^+]) -1

3640) What is the calculation for total body water (TBW)?

a) Kg x 0.6

3641) Give the calculation for total body water deficit.

a) Deficit in liters = TBW (1-[140/current sodium])

3642) How much do the sodium levels generally increase with each liter of free water deficit in hypernatremia?

a) 3-5 meq

3643) What is the treatment for hypernatremia?

a) Fluid administration (1/2 NS), Free water deficit replacement, and Diuretics (if hypervolemic)

3644) What autosomal dominant electrolyte condition can lead to rapidly progressing extremity weakness, that resolves over time, and is commonly seen in young males?

a) Hypokalemic periodic paralysis

3645) What is the most common electrolyte abnormality that causes weakness?

a) Hypokalemia

3646) At what level of hypokalemia do symptoms such as weakness, fatigue, paresthesias, dysrhythmias, ileus, and cramps typically occur?

a) < 2.5 mEq/L

3647) What ECG changes are seen with hypokalemia?

a) PVC's, PAC's, Decreased T waves, U waves, ST-segment depressions, and Dysrhythmias

3648) What electrolyte abnormality is often associated with hypokalemia?

a) Hypomagnesemia

3649) List the treatment for hypokalemia.

a) Oral replacement before IV, and correct acid-base abnormalities

3650) What is the fastest rate K⁺ can be given IV without a central line?

a) 10 mEq/hr

3651) How much is the potassium level expected to increase in acute hypokalemia per 10 mEq/L of potassium given?

a) 0.1 mEq/L per 10 mEq dose given

3652) What ECG changes are seen with hyperkalemia?

a) Peaked T waves, Wide QRS, Flat P waves, Prolonged PR, QRS and QT intervals

3653) What ECG change is significant for very high levels of potassium?

a) Sign waves due to a widened QRS

3654) List causes of hyperkalemia.

a) Hemolysis, Renal failure, Digoxin toxicity, Acidosis, Rhabdomyolysis, Spironolactone, and Increase intake

3655) What is the most common cause of hyperkalemia?

a) Lab error from hemolysis (REPEAT LABS)

3656) List the medical treatments used to treat hyperkalemia.

a) CBIGK: Calcium gluconate, Calcium chloride, Bicarbonate (fastest), B-agonist (albuterol) Insulin and Glucose (D50), and Kayexalate

3657) What treatment is recommended for refractory hyperkalemia or severe hyperkalemia with renal failure?

a) Dialysis

3658) What treatment for hyperkalemia should you avoid in hyperkalemia with digoxin toxicity?

a) Calcium

3659) List the causes of hypercalcemia.

a) Hyperparathyroidism, Addison's, Multiple myeloma, Paget's disease, Sarcoidosis, Thiazide diuretics, Vitamin D, or Milk alkali syndrome

3660) What is the most common cause of hypercalcemia?

a) Hyperparathyroidism

3661) List the equation for calcium correction in hypoalbuminemia.

a) Corrected Ca$^+$ = [0.8 x (NL albumin- Pt albumin)] = serum Ca$^+$

3662) What ECG changes are seen with hypercalcemia?

   a) Shortened QT, Bundle branch block, or Heart block

3663) List the symptoms caused by hypercalcemia.

   a) Kidney stones, Polyuria, Altered mental status, Abdominal pain, Bone pain, Hyporeflexia, and Constipation

3664) What are the treatments for hypercalcemia?

   a) IV Normal saline first, then Loop diuretics (Lasix), Bisphosphonates, or Dialysis

3665) List the causes of hypocalcemia.

   a) Hypoparathyroidism, Renal failure, Vitamin D deficiency, Drugs, Digeorge syndrome, Hypomagnesemia, and Pancreatitis

3666) What signs and symptoms can be seen with hypocalcemia?

   a) Paresthesias, Hyperreflexia, Seizures, Carpal spasms, and Facial spasms

3667) Name the physical exam finding associated with hypocalcemia that is twitching of the corner of the mouth while tapping the facial nerve.

   a) Chvostek's sign

3668) Name the physical exam finding associated with hypocalcemia that is a carpal spasm that occurs when the BP cuff is inflated.

   a) Trousseau's sign

3669) What ECG changes are seen with hypocalcemia?

   a) Prolonged QT and Flattened T waves

3670) What is the treatment for hypocalcemia?

   a) Calcium gluconate, Magnesium, and Stop loop diuretics

3671) What electrolyte disorder is primarily caused by renal failure or ingestion, and leads to weakness, hyporeflexia, respiratory depression, and heart blocks?

   a) Hypermagnesemia

3672) List the treatments used for hypermagnesemia.

   a) IV Calcium +/- Dialysis

3673) What conditions can lead to hypomagnesemia?

   a) Alcoholism, Malnutrition, and Diuretics

3674) What is the most common cause of hypomagnesemia?

   a) Alcoholism

3675) What is the relationship between calcium and phosphorus during renal resorption?
   a) Inverse: ↑Ca⁺ → ↓Phosphate; ↓Ca⁺ → ↑Phosphate

3676) What hormone regulates absorption of Ca⁺ and phosphorus?
   a) Parathyroid hormone (PTH)

3677) What is the treatment of hyperphosphatemia?
   a) Oral phosphate-binding gel

3678) What level of glucose defines hypoglycemia in adults, pediatrics, and infants?
   a) Adult: < 60
   b) Pediatrics: < 60
   c) Infants: < 50

3679) What symptoms can be seen with hypoglycemia?
   a) Sweating, Tremor, Nausea, Confusion, Coma, and Seizure

3680) What lab test can be ordered to distinguish endogenous vs exogenous insulin causing hypoglycemia?
   a) C-peptide (↑ with endogenous insulin)

3681) List the IV glucose solution treatments for hypoglycemia for each of the adult, pediatric, and neonate patients.
   a) Adults: D50
   b) Pediatrics: D25
   c) Neonates: D10

3682) What medication can be administered for hypoglycemia if there is no IV established?
   a) Intramuscular Glucagon

3683) What medication can be used to treat sulfonylurea inducece hypoglycemia ?
   a) Octreotide

3684) What care plan is needed for hypoglycemia in a patient on long-acting hypoglycemic agents such as a sulfonylurea and Repaglinide?
   a) D10 drip and Observation

3685) What diabetic medication can cause lactic acidosis after IV dye administration?
   a) Metformin

3686) What medication should be given in alcoholics or malnourished patients before giving glucose to prevent Wernicke's encephalopathy?

    a) Thiamine

3687) What type of diabetic emergency is seen in type 1 diabetics with, dehydration, and blood glucose> 250?

    a) Diabetic ketoacidosis (DKA)

3688) What is the specific type of compensatory hyperventilation seen in DKA?

    a) Kussmaul breathing

3689) What is the major ketone produced from the fat breakdown that can help with the diagnosis of DKA?

    a) Beta-hydroxybutyrate (but only acetoacetate is measured)

3690) What type of diabetic emergency is seen in type 2 diabetics with coma, confusion, dehydration, and blood glucose between 500-1000?

    a) Hyperosmolar hyperglycemic state (HHS) previously known as Hyperosmolar hyperglycemic nonketotic syndrome (HHNK)

3691) What are some medication conditions that lead to DKA and HHS?

    a) Noncompliance of insulin, Infections, MI, CVA, Trauma, Pancreatitis, Dehydration, and Hyperthyroidism

3692) What is the primary treatment for DKA and HHNS?

    a) IV regular insulin drip, IV hydration, +/- Antibiotics for infection

3693) What is the dosing for IV insulin infusion for DKA and HHNS?

    a) 0.1 units/kg/hr

3694) What CNS abnormality can occur with too much fluid administration in DKA/HHS and is more commonly seen in pediatrics?

    a) Cerebral edema

3695) What types of electrolyte abnormalities can be seen in DKA and HHS?

    a) Hypokalemia, Hypophosphatemia, and Pseudohyponatremia

3696) What is the calculation for the corrected sodium with hyperglycemia?

    a) Add 1.6 mEq/L for every 100 mg/dl increase of glucose over 100

3697) Why should you give potassium before starting the insulin drip when the level is between 3-5 mEq/L?

a) Because insulin drives K into cells

3698) Can binge drinking and alcohol abuse cause starvation ketoacidosis?

a) Yes

3699) What is beer potomania?

a) Hypo-osmolality syndrome causing hyponatremia

3700) What is the treatment for alcoholic ketoacidosis?

a) Dextrose 5% + Normal saline, Thiamine, and +/- Potassium

3701) What is the most common cause of hyperthyroidism?

a) Graves' disease

3702) List causes of hyperthyroidism.

a) Grave's disease, Toxic thyroid adenoma, Thyroiditis, Pituitary adenoma, or Excess iodine

3703) What is the most common cause of hyperthyroidism?

a) Graves' disease

3704) List the symptoms for hyperthyroidism.

a) Anxiety, Sweating, Diarrhea, Tachycardia, Thyroid bruit, Exophthalmos, Lid lag, Weight loss, Hair loss, and Pretibial myxedema

3705) Describe pretibial myxedema seen in hyperthyroidism.

a) Bilateral elevated yellow waxy dermal nodules

3706) What are the TSH, T_3 and T_4 lab abnormalities to diagnose hyperthyroidism?

a) ↓TSH, with ↑T_3 and T_4,

3707) What life-threatening condition can result from uncontrolled hyperthyroidism, and presents with sudden onset tachycardia, hyperthermia, anxiety, disorientation, and diaphoresis?

a) Thyroid storm

3708) What are the medical treatments for thyroid storm and hyperthyroidism?

a) IVF + Beta-blockers (Propranolol) 1st, then PTU or Methimazole, Lugol's solution (iodine), Lithium (if iodine allergy), Reserpine (if propanol resistant), and Radioactive iodine

3709) What medication should be given first for tachycardia due to hyperthyroidism?
   a) Beta-blocker (Propranolol)
3710) Which medications used for hyperthyroidism and thyroid storm prevent the production of TSH?
   a) PTU and Methimazole
3711) Which medications used for hyperthyroidism and thyroid storm block the peripheral effects and conversion of T4 to T3?
   a) Propranolol or Reserpine
3712) Which medications used for hyperthyroidism and thyroid storm inhibit the release of T3 and T4?
   a) Iodine, Lugol's solution, and Lithium
3713) List the causes of hypothyroidism.
   a) Hashimoto's, Treatment of Graves' disease (radioblation/thyroidectomy), Iodine deficiency, Lithium, Amiodarone, and Pituitary disorder.
3714) List the symptoms of hypothyroidism.
   a) Weakness, Cold intolerance, Hypothermia, Weight gain, Dry skin, Myxedema, and Heavy periods
3715) What is the most common cause of hypothyroidism?
   a) Hashimoto's disease
3716) What are the TSH, T_3, and T_4 lab abnormalities to diagnose hypothyroidism?
   a) ↑TSH with ↓ T_3 and T_4
3717) What is the life-threatening condition seen with untreated hypothyroidism, with hypothermia, altered mental status, hypotension, bradycardia, hypoglycemia, and generalized non-pitting periorbital edema?
   a) Myxedema Coma
3718) List precipitating factors of myxedema coma.
   a) Infections, trauma, sedation, MI, CVA, and Cold exposure
3719) What is the treatment for myxedema coma?
   a) IV T_4 (levothyroxine), IV T_3 (liothyronine), Rewarming, and Steroids
3720) What hormone in the adrenal gland effects Na resorption and K excretion?

a) Aldosterone

3721) What disease causes primary adrenal failure, hyponatremia, hyperkalemia, fever, hypotension, dehydration, and vomiting?
a) Addison's disease

3722) What skin condition can be seen in Addison's disease?
a) Hyperpigmentation (due to ACTH)

3723) What two hormones are lacking in primary adrenal insufficiency?
a) Cortisol and Aldosterone

3724) What is the most common cause of primary adrenal insufficiency worldwide?
a) Tuberculosis

3725) What is the most common cause of adrenal insufficiency in the US?
a) Steroid withdrawal

3726) What bacteria causes meningitis and can lead to bilateral adrenal failure?
a) Neisseria meningitidis

3727) What lab do you order to help diagnose adrenal failure?
a) Serum cortisol level or Corticotropin stimulation test

3728) What is the medical treatment for adrenal crisis (insufficiency)?
a) Dextrose 5% with Normal saline and Hydrocortisone

3729) What condition is caused by excess cortisol, and causes truncal obesity, hirsutism, moon facies, buffalo hump, and purple striae?
a) Cushing syndrome

3730) List causes of Cushing syndrome.
a) Prolonged steroid use, Adrenal neoplasms, ACTH secreting carcinomas or pituitary tumors

3731) What syndrome due to excessive ADH secretion, causes polydipsia, fluid retention, and dilutional hyponatremia?
a) Syndrome of Inappropriate secretion of Antidiuretic Hormone (SIADH)

3732) What serum and urine abnormalities are seen with SIADH?
a) Serum: Hypoosmolar (euvolemic)
b) Urine: Hyperosmolar (concentrated)

3733) What medication can be given to decrease the free water from fluid overload in the treatment of SIADH?
   a) Furosemide
3734) List the two types of Diabetes insipidus (DI) from the lack of ADH activity.
   a) Central and Nephrogenic
3735) What urine abnormalities are seen with DI?
   a) Dilute urine
3736) What type of DI is due to a failure to secrete ADH, and can be seen with cranial neoplasms, and after head trauma or pituitary surgery?
   a) Central
3737) What is the treatment of central DI?
   a) Desmopressin (DDAVP)
3738) What is the pathophysiologic problem that causes nephrogenic DI?
   a) The kidneys do not respond to ADH
3739) What medication can cause nephrogenic DI?
   a) Lithium
3740) What is the treatment of nephrogenic DI?
   a) Hydrochlorothiazide
3741) What adrenal disease is a tumor of the adrenal medulla secreting excess norepinephrine causing an uncontrolled hypertensive emergency, palpitations, headache, and diaphoresis?
   a) Pheochromocytoma
3742) How do you diagnosis a pheochromocytoma?
   a) ↑ serum / urine catecholamine (metanephrine), and 24-hour urine for VMA (catecholamine)
3743) What is the medical treatment for a hypertensive crisis due to a pheochromocytoma?
   a) Alpha-blocker (1st) +/- Beta-blocker (to control HR)
3744) What are the main alpha-blockers used to treat hypertension due to a pheochromocytoma?
   a) Phentolamine (nonselective alpha blockers) or Phenoxybenzmine

3745)   What type of neuroendocrine tumor from the distal small
        bowel can cause flushing, diarrhea, hypotension, hypoglycemia,
        edema, wheezing, and muscle cramping?
   a)   Carcinoid tumor
3746)   What are the two hormones secreted from a carcinoid tumor
        causing carcinoid syndrome?
   a)   Serotonin and Prostaglandin

Hematology & Oncology

Oncology

3747) What is the second leading cause of death in the US?
   a) Cancer

3748) List the three cancers in men with the highest mortality.
   a) Lung, Prostate, and Colorectal

3749) Starting with the most common, list the three cancers in men with the highest incidence.
   a) 1) Prostate 2) Lung 3) Colorectal

3750) List the three cancers in women with the highest mortality.
   a) Lung, Breast, and Colorectal

3751) Starting with the most common, list the three cancers in women with the highest incidence.
   a) 1) Breast 2) Lung 3) Colorectal

3752) List the top three most common cancers in pediatrics.
   a) 1) Leukemia 2) CNS 3) Lymphoma

3753) List symptoms in adults that raise suspicion for cancer.
   a) Weight loss, Fatigue, Night sweats, Blood in the stool, Persistent vaginal bleeding, Persistent cough, Head, Neck, and Upper extremity swelling, or an Abnormal mole.

3754) List symptoms in pediatric that raise suspicion for cancer.
   a) Pale, Fatigued, Recurrent fever, Weight loss, Night sweats, Bone pain, Severe headache, Mass in the abdomen, and White dot in the eye.

3755) What autoimmune disorder can be associated with a thymoma?
   a) Myasthenia gravis

3756) What cardiac condition causing pain and a cardiac rub, can develop as a complication from radiation treatment to the chest?
   a) Radiation pericarditis

3757) What cardiac condition needs to be evaluated in a cancer patient who presents with muffled heart sounds, increased jugular venous pressure and hypotension?
   a) Neoplastic cardiac tamponade

3758) What condition is caused by a bronchogenic carcinoma in the chest that leads to obstruction of the venous system, swelling of the head and upper extremities, and dyspnea?
   a) Superior vena cava (SVC) obstruction
3759) What is the first sign that develops in SVC syndrome/obstruction from a tumor?
   a) Unilateral facial swelling
3760) What is the treatment for SVC syndrome?
   a) SVC stenting, Radiation, and Chemotherapy
3761) What emergency spinal cord condition in a cancer patient needs to be ruled out when they present with leg weakness, numbness, trouble urinating, and back pain at night when supine?
   a) Spinal cord compression / Cauda Equina Syndrome
3762) What emergent imaging of the spine is required to diagnose spinal cord compression?
   a) MRI
3763) What are the three most common cancers that metastasis to the bone?
   a) Lung, Breast, and Prostate
3764) What location of the spine is the most common site of metastasis and spinal cord compression?
   a) Thoracic
3765) List the treatments for spinal cord compression from metastasis.
   a) Surgery, Steroids, and Immediate radiation
3766) What electrolyte abnormality is the most common disorder associated with cancer that causes nausea, constipation, lethargy, and confusion?
   a) Hypercalcemia
3767) What metabolic abnormality can occur from radiation or chemotherapy caused by the breakdown of tumors?
   a) Hyperuricemia
3768) List the treatments for hyperuricemia.
   a) Urinary alkalinization (7.0-7.5), IV Saline, and Allopurinol
3769) What syndrome can develop from small cell carcinoma and brain tumors that lead to hyponatremia?
   a) SIADH

3770)   What electrolyte abnormalities can be seen with tumor lysis syndrome?
   a)   Hyperkalemia, Hyperphosphatemia, Hyperuricemia, and Uremia, and Hypocalcemia
3771)   What is the most common electrolyte abnormality seen with tumor lysis syndrome?
   a)   Hyperkalemia
3772)   What is the recommended treatment for tumor lysis syndrome?
   a)   IV Hydration, Dialysis, and Rasburicase (for hyperuricemia)
3773)   List the causes of hyperviscosity syndrome.
   a)   Dysproteinemia (Waldenstrom macroglobulinemia, Multiple Myeloma), Leukocytosis (leukemia), and Polycythemia
3774)   What is the most common cause of hyperviscosity syndrome?
   a)   Waldenstrom macroglobulinemia
3775)   List the symptoms seen with hyperviscosity syndrome.
   a)   Fatigue, Confusion, Dyspnea, Chest pain, Visual loss, and Bleeding
3776)   What findings are seen on the funduscopic exam with hyperviscosity syndrome?
   a)   Sausage linked retinal vessels
3777)   What are the treatments for hyperviscosity syndrome?
   a)   IV Hydration, Plasmapheresis, Phlebotomy, FFP, and Vitamin K (if bleeding)
3778)   What type of plasma cell malignancy causes bone pain, fatigue, weakness, renal failure, hypercalcemia, and lytic bone lesions?
   a)   Multiple myeloma
3779)   What are the criteria to diagnose neutropenia?
   a)   Absolute neutrophil count < 500 or < 1000 with an anticipated drop to less than 500 within 48 hours
3780)   What are the criteria for neutropenic fever?
   a)   Single fever > 101° F (38.3° C) or Fever 100.4° F > 1 hour
3781)   What is the workup for neutropenic fever?
   a)   CBC, BMP, LFT, Urinalysis and culture, Chest X-ray, Blood cultures x2, Central line/port culture, +/- a Lumbar puncture
3782)   What antibiotics should be used in neutropenic fever?

a) Vancomycin and Broad spectrum beta-lactamases

3783) What life-threatening disease caused by cancers, sepsis, and trauma, leads to both bleeding and thrombosis, with end-organ failure by the extrinsic pathway?
a) Disseminated intravascular coagulation (DIC)

3784) What lab abnormalities help diagnose DIC?
a) Thrombocytopenia, Low fibrinogen, Increased fibrin split products, Increased fibrin degradation products, Elevated D-Dimer, and Prolonged PTT and PT.

3785) What platelet count should levels be above in DIC?
a) > 50,000

3786) What is the treatment of DIC?
a) Fresh frozen plasma and +/- Heparin and Platelets

3787) What oncologic condition from brain metastasis causes headaches with increased intracranial pressure, worse in the morning, and are better with vomiting?
a) Leptomeningeal carcinomatosis

3788) How is leptomeningeal carcinomatosis diagnosed?
a) CSF fluid analysis

3789) What is the treatment for leptomeningeal carcinomatosis
a) Radiation +/- Intrathecal chemotherapy

3790) List the medications that can be used for post-chemotherapy nausea and vomiting.
a) Ondansetron, Promethazine, Metoclopramide

3791) What is the most common complication of a stem cell transplant?
a) Graft verse host disease

3792) What oncological condition causes hypertension, diarrhea, rapid eye movements, and muscle jerking (opsoclonus-myoclonus syndrome), and is associated with neuroblastoma tumors?
a) Paraneoplastic syndrome

3793) What is the common solid tumor in pediatrics?
a) Brain tumors

3794) What is the most common type of leukemia in pediatrics and makes up ¾ of all pediatric malignancies?
a) Acute lymphocytic leukemia (ALL)

3795) What type of fracture commonly seen in proximal long bones, occurs out of proportion to the mechanism and is caused by solid tumors?
a) Pathologic fracture
3796) What malignant stem cell disorder of the bone marrow leads to increased WBC, RBC, Hb, Hct, platelet, and leukocyte alkaline phosphatase levels, causing headache, fatigue, blurry vision, bone pain, and dizziness?
a) Polycythemia vera
3797) What is the treatment for polycythemia vera?
a) Aspirin 1st then Phlebotomy

Hematology
3798) What diagnoses should be considered for cyanosis that is unresponsive to oxygen therapy?
a) Carboxyhemoglobinemia, Methemoglobinemia, and Cardiac shunts
3799) What hemoglobinopathy can be caused by sulfonamides, nitrates, aniline dyes (material dyes), Pyridium, and Benzocaine/oral gel?
a) Methemoglobinemia
3800) What is the symbol for ferrous iron that normally binds to Hb and ferric iron that cannot bind Hb?
a) Normally binds to Hb: Fe^{++}
b) Unable to bind Hb: Fe^{+++}
3801) What is the treatment of methemoglobinemia?
a) Methylene blue
3802) List the causes of anemia with an elevated MVC.
a) B12 and Folate deficiency, Alcohol abuse, Chemotherapy, and Aplastic anemia
3803) List the causes of anemia with a low MVC.
a) Iron deficiency, Chronic disease, Hemolysis, and Thalassemia
3804) What does a positive coombs test with anemia mean?
a) Autoantibodies to RBCs causing destruction
3805) How much does one unit of PRBC usually increase Hb level?
a) 1.5-2.0 g/dL
3806) What is the total human blood volume?

a) 70 mL/kg = 5 liters

3807) What blood type is the universal donor?
a) Type O negative

3808) Can type O patients receive any type of blood?
a) No

3809) What blood type is the universal recipient?
a) Type AB

3810) What electrolyte abnormality can result from citrate toxicity from a massive blood transfusion?
a) Hypocalcemia

3811) What is the most common complication of massive blood transfusion?
a) Hypothermia

3812) List the different type's of blood transfusion reactions.
a) Acute hemolytic transfusion reactions, Febrile nonhemolytic transfusion reaction, Allergic transfusion reaction, and Delayed hemolytic reaction

3813) What is the treatment for most of all transfusion reactions?
a) Discontinuation of transfusion (except allergic)

3814) What transfusion reaction is usually within 15min of starting the transfusion, and causes erythema, urticaria, and bronchospasm without a fever?
a) Allergic transfusion reaction

3815) What type of transfusion reaction presents with fever, chills, low back pain, dyspnea, bleeding, pain at IV site, and acute tubular necrosis?
a) Acute hemolytic transfusion reaction

3816) What is the most common type of transfusion reaction that presents with fever and chills shortly after the transfusion is started?
a) Febrile nonhemolytic transfusion reaction

3817) What is the time frame for a delayed hemolytic reaction to occur after a transfusion?
a) Within 7-10 days

3818) Give the risk of acquiring hepatitis B from a transfusion.
a) 1:200,000

3819) Give the risk of acquiring hepatitis C from a transfusion.
   a) 1:2,000,000
3820) Give the risk of acquiring HIV from a transfusion.
   a) 1:2,000,000
3821) On average how much will 1 unit of platelets from whole blood increase the platelet count?
   a) 10,000
3822) What type of platelet dysfunction causes non-palpable purpura, epistaxis, and bruising, and occurs during the recovery of a viral illness?
   a) Idiopathic thrombocytopenic purpura (ITP)
3823) At what platelet count level should treatment with a platelet transfusion be initiated for thrombocytopenia, with and without active bleeding?
   a) Without bleeding: 20,000
   b) With bleeding: 30-50,000
3824) At what platelet count in ITP can intracranial bleeding happen spontaneously?
   a) <10,000
3825) What are the treatment options for ITP?
   a) Steroids, IVIG, Anti-Rheumatoid immunoglobulin, or RhoGAM (only if Rh+)
3826) What definitive treatment may be necessary for those with recurrent ITP?
   a) Splenectomy
3827) What is the pentad of symptoms seen with thrombotic thrombocytopenic purpura (TTP)?
   a) Fever, Anemia, Thrombocytopenia, Renal failure, and Neurological symptoms (pneumonic FAT RN)
3828) What is the most common cause of TTP?
   a) Pregnancy
3829) What are the treatments for TTP?
   a) Steroids and Fresh frozen plasma (FFP), or +/- Plasmapheresis
3830) Is a platelet transfusion recommended in TTP?
   a) No, it can lead to increased destruction and thrombosis of the platelets

3831) What gene is lost leading to bleeding in TTP?
   a) ADAMTS-13
3832) What bleeding pathway does prothrombin time (PT) measure?
   a) Extrinsic pathway (2,7,9,10)
3833) What vitamin does Warfarin inhibit, affecting the extrinsic pathway and prolonging the PT?
   a) Vitamin K
3834) List the treatments for Warfarin hypercoagulation with active bleeding.
   a) Vitamin K IV, FFP, and Prothrombin complex
3835) What bleeding pathway does partial thromboplastin time (PTT) measure?
   a) Intrinsic pathway
3836) What is the reversal agent and dose for heparin?
   a) Protamine sulfate (1mg reverses 100 units of Heparin)
3837) List the common causes leading to a sickle cell crisis.
   a) Infection, Cold, Dehydration, or High altitude
3838) What is the most common cause of death in sickle cell crisis?
   a) Sepsis (pneumonia)
3839) What is the most common symptom from a vaso-occlusive crisis in sickle cell disease?
   a) Musculoskeletal pain
   b) 2nd most common: Abdominal pain
3840) What spleen injury can occur in sickle cell patients?
   a) Autosplenectomy
3841) What types of bacteria are sickle cell patients predisposed to?
   a) Encapsulated organisms (N. meningitidis, H. influenzae, S. pneumonia), Mycoplasma, E. coli, Salmonella, and Staphylococcus
3842) What is the leading cause of death in sickle cell patients, and presents with chest pain, fever, wheezing, and tachypnea?
   a) Acute chest syndrome
3843) What are the recommended treatments for acute chest syndrome?
   a) Oxygen, Antibiotics, Incentive spirometry, Bronchodilator, Pain control, and Transfusion

3844)   What sickle cell crisis is due to the failure of bone marrow erythropoiesis and seen with a low reticulocyte count < 3%?

a)   Aplastic crisis

3845)   What virus can lead to an aplastic crisis in sickle cell disease?

a)   Parvovirus

3846)   What is the treatment for an aplastic crisis in sickle cell disease with a hemoglobin count < 10?

a)   PRBC transfusion

3847)   List other organ injuries that can occur in a sickle cell crisis.

a)   Ischemic or hemorrhagic CVA, seizures, and Renal failure

3848)   What is the leading cause of death in sickle cell patients?

a)   Infections

3849)   What is the treatment for CVA in a sickle cell patient?

a)   Transfusion

3850)   What are the signs of acute splenic sequestration crisis in sickle cell patient?

a)   Shock, Abdominal pain, and High reticulocyte count

3851)   What is the treatment for acute splenic sequestration crisis in a sickle cell patient?

a)   Transfusion (replaces RBC), Exchange transfusion (removes sickled cells while replacing) and Splenectomy

3852)   What is the difference between a simple transfusions and exchange transfusion?

a)   Exchange transfusion: removes sickled cells and replaces RBC

b)   Simple transfusion: replaces RBC

3853)   What is the most common variant of sickle cell disease?

a)   Sickle cell trait

3854)   What is the most common symptom seen in patients with sickle cell trait?

a)   Hematuria

3855)   What type of hemophilia is the most common and is from a factor VIII deficiency?

a)   Hemophilia A

3856)   List the treatments for Hemophilia A.

a)   Desmopressin (DDAVP) or Factor VIII recombinant-plasma derived

3857) What type of hemophilia is from a factor IX deficiency?
   a) Hemophilia B
3858) List the treatments for Hemophilia B.
   a) Factor IX replacement
3859) What is the calculation to determine factor dosing and replacement for hemophilia A and B patients with a bleed?
   a) Kg x 0.5 x % change in factor
3860) What factor replacement percentage is the target for hemophilia A and B patients with Hemarthrosis, GI, and CNS bleeds?
   a) Hemarthrosis: 50% (25 U/kg)
   b) GI: 100% (50 U/kg)
   c) CNS: 100% (50 U/kg)
3861) What is the most common inherited coagulation disorder that leads to a prolonged bleeding time, increased PTT, and is treated with DDAVP?
   a) Von Willebrand's Disease
3862) What is the most common type of Von Willebrand's disease?
   a) Type 1
3863) What autosomal dominant protein deficiencies are vitamin K-dependent proteins that increase the risk of thrombosis when absence?
   a) Protein C & S deficiency
3864) What is the treatment for thrombosis prevention and treatment in patients with protein C & S deficiencies?
   a) Anticoagulants
3865) What are the mutation types of protein C & S deficiencies and which is the most common?
   a) Type 1 quantitative disorder (most common)
   b) Type 2 dysfunctional disorder
3866) What skin condition can develop in patients with protein C & S deficiency on Warfarin, and presents with painful red lesions all over the body?
   a) Warfarin-induced skin necrosis
3867) What is the treatment of Warfarin-induced skin necrosis?
   a) Low molecular weight heparin products

3868) What is the most common inherited clotting disorder, whose mutation makes it resistant to protein C inhibition?

a) Factor V Leiden

3869) What autosomal dominant gene mutation leads to thrombosis and pregnancy complications such as recurrent miscarriages?

a) Prothrombin 2021A mutation

3870) What inherited clotting disorder is due to increased levels of enzymes causing a toxic effect on the vessels leading to increased thrombosis?

a) Hyperhomocysteinemia

3871) What are the treatments for hyperhomocysteinemia used to lower homocysteine levels?

a) Folate + Pyridoxine + Vitamin B12

3872) What autosomal dominant protein deficiency is there a loss of direct thrombin inhibition and an increased risk of thrombosis?

a) Antithrombin III deficiency

3873) What autoimmune acquired clotting disorder is associated with lupus and leads to venous and arterial thrombosis, miscarriages, strokes, and skin conditions?

a) Antiphospholipid syndrome

3874) How is antiphospholipid syndrome diagnosed?

a) Antiphospholipid antibody

3875) What type of acquired clotting disorder can develop in patients on Heparin products and presents with a > 50% decrease in the platelet count?

a) Heparin-induced thrombocytopenia (HIT)

3876) What is the treatment for HIT in the ED?

a) Admission, Discontinue heparin products, and Start a new anticoagulant (Fondaparinux)

3877) What medication causes an elevated INR that is monitored for therapeutic treatment?

a) Warfarin

3878) What medications can be used for bleeding in patients with liver failure?

a) FFP, Vitamin K, or Cryoprecipitate

3879) What vitamin deficiency causes bleeding gums, gingivitis, and leads to poor wound healing?
   a) Vitamin C deficiency

Immunology

3880)   What autoimmune condition presents with pain in the fingers and toes with bluish or white color changes when exposed to cold environments?
   a)   Raynaud's phenomenon
3881)   What is the treatment for Raynaud's syndrome?
   a)   Calcium channel blockers (Nifedipine)
3882)   What syndrome is seen with Calcinosis, Raynauds, Esophageal dysmotility, Sclerodactyly, and Telangiectasias?
   a)   CREST syndrome
3883)   What antibody is seen in CREST syndrome?
   a)   Anti-centromere and Anti-Scl-70
3884)   What skin condition is a progressive autoimmune systemic sclerosis seen most commonly in women?
   a)   Scleroderma
3885)   What condition is seen with carditis, polyarthritis, chorea, subcutaneous nodules, erythema marginatum, murmur, fever, and positive antistreptolysin O (ASO) titer?
   a)   Rheumatic Fever
3886)   What is the most common valvular complication see in rheumatic fever?
   a)   MItral valve stenosis
3887)   How many major and minor criteria do you need to diagnose rheumatic fever?
   a)   2 Major or 1 major and 2 minor
3888)   What are the major Jones criteria to diagnose rheumatic fever?
   a)   Carditis, Polyarthritis, Chorea, Subcutaneous nodules, and Erythema marginatum
3889)   What are the minor Jones criteria to diagnose rheumatic fever?
   a)   Fever, Elevated ESR or CRP, Arthralgia's, Prolonged PR interval on ECG, and a Positive antistreptolysin O (ASO) titer
3890)   What is the most common symptom seen in acute rheumatic fever?
   a)   Migratory polyarthritis
3891)   What is the treatment for rheumatic fever?

a) Antibiotics and NSAIDs

3892) What condition is seen with fever, polyarthralgia, polyarthritis, and rash 1-2 weeks after starting a new medication?
a) Serum sickness

3893) What medications typically lead to serum sickness?
a) Sulfonylureas, Penicillins, and Anticonvulsants

3894) What type of hypersensitivity reaction is seen with IgE-mediated anaphylaxis?
a) Type 1

3895) What type of hypersensitivity reaction occurs when a cytotoxic antibody causes an acute hemolytic transfusion reaction?
a) Type 2

3896) What type of hypersensitivity reaction is see with the immune complex-mediated serum sickness?
a) Type 3

3897) What type of hypersensitivity reaction is see with cell-mediated erythema multiforme and Steven-Johnson syndrome?
a) Type 4

3898) What medical emergency can cause rapid facial swelling in a patient on an ACE inhibitor?
a) Angioedema

3899) What is the most common drug leading to angioedema?
a) Angiotensin-converting enzyme inhibitors (ACE inhibitors)

3900) What enzyme level is elevated in ACE inhibitor angioedema?
a) Bradykinin level

3901) List the medications used for an angioedema allergic reaction.
a) Steroids, Diphenhydramine, and Ranitidine (H2 blockers) +/- Epinephrine

3902) What type of angioedema presents in a young patients, may be recurrent without any inciting factors or medications on board?
a) Hereditary angioedema

3903) What cell deficiency is present in hereditary angioedema?
a) C1 esterase inhibitor

3904) What is the 1st line treatment for hereditary angioedema?
a) C1 esterase inhibitor (Icatibant (bradykinin B2 receptor antagonist) or Ecallantide (kallikrein inhibitor))

3905) What is the 2nd line treatment for hereditary angioedema?
   a) Fresh frozen plasma (FFP) and Steroids
3906) What medications can be given to lower recurrent hypersensitivity reactions to contrast dye?
   a) Pre-medicate with Steroids and Diphenhydramine
3907) What is the treatment for giant cell arteritis/temporal arteritis?
   a) High dose corticosteroids
3908) What are the criteria for diagnosing temporal arteritis (giant cell arteritis)?
   a) > 50-year-old, New-onset localized headache, Elevated ESR > 50, and Abnormal artery biopsy
3909) What are the symptoms seen with systemic juvenile idiopathic arthritis/Still's disease?
   a) Fever, Arthritis, and Rash
3910) What is the most common type of juvenile immune/rheumatoid arthritis or Still's disease seen in pediatric patients?
   a) Pauciarticular
3911) What is the treatment of Still's disease?
   a) NSAID's, Steroids and/or Methotrexate
3912) What condition is seen more in African American females, and presents with fever, joint pains, butterfly facial rash, and renal disease?
   a) Systemic Lupus Erythematosus (SLE)
3913) What thrombolysis syndrome can be associated with Systemic Lupus Erythematosus?
   a) Antiphospholipid syndrome
3914) What is the general treatment for systemic lupus erythematosus?
   a) Steroids
3915) What is the common finding on chest X-ray with lupus?
   a) Bilateral hilar adenopathy
3916) What is the treatment for antiphospholipid syndrome causing thrombosis, strokes, miscarriages, MI, and DVTs?
   a) Lifelong anticoagulation
3917) What is the most common chest radiograph abnormality seen with sarcoidosis?
   a) Hilar lymphadenopathy

3918) What specific types of granulomas are present with sarcoidosis?
   a) Non-caseating granulomas
3919) What is the gene that is associated with seronegative spondyloarthropathies (SS)?
   a) HLA-B27
3920) List the different types of seronegative spondyloarthropathies.
   a) Ankylosing spondylitis, Reactive arthritis, Psoriatic arthritis, and Enteropathic arthritis
3921) What arthritis is seen weeks after a sexually transmitted disease or gastrointestinal infections?
   a) Reactive arthritis
3922) What seronegative spondyloarthropathy (SS) condition is caused by an infection such as chlamydia, and presents with a classic triad of urethritis, conjunctivitis, and arthritis?
   a) Reactive arthritis (Reiter's syndrome)
3923) List the two types of GI induced enteropathic seronegative conditions.
   a) Crohn's and Ulcerative colitis
3924) What seronegative spondyloarthropathy (SS) condition is a progressive inflammation and fusion of the spine, starting with the sacral iliac joints?
   a) Ankylosing spondylitis
3925) What genotype is seen with ankylosing spondylitis?
   a) HLA-B27

Dermatology

3926) What is the largest organ system of the body?
   a) Skin

3927) Name the three layers of the skin.
   a) Epidermis, Dermis, and Subcuticular tissue

3928) List the size for each of the following primary lesions: macule, papule, patch, plaque, nodule, vesicle, petechiae, and purpura.
   a) Macule: flat < 1.5 cm
   b) Patch: flat > 1.5 cm
   c) Papule: raised < 1.5 cm
   d) Plaque: raised > 1.5 cm
   e) Nodule: raised > 1.5 cm
   f) Vesicle: fluid < 1.0 cm
   g) Petechiae: < 3 mm
   h) Purpura: > 3 mm

3929) What medication type is the most common offending agent leading to an allergic rash?
   a) Antibiotics

3930) What skin condition is defined by erythema with sharp demarcation from uninvolved skin?
   a) Erysipelas

3931) What is the treatment of erysipelas (superficial dermal infection)?
   a) Antibiotics (Penicillins)

3932) What premalignant condition is usually a single, dry, rough, raised lesion?
   a) Actinic keratosis

3933) What is the most common skin cancer characterized by isolated, hard, pearly, nodules with central ulceration, and rarely becomes invasive?
   a) Basal cell carcinoma

3934) What malignant skin lesions are rapidly growing indurated erythematous plaques on sun-exposed areas and metastasizes early?
   a) Squamous cell carcinoma

3935) What is the treatment for squamous cell carcinoma?
a) Excision and Radiation

3936) What are the five irregularities used to help identify melanoma?
a) Asymmetry, Irregular Borders, Color changes, Large Diameter, and Enlarging

3937) What malignant skin lesion has the highest mortality?
a) Melanoma

3938) What finding on a skin biopsy of melanoma suggests a worse prognosis?
a) The greater the depth

3939) What dermatologic condition is an inflammatory reaction with painful, raise, violaceous nodules on the pretibial area?
a) Erythema nodosum

3940) What are common causes of erythema nodosum?
a) Pregnancy, Sarcoidosis, Birth control, and Infections

3941) What skin condition caused by allergic reactions, stress, exercising, and weather and are vascular raised pruritic lesions?
a) Urticaria

3942) What are the recommended medication treatments for urticaria?
a) Steroids and Antihistamines (H-1 and H-2 blockers)

3943) What is the term used for non-blanching vasculitic ecchymotic areas of the skin around 2 mm?
a) Petechiae

3944) What skin condition is characterized by macular papular areas with a central clearing "target lesions" from a hypersensitivity reaction and does not involve the mucous membranes?
a) Erythema multiforme

3945) What hypersensitivity reaction to medications causes separation of the epidermis and dermis, positive Nikolsky sign, and involves the mucous membranes and 10-30% of the body surface?
a) Stevens-Johnson's syndrome

3946) What is another name for Steven-Johnson's syndrome?
a) Erythema multiforme Major

3947) What is the treatment for Steven Johnson syndrome?

a) Steroids and Remove offending agent, +/- Plasmapheresis or Immunomodulators

3948) What sign is characterized by the spreading of a bulla and disruption of the epidermis with lateral pressure?
a) Nikolsky's sign

3949) List the conditions that can have a positive Nikolsky's sign.
a) Bullous pemphigoid, Toxic epidermal necrolysis, Staphyloccal scalded skin syndrome and Porphyrias

3950) What condition develops with progressing Steven Johnson syndrome, erythema, erupting bullae, involves > 30% of the body surface, and has a positive Nikolsky sign?
a) Toxic epidermal necrolysis (TEN)

3951) What are the most common medications leading to erythema multiforme, Steven Johnson's, and TEN?
a) Penicillins, Phenytoin, Sulfonamides, Furosemide, Barbiturates, NSAIDs, and Aspirin

3952) What special units treat patients with TEN?
a) Burn units

3953) What skin condition is seen with a history of asthma, and is an erythematous, itchy, dry scaly rash on the extremities with lichenification of the skin?
a) Eczema (atopic dermatitis)

3954) What type of eczema is from chronic dry skin irritation and presents with round erythematous dry areas?
a) Nodular eczema

3955) Give the treatments for eczema.
a) Topical steroids, Antihistamines, and Moisturizers

3956) What skin conditions can be from direct contact with an irritant such as metals or poison ivy, and leads to erythema, itching, and burning?
a) Contact dermatitis

3957) Give the treatments for contact dermatitis.
a) Steroids, Antihistamines, and Remove offending agent

3958) What type of dermatitis, causes diffuse erythema and leads to extensive exfoliation?
a) Exfoliative dermatitis

3959) Give the treatment for exfoliative dermatitis.

a) Admission and IV Steroids for severe cases

3960) What skin condition has white waxy scales with erythematous bases, on the scalps, eyebrows, groin, and hairy skin areas and is due to a fungus?

a) Seborrheic dermatitis

3961) What fungus causes seborrheic dermatitis?

a) Malassezia furfur (Pityrosporum ovale)

3962) Give the treatment for seborrheic dermatitis.

a) Antidandruff shampoos (Selsun Blue) or Ketoconazole shampoo

3963) What chronic skin condition has papulosquamous eruptions and erythematous plaques with white scales on the extensor surfaces of elbows, knees, and scalp?

a) Psoriasis vulgaris

3964) Give the treatment for psoriasis.

a) Steroids, Methotrexate, Emollients, and UV light therapy

3965) What chronic skin condition has purple, polygonal, pruritic, papules on the extremities and buccal mucosa?

a) Lichen planus

3966) What are the buccal lesions called with lichen planus?

a) Wickham's striae

3967) Give the treatment for lichen planus.

a) Steroids (topical and systemic)

3968) What skin condition starts with a single patch and erupts to a diffuse pruritic erythematous rash in a "Christmas tree" pattern?

a) Pityriasis rosea

3969) What life-threatening skin condition is an autoimmune intraepithelial blistering disease that affects the mucous membranes and skin with tender bullae and has a positive Nikolsky sign?

a) Pemphigus vulgaris

3970) Give the treatment for pemphigus vulgaris.

a) Admission, IV Steroids, and Immunosuppressants

3971) What autoimmune blistering skin condition has diffuse urticarial lesions that develop into tense bullae with a negative Nikolsky sign?

a) Bullous pemphigoid

3972) Which skin disease has IgG autoantibodies against the basement membrane and is sub-epidermal?

a) Bullous pemphigoid

3973) Give the treatment for bullous pemphigoid.

a) Steriods (topical or systemic) or Immunosuppressants

3974) What sign on skin exam differentiates bullous pemphigoid and pemphigus vulgaris?

a) Nikolsky test

3975) What skin infection is caused by an exotoxin, is seen in young children < 2 after a URI and fever, and has extensive bullae, positive Nikolsky sign?

a) Staphylococcal scalded skin syndrome (SSSS)

3976) What is the treatment of SSSS?

a) Nafcillin or Vancomycin

3977) What skin condition from strep and staph causes small round honey crusted vesicles usually on the face?

a) Impetigo

3978) What bacteria causes bullous impetigo?

a) Staph

3979) Give the treatment for localized and diffuse impetigo.

a) Localized: Topical Mupirocin

b) Diffuse: Systemic Dicloxacillin

3980) What red, rough, papular, blanching rash develops in patients with a sore throat, adenopathy, and strawberry tongue?

a) Scarlet fever rash

3981) What is the pathognomonic finding of linear petechiae in the extremity flexure folds after a scarlet fever rash?

a) Pastia's lines

3982) What bacteria leads to scarlet fever?

a) Group A beta-hemolytic streptococci

3983) Give the treatment of scarlet fever.

a) Penicillins

3984) What diffuse pruritic rash commonly in pediatric patients, starts on the trunk or scalp as faintly raised vesicles on an erythematous base that crust over when healing?

a) Varicella rash

3985) What patient populations may require antiviral treatment for varicella?

a) > 12 years old, Pregnant, and Immunocompromised

3986) Which medication is contraindicated in patients with a varicella infection?

a) Steroids

3987) What is the recommended treatment for an unvaccinated pregnant patient with varicella?

a) Antiviral and Varicella IG

3988) What skin condition is seen more in the elderly causes prodromal burning pains followed by a unilateral vesicular red raised skin eruption that follows the dermatomes?

a) Herpes zoster (shingles)

3989) Give the treatments used for shingles.

a) Antiviral (Acyclovir), Steroids, Analgesics, and Antihistamines

3990) What is the window for treating shingles after skin eruption?

a) < 72 hours

3991) What persistent condition can happen after an acute herpes zoster infection and is associated with a dermatomal hypersensitivity?

a) Post-herpetic neuralgia

3992) What diffuse head to toe spreading erythematous maculopapular "morbilliform" rash occurs in pediatric patients with associated cough, conjunctivitis, and fever?

a) Rubeola (measles)

3993) What virus causes to Rubeola?

a) Myxovirus

3994) What are the 3 C's associated with Rubeola?

a) Cough, Coryza, and Conjunctivitis

3995) What are the pathognomonic bluish-gray 1 mm macules seen on oral mucosa with measles?

a) Koplik spots

3996) What pink maculopapular rash spreads from the face to the trunk, follows fever, sore throat, headaches, and lymphadenopathy in the unvaccinated and pediatric populations?

a) Rubella (German Measles)

3997) What are the pathognomonic petechial macules on the posterior palate called with Rubella?
a) Forchheimer spots

3998) What virus causes Rubella?
a) Rubivirus

3999) What is the treatment for Rubeola and Rubella?
a) Supportive

4000) What type of rash is a generalized maculopapular rash that develops in a patient with viral pharyngitis due to EBV who is given Amoxicillin?
a) Infectious mononucleosis rash

4001) Describe the rash typically seen in a patient allergic to amoxicillin.
a) Diffuse maculopapular erythematous pruritic rash

4002) What rash caused by an STD presents with scaly diffuse, round, red-brown macules that are non-pruritic?
a) Secondary syphilis rash

4003) What type of rash caused by a disseminated STD, causes diffuse tender palpable pustules on an erythematous base with associated polyarthralgia?
a) Gonorrhea rash

4004) What is the classic rash associated with Lyme disease that is an annular, raised, warm, erythematous area described as a "bull's-eye" or "target" pattern?
a) Erythema chronicum migrans

4005) What tick-borne infection causes fever, myalgias, and pink macules and petechiae that first appears on the extremities and spread centrally?
a) Rocky Mountain spotted fever rash

4006) What type of rash can develop with a Neisseria meningitides infection?
a) Diffuse maculopapular petechial rash

4007) Describe the skin findings with herpes simplex.
a) Painful vesicles on an erythematous base

4008)　　What type of skin condition is an umbilicated flesh-colored, dome-shaped lesion that is transferred sexually by skin-to-skin contact in adults?

　　a)　Molluscum contagiosum

4009)　　What type of virus is molluscum contagiosum?

　　a)　Poxvirus

4010)　　What treatments are there for molluscum contagiosum?

　　a)　Curettage and Liquid nitrogen

4011)　　Describe the tinea (ringworm) fungal pattern rash?

　　a)　Red, raised, scaly, annular, pruritic rash

4012)　　List the terms used for tinea infections of the head, body, feet, groin, and nails.

　　a)　Head: Capitis

　　b)　Body: Corporis

　　c)　Feet: Pedis

　　d)　Groin: Cruris

　　e)　Unguium: Nails

4013)　　What finding on the woods lamp exam of a rash suggests tinea as the cause?

　　a)　Blue-green fluorescence

4014)　　What fungi cause ringworm?

　　a)　Microsporum and Trichophyton

4015)　　What is the treatment of tinea capitis or unguium?

　　a)　Oral fluconazole/antifungal

4016)　　What is the treatment of tinea corporis, cruris, and pedis?

　　a)　Topical antifungal cream

4017)　　What is the term for a raised boggy swollen mass with pustules seen with a tinea capitis infection on the scalp?

　　a)　Kerion

4018)　　What is the medication used to treat a kerion?

　　a)　Oral steroids

4019)　　What fungal rash causes a diffuse round hypo and hyperpigmentation macules and patches on the trunk and has microscopic findings of "Spaghetti and meatballs"?

　　a)　Tinea versicolor

4020)　　What fungus causes tinea versicolor?

a) Malassezia furfur (Pityrosporum ovale)

4021) What is the treatment for tinea versicolor?
a) Selenium sulfide shampoo or lotion

4022) What fungus causes erythematous scaling patches with satellite lesions and can affect the mucous membranes, axilla, groin, and skin folds?
a) Candidiasis

4023) What is the treatment for localized and diffuse Candidiasis?
a) Topical or systemic antifungal (Fluconazole or Clotrimazole)

4024) What rash has fine scaly sharp demarcated macules in the groin and axilla of obese and diabetic patients?
a) Erythrasma

4025) What bacteria causes erythrasma?
a) Corynebacterium minutissimum

4026) What is the treatment for Erythrasma?
a) Erythromycin

4027) What fungal rash presents in farmers and gardeners with infected pustules, nodules, and ulcers with surrounding ecchymotic tissue?
a) Sporotrichosis

4028) What is the most common type of sporotrichosis infection?
a) Lymphocutaneous nodule type

4029) What is the treatment of sporotrichosis?
a) Itraconazole (3-6 months)

4030) What rash coincides with an acute febrile illness and appears as a butterfly pattern on the face with a diffuse lacy reticular rash on the trunk?
a) Erythema infectiosum (Fifths disease/Slapped cheek)

4031) What virus causes Fifths disease?
a) Parvovirus B19

4032) What is the treatment for erythema infectiosum?
a) Supportive (resolves within 5-7 days)

4033) What pediatric blanching, erythematous, palpable rash seen on the trunk and head, follows the resolution of a fever?
a) Roseola (exanthema subitum)

4034) What virus is associated with Roseola?

a) Herpesvirus (HHV6)

4035) What is the treatment for Roseola?

a) Supportive

4036) What viral pediatric rash presents with fever, sore throat, and painful oral erythematous vesicles and red papules on the hands and feet?

a) Hand-Foot-Mouth disease

4037) What main virus causes hand-foot-mouth disease?

a) Coxsackievirus (Enterovirus)

4038) What is the cause of a diffuse, pruritic, red, raised, crusting papules with overlying excoriation marks seen in the trunk, webs of the fingers, groin, and flexor regions of extremities that is worse at night?

a) Scabies rash

4039) What type of scabies is highly contagious, with diffuse crusting scabs, hyperkeratosis, and is seen more in elderly and nursing home patients?

a) Norwegian scabies

4040) What is the treatment for scabies?

a) Permethrin or Ivermectin, then wash all clothes and repeat in 1 week if required

4041) What medication that treats scabies and lice can cause seizures in children?

a) Lindane

4042) What type of infestation can have diffuse red raised pruritic areas on the body with white nits in the hair?

a) Lice (pediculosis)

4043) What is another name for a pediculosis groin infestation and is associated with an STD?

a) "Crabs"

4044) What is the treatment for lice?

a) Permethrin/Pyrethrin and remove knits in hair

4045) What worm infection causes an erythematous, meandering, pruritic tracts on the skin after skin inoculation walking on the beach in a tropical area?

a) Cutaneous larva migrans (hookworm)

4046) What is the treatment for hookworm?

 a) Albendazole, or Ivermectin

4047) What pediatric palpable purpuric rash is seen on the extremities and buttocks, after a recent viral infection, has associated arthralgias, hematuria, and abdominal pain?

 a) Henoch-Schonlein purpura rash

4048) What vasculitis condition causes erythematous, ecchymotic, painful subcutaneous nodules along the blood vessels?

 a) Polyarteritis nodosa

4049) What type of vasculitis rash presents with diffuse petechiae or non-palpable purpura usually on the extremities with anemia, fever, and renal disease?

 a) Thrombotic thrombocytopenic purpura rash

4050) What condition leads to a diffuse maculopapular rash with extremity swelling, erythema, and desquamation after having a fever for five days?

 a) Kawasaki syndrome (Mucocutaneous Lymph Node Syndrome)

4051) What skin condition in HIV and immunocompromised patients presents with painless, non-pruritic, purple plaques on the lower extremities?

 a) Kaposi's sarcoma

Chronic Pain Syndromes

4052) Which chronic pain condition has diffuse muscular pain, stiffness, constant fatigue, and is diagnosed with > 11 of 18 positive trigger points?
   a) Fibromyalgia

4053) What medications can be used to treat fibromyalgia?
   a) NSAIDs, Tylenol, Muscle relaxants, Tramadol, Gabapentin, and Amitriptyline

4054) What chronic pain condition is seen with diabetes causing symmetric numbness and burning pain in the lower extremities?
   a) Diabetic neuropathy

4055) What chronic pain condition is seen after amputations of extremities and causes cramping, burning, and aching in the amputated limb with peri-incisional sensory loss?
   a) Phantom limb pain

4056) What chronic pain condition can result from HIV causing pain and paresthesias in the feet?
   a) HIV related neuropathy

4057) What chronic pain condition can develop after a shingles flare?
   a) Postherpetic neuralgia

4058) What chronic back pain condition causes sharp, shooting, burning, electric shock like pain down the leg to the foot and is associated with herniated discs?
   a) Sciatica

4059) What type of chronic back pain is a constant, dull pain that does not follow nerve distributions, and is diagnosed by trigger points in the area of pain and decrease ROM of the affected muscle?
   a) Myofascial back pain syndrome

4060) What chronic pain syndrome occurs after trauma or surgeries causes burning, persistent pain and allodynia, and presents with edema, pallor, coldness, and local sweating of an extremity?
   a) Complex regional pain syndrome (CRPS)

4061) List the early and late signs seen with CRPS.
   a) Early: edema, warmth, and local swelling
   b) Late: cold, pale, cyanosis, and atrophic changes

4062) What type of CRPS occurs because of prolonged immobilization or disuse of an extremity?
   a) Reflex Sympathetic Dystrophy (Type 1)
4063) Which type of CRPS is due to a peripheral nerve injury?
   a) Type 2
4064) What type of migraine develops over time into a chronic pain syndrome?
   a) Transformed migraine
4065) What type of pain can follow a stroke with throbbing, shootings pains, with loss of hot and cold differentiation on the same side of weakness?
   a) Poststroke pain
4066) List common pain complaints seen with drug-seeking behavior.
   a) Back pain, Headache, Extremity pain, and Dental pain
4067) List behaviors associated with drug-seeking patients.
   a) Demanding, Intimidating, and Flattering
4068) List common characteristics of drug-seeking patients.
   a) Inconsistent history and physical, Fictitious illness, Asks for narcotics, Repeat visits for new pain complaints, and Lies about previous narcotic prescriptions and hospital visits
4069) List common fraudulent techniques of drug-seeking patients.
   a) History of abnormal X-rays or notes from PCP, Loss of pain prescriptions, "Impending" surgery history, or Fictitious hematuria with complaints of kidney stones

Administration / EMS

4070) Which United States EMS act established federal funding and grants for an EMS system?

    a) EMS System act of 1973

4071) Which type of EMS personnel is the first professional or trained person on the scene and can provide CPR?

    a) First responder (Police, Fire, and EMT basic)

4072) Which type of EMS personnel can provide oxygen, CPR, AED, extrication, and hemorrhage control?

    a) EMT Basic

4073) How many hours of training are required for EMT basic certification?

    a) 100-150

4074) Which type of EMS personnel can provide CPR, oxygen, AED, IV insertion, medication administration, and ECG interpretation?

    a) EMT Intermediate

4075) How many hours of training are required for EMT intermediate certification?

    a) 400-500

4076) Which type of EMS personnel can provide CPR, advanced airway, cricothyrotomy, IO placement, cardiac monitoring, oxygen, AED, IV insertion, medication administration, and ECG interpretation?

    a) EMT Paramedic

4077) How many hours of training are required for EMT paramedic certification?

    a) > 1,000

4078) What are the EMS staffing and supplies requirements for a basic life support (BLS) transportation system?

    a) EMT Basic, Oxygen, AED, Ventilation devices, Splinting equipment, and Wound dressings

4079) What are the EMS staffing and supplies requirements for an advanced life support (ALS) transportation system?

    a) EMT Paramedics, Oxygen, AED, Advance airway devices, Cardiac monitor, IV Supplies, IV Fluids, and Medications

4080)   What type of transfer transportation is suggested and best for intubated patients receiving critical care treatment in the ED?
a)   Air or Ground MICU

4081)   What order can be given to the local EMS services when a hospital is full and the ED's are boarding patients?
a)   EMS Diversion

4082)   Are EMS systems run by the city and state allowed to refuse patients medical care if they don't have insurance?
a)   No

4083)   What law in 1986 was passed to combat patient dumping practices?
a)   Comprehensive Omnibus Budget Reconciliation Act (COBRA)

4084)   What law that is part of COBRA requires the emergency department to provide a medical screening regardless of being able to pay, and stabilizing care before transferring a patient to another facility?
a)   Emergency Medical Treatment and Active Labor Act (EMTALA)

4085)   Can an unstable patient be transferred under EMTALA if the definitive care for the patient cannot be provided at the current facility?
a)   Yes- only if the transferring physician certifies it is medically necessary and the receiving facility agrees to accept.

4086)   What four components need to be met in a medical malpractice case?
a)   Negligence, Breach of duty, Damages, and Causation

4087)   Which of the four medical malpractice components is defined as the omission to do something that is reasonable, and is guided by ordinary considerations that regulate human affairs?
a)   Negligence

4088)   Which of the four medical malpractice components is defined as a contract created by the formation of a physician-patient relationship, where the physician must act in accordance with the "standard of care" in treating the patient?
a)   Duty

4089)   Define the "standard of care".

a) Care that a similarly trained physician in emergency medicine would exercise under similar circumstances

4090) Which of the four medical malpractice components is defined as an actual loss, injury, or deterioration sustained by the patient due to a breach of duty and physician negligence?
a) Damages

4091) Define the "fact" and "foreseeability" branches of Legal causation.
a) Fact: Event A was the cause of event B
b) Foreseeability: Patients damages are the result of the physician's substandard care of practice

4092) Failure to diagnose what pathology is the single largest category of settlements for emergency medicine physicians?
a) Myocardial infarction

4093) What two conditions are required to obtain informed consent for a non-emergent procedure?
a) Patient possesses decision-making capacity
b) Patient can make a voluntary choice free of undue influence

4094) What four components makeup decision-making capacity?
a) *Understanding*: Understand information presented about treatment
b) *Appreciation*: Weigh the risks and benefits of the treatment options
c) *Reasoning*: Reasoning about the situation and consequences of the decision made
d) *Communication*: Communication of choice

4095) Who determines competence for a patient in making decisions?
a) The Court

4096) Which type of consent is where a patient goes to a hospital for a condition and signs a form authorizing evaluation and treatment of a problem?
a) Expressed consent

4097) Which type of consent is used when an emergency medical condition exists and the patient is incompetent or unable to answer for themselves?
a) Implied consent

4098) Does implied consent for treatment for a patient without a parent present also pertain to minors during an emergency?
a) Yes

4099) What situations denote a minor being emancipated?
a) Marriage, Military enlistment, or Self-supporting and living on their own

4100) List the medical conditions or complaints that parental consent is not required for a minor to receive medical treatment and evaluation.
a) STDs, Pregnancy, Substance abuse, Child abuse, and Psychiatric conditions

4101) Which type of consent would be used in a patient in respiratory failure who requires intubation or a critical care action and treatment?
a) Emergent consent

4102) What five issues should be addressed in the ED chart for a patient leaving against medical advice (AMA)?
a) Capacity, Discussion, Alternative treatment, Family involvement (if possible), and Patient signature

4103) What medical ethics principle is defined as telling the truth between the patient and the physician?
a) Veracity

4104) What medical ethics principle is defined as the patient's right and freedom to make an informed choice and care plan and right to patient privacy?
a) Autonomy

4105) What medical ethics principle is defined as the principle of doing good and promoting the well-being of others while responding to those in need?
a) Beneficence

4106) What medical ethic principle is defined as "do no harm" and to protect others from danger, pain, and suffering?
a) Non-maleficence

4107) What medical ethic principal involves fairness, respect for human equality, and equitable allocation of scarce resources?
a) Justice

4108) What does the acronym HIPPA stand for?
   a) Health Insurance Portability and Accountability Act
4109) What US law deals with protecting the health care privacy and confidentiality of individuals?
   a) HIPAA
4110) What three purposes are the uses of protected health information allowed to be used under HIPAA?
   a) Treatment, Payment, and Operations
4111) Is it a breach of HIPAA to notify law enforcement when someone is suicidal or homicidal?
   a) No
4112) Which US law prohibits physician self-referral of Medicare or Medicaid patients to an entity providing health services, if the physician has a financial relationship with that entity?
   a) Stark Law
4113) Is there an obligation to administer treatment to a patient that is futile?
   a) No (medically and ethically)
4114) Describe the "do-not-resuscitate" order for a patient's code status.
   a) Provide medical treatment until cardiac or respiratory arrest
4115) Is it recommended to give medical advice over the phone without asking the patient to also come to the emergency department for evaluation?
   a) No
4116) What is the calculation to determine specificity?
   a) Specificity = TN / (TN + FP)
   b) TN: True negative and FP: False positive
4117) How is sensitivity calculated?
   a) Sensitivity = TP / (TP + FN)
   b) TP: True positive and FN: False negative
4118) What is the calculation for determining a positive likelihood ratio?
   a) LR = Sensitivity / (1-Specificity)

Abuse and Assault

4119) Who is most often the perpetrator in sexual assault cases?

a) Someone known to the victim

4120) What specific physical exam needs to be performed in sexual assault cases?

a) Sexual assault exam

4121) What must be obtained from the patient or guardian prior to performing a sexual assault exam?

a) Informed consent

4122) What time frame is evidence collection supposed to be performed on the sexual assault exam to improve accuracy?

a) < 72 hours

4123) What prophylactic treatments and vaccinations should be offered after sexual assault?

a) Pregnancy prevention (Plan B), Sexually transmitted disease, HIV prophylactic treatment (case by case), and Hepatitis vaccinations if not up to date

4124) What time frame after a sexual assault is emergency contraception most affective?

a) Within 72 hours

4125) What areas of the body is it common to find defensive injuries in sexual assault?

a) Oral cavity, Breasts, Thighs, and Buttocks

4126) On vaginal exam, what specific genital injuries suggest sexual assault?

a) Posterior fourchette tear, Labia minora bruising, Hymen tear, and Fossa navicularis injury

4127) What stain can be used to help identify sexual trauma in assault cases?

a) Toluidine blue stain

4128) What type of abuse is mandatory to report to authorities?

a) Geriatric and Pediatric abuse

4129) What is best for the safety of a pediatric or geriatric patient that does not have a safe location to go after discharge in sexual or physical abuse cases?

    a) Hospital admission

4130) What services are required to be involved in pediatric abuse or neglect?

    a) Child protective services and/or Law enforcement agencies

4131) List the concerning features in a patient's history that may be associated with child abuse.

    a) Absent history about injury, Unusual interaction between the parent and child, History of domestic violence, and Parental substance abuse history

4132) List the risk factors for child abuse.

    a) Multiple gestation, Prematurity, Young parents, Low socioeconomic status, Parental substance abuse, Male gender, and Parental mental illness

4133) What are the pediatric pathognomonic findings consistent with child abuse?

    a) Torn tongue frenulum, Posterior rib fractures, Bucket handle fractures, Multiple healing bruises, Buttock and Genital burns from immersion, Stocking glove burns, and Cigarette burns

4134) What is the diagnostic term used to describe a child of abuse who presents as an inconsolable crying baby and is found to have retinal hemorrhages and a subdural hemorrhage?

    a) Shaken baby syndrome

4135) What is the most common finding of pediatric sexual abuse on the physical exam?

    a) 80% have no abnormalities

4136) List clinical features associated with "failure to thrive" due to neglect in a pediatric patient.

    a) Poor hygiene, Little subcutaneous fat, Increased muscle tone in lower extremities, Avoidance of eye contact, and Infants with alopecia over occiput

4137) Is it required to report spousal domestic violence if the patient declines?

a) No (in most states)

4138) What is the most common explanation of multiple injuries at different sites with partner violence?
   a) Falls

4139) List characteristic injuries seen with abuse.
   a) Fingernail scratches, Broken fingernails, Bite marks, Cigarette burns, Bruises in different stages, Nightstick fractures, Rope burns or Ligature marks

4140) List the risk factors of increased mortality in domestic violence.
   a) Child abuse, Firearm use, Public abuse, Sexual abuse, Increased severity of violence, Stalking, Homicidal/Suicidal threats by abuser, Substance abuse by the abuser, or the Partner (victim) ends the relationship

4141) What specific factor increases the risk for domestic violence in women?
   a) Pregnancy

4142) What complications can occur due to abdominal trauma in pregnancy with partner violence and is seen seen in up to 45% of women who are pregnant?
   a) Preterm labor, Placental abruption, and Direct fetal injury

4143) Which gender is more likely to be victim of domestic violence?
   a) Female

4144) What safety options are available for a domestic violence victim if they feel unsafe going back to the home or do not have a safe location to go to at discharge?
   a) Provide information on locations that are safe to stay (battered women's shelters) or Hospital admission

4145) What should you do when you suspect partner violence and the partner (perpetrator) is answering all the victim's questions?
   a) Separate them

Imaging

4146) What primary imaging study is used for screening ED patients for stroke?
   a) CT brain without contrast

4147) What type of contrast is recommended for trauma patients receiving CTs?
   a) Water-soluble contrast

4148) What medications can be given to patients with a contrast dye allergy who require a contrast dye study?
   a) Steroids and Diphenhydramine

4149) Which imaging studies are non-ionizing?
   a) Ultrasound and MRI

4150) What type of MRI imaging delineates tissues and is used for anatomy scans?
   a) T1

4151) What type of MRI imaging reveals bright fluid allowing edema to be seen, and is used for pathology scans?
   a) T2

4152) Which pathologies should MRI be used to identify in the ED?
   a) Spinal cord compression, Spinal cord infection, Epidural hematoma, Osteomyelitis, Acute stroke, and Posterior cranial fossa pathology

4153) What imaging modality is the study of choice for evaluating biliary disease?
   a) Ultrasound

4154) List the indications for ultrasound (US) use in the ED.
   a) Focused assessment with sonography in trauma (FAST) exam, Rule out hydronephrosis, Rule out DVT, Gallbladder pathology, Common bile duct pathology, Cardiac tamponade, AAA, Aortic dissection, PEA, Fractures, Foreign body location, Fetal heart tones, Intrauterine pregnancy (IUP) confirmation, Nerve blocks, Abscesses, Cellulitis, Cysts, Performing Central and peripheral line placement, Thoracentesis, and Paracentesis

4155) What sign is positive when the point of maximal tenderness is elicited from the transducer pressing directly over the gallbladder, suggesting cholecystitis?
a) Sonographic Murphy's sign

4156) What gallbladder wall thickness on US is considered abnormal for suspected cholecystitis?
a) > 5 mm

4157) What is the normal diameter of the common bile duct on US?
a) 5-7 mm

4158) What are the US findings on a gallbladder scan that suggests cholelithiasis?
a) Hyperechoic mass with hypoechoic shadowing behind it

4159) List the four views that make up the FAST ultrasound exam used during trauma evaluation.
a) Subxiphoid (Cardiac)
b) Morison's pouch (Hepatic window)
c) Splenorenal recess or Subdiaphragm
d) Pelvic (Pouch of Douglas and Rectovesicular space)

4160) What indicates a positive finding on a FAST exam?
a) Free fluid

4161) What 3 views in addition to the traditional FAST exam make up an extended FAST exam?
a) Supradiaphram views (bilaterally), Anteromedial lung windows (bilaterally), and IVC visualization

4162) Which view in an extended FAST exam can help rule out pneumothorax?
a) Anteromedial lung window

4163) What mode on the US is used to confirm lung sliding and diagnosing a pneumothorax?
a) M-mode

4164) What sign on ultrasound M-mode confirms lung sliding?
a) Seashore sign

4165) What sign on ultrasound M-mode suggests abnormal lung sliding and pneumothorax?
a) Barcode sign/Stratosphere sign

4166) What area on the FAST exam is typically the first to show free fluid as an anechoic stripe in the paracolic gutter?

    a) Morison's pouch

4167) Which is the first area to show free fluid on the splenorenal view of the FAST exam between the splenorenal fossa and subdiaphragmatic space?

    a) Subdiaphragmatic space

4168) List the three different US probes used in the ED and their associated US frequencies.

    a) Linear: High frequency

    b) Curvilinear: Low frequency

    c) Phased array: Low frequency

4169) What is the transducer orientation when the transducer indicator is towards the head?

    a) Sagittal

4170) Which US probe is used for superficial skin and vascular issues?

    a) Straight probe

4171) Which US probe is used for cardiovascular issues?

    a) Phased array probe

4172) List the two US cardiac views used to evaluate the valves and the aorta.

    a) Parasternal long and short axis

4173) What is the specific sign found on cardiac US that suggests right ventricle (RV) dilation?

    a) "D" sign

4174) What location and direction should the transducer be placed to obtain the four-chamber cardiac apical view on US?

    a) Placed at the PMI with the transducer directed toward the right shoulder

4175) What are the US findings indicating a pericardial effusion?

    a) Anechoic fluid in the pericardial sac

4176) What is the radiologic term for two structures that have similar brightness on US?

    a) Isoechoic

4177) List structures that are hyperechoic on US.

    a) Bones, Tendons, Nerves, and Gallstones

4178) List structures that are hypoechoic on US.
   a) Fat, Spleen, or Liver
4179) List structures that are anechoic on US.
   a) Arteries, Veins, and Fluid
4180) What measurement on abdominal ultrasound of the aorta measured from the outside walls is considered abnormal for suspected AAA?
   a) > 3 cm
4181) Which transducer is used to identify an AAA?
   a) Low frequency curvilinear
4182) What diameter size of an AAA has an increased risk of sudden rupture?
   a) > 5 cm
4183) Is the US sensitive to detect an abdominal aortic dissection?
   a) No
4184) What are the uses of bedside US in the ED for evaluating a pregnant patient?
   a) Identify Fetal heart tones, IUP, and Ectopic pregnancy
4185) What are the two US techniques used for identifying fetal heart tones, IUP, and ectopic pregnancy?
   a) Transvaginal and Transabdominal
4186) What US mode is the best for evaluating the fetal heart rate?
   a) M-mode
4187) In which obstetric US view is it recommended having a full bladder to increase visualization?
   a) Transabdominal
4188) What is the earliest sonographic finding of pregnancy?
   a) Gestational sac
4189) What is the first reliable sign of an IUP on the transvaginal US that can be seen around 5-6 weeks?
   a) Yolk sac
4190) What is the term for the US finding showing a gestational sac and yolk sac present confirming pregnancy?
   a) Double decidual sign
4191) What beta-human chorionic gonadotropin (β-hCG) level is termed the discriminatory zone to determine IUP on the transvaginal US?

a) > 1000 mIU/mL

4192) Presence of what findings on the transabdominal or transvaginal US suggests intrauterine fetal demise?

a) No fetal heart tones

4193) What are the structures measured on US to determine fetal growth during each of the 1st, 2nd and 3rd trimesters?

a) 1st: Crown-Rump length
b) 2nd: Biparietal diameter
c) 3rd: BPA and Femur length

4194) Which transducer is used to rule out renal pathology such as hydronephrosis?

a) Curvilinear low-frequency transducer

4195) What is the US appearance of the renal sinus that suggests hydronephrosis from ureteral obstruction?

a) Bear-claw

4196) What are the findings on ophthalmic US with the linear transducer, that suggest a retinal detachment or vitreous hemorrhage?

a) Free-floating retina or vitreous in the posterior eye

4197) What are the US findings with an abscess?

a) Hyperechoic or Hypoechoic fluid collection

4198) What is the finding on US for cellulitis?

a) Cobblestone appearance

Wound Management

4199) What is the infectious rate of lacerations?
a) < 5%

4200) What vaccination should be updated with all lacerations, if it has been greater than 5 years with a dirty wound or 10 years with a clean wound since the last vaccination?
a) Tetanus

4201) What types of wounds are at an increased risk of developing tetanus infections?
a) >24 hours old, Burns, IV Drug users, Postpartum, Crush injury, and Dirty wounds

4202) Which type of soft tissue injury is more likely to cause a wound infection due to greater tissue damage?
a) Crush/Blunt injuries

4203) What is the normal distance for the two-point discrimination test that suggests intact digital nerves?
a) < 6mm

4204) The combination of Lidocaine and Epinephrine local anesthetics are not recommended for use in which parts of the body due to the increased risk of ischemia?
a) Nose, Fingers, Toes, and Ears

4205) What two liquids are safe for irrigating wounds?
a) Saline and Tap water

4206) What amount of pressure is recommended for the irrigation of an uncontaminated wound?
a) 0.5 psi

4207) What amount of pressure is recommended for the irrigation of a contaminated wound?
a) 7 psi

4208) How much fluid per centimeter of the wound is recommended for irrigation?
a) 60 mL per centimeter (minimum of 200 mL)

4209) Are povidone-iodine, detergents, or peroxide supposed to be used on open wounds?
a) No (Toxic to tissue)

4210) Which two types of suture material decrease the risk of infection in laceration repairs?
   a) Nylon and Polypropylene
4211) What type of suture is recommended for intradermal, galea, muscle, fascia, and cartilage repairs?
   a) Absorbable (vicryl)
4212) Give the recommended size of sutures used to repair each of the following body sites: scalp, face, hands, fingers, trunk, and proximal extremities.
   a) Scalp: 3-0 or 4-0
   b) Face: 6-0
   c) Hands/Feet: 5-0
   d) Fingers/Toes: 5-0
   e) Trunk: 4-0
   f) Proximal extremities: 4-0
4213) Give the time frame when sutures and staples are to be removed at the following body sites: scalp, face, extremities, joints, and trunk.
   a) Scalp: 7-10 days
   b) Face: 3-5 days
   c) Extremities: 10-14 days
   d) Joints: 14 days
   e) Trunk: 10-14 days
4214) List the different types of suture techniques.
   a) Interrupted (Most Common), Simple running, Figure 8, Vertical mattress, and Horizontal mattress
4215) Explain why vertical and horizontal mattress suture is used to approximate wide lacerations.
   a) To displace the pressure on the skin while approximating the wound
4216) What type of sutures are recommended to help approximate deep and wide lacerations?
   a) Deep dermal
4217) Within what period of time is it recommended to perform a delayed closure of a wound to decrease the risk of infection?
   a) > 12 hours

4218) When is a wound that was treated with delayed primary closure usually repaired if no infection supervenes?
   a) 3-5 days
4219) What wound width can Cyanoacrylate tissue adhesives (skin glue) be used on?
   a) Wounds < 5 mm wide
4220) What wound length can Cyanoacrylate tissue adhesives (skin glue) be used on?
   a) Wounds < 5 cm long
4221) Which areas is it not recommended to use skin glue to close a wound?
   a) Mucous membranes, Infected areas, Joints, Wounds exposed to body fluids, and Areas with dense hair
4222) What types of eye lacerations need to be referred to an ophthalmologist?
   a) Inner eyelid, Lid margins, Lacrimal duct, Tarsal plate injuries, and Injuries associated with ptosis
4223) What structures are the most important to align and repair in lip injuries?
   a) Vermilion border and Orbicularis oris muscle
4224) Do most intraoral lacerations need to be repaired?
   a) No
4225) Is it recommended to give prophylactic antibiotics after repairing intraoral lacerations?
   a) Yes (Penicillin or Clindamycin)
4226) What nerve is injured when you see loss of wrist extension (wrist drop) on exam?
   a) Radial
4227) What nerve is injured when you see loss of thumb adduction and an inability to flex the wrist on exam?
   a) Median
4228) What nerve is injured when there is an inability to abduct and adduct the fingers on exam?
   a) Ulnar
4229) What nerve is injured when you see loss of ability to evert the foot?

a) Superficial peroneal

4230) What nerve is injured when you see loss of ability to invert the foot and dorsiflex the ankle?

a) Deep peroneal and/or Common peroneal

4231) What nerve is injured when you see loss of ability to plantar flex the ankle?

a) Tibial nerve

4232) What position are hand, arm, toe, and foot lacerations supposed to be examined in to avoid missing a tendon, artery, or nerve injury?

a) The position that the injury occurred in

4233) What type of extremity tendon laceration can be repaired in the ED?

a) Extensor tendons

4234) What extremity tendon lacerations need to be referred to orthopedic surgery for repair?

a) Flexor tendons

4235) What type of stitch is recommended to repair extensor tendons?

a) A figure of eight stitch

4236) What is the treatment of a subungual hematoma?

a) Trephination

4237) What size of subungual hematoma is it recommended removing the nail or trephinating it?

a) > 50%

4238) What type of bacteria is associated with farming accidents and lacerations?

a) Clostridium perfringens

4239) What type of bacteria is seen with freshwater lacerations?

a) Aeromonas hydrophila

4240) What type of bacteria is associated with lacerations sustained from high-pressure water systems used for cleaning surfaces?

a) Acinetobacter calcoaceticus

4241) What imaging is the most sensitive for determining the presence of a foreign body in a wound?

a) CT

4242) List the different types of foreign bodies that can be seen on plain radiographs.
   a) Metal, Bone, Teeth, Pencil graphite, Glass, Gravel, Sand, Aluminum, and some Plastics
4243) Give the three different techniques for removing fishhooks.
   a) String-pull method, Needle cover technique, and Advance and Cut technique
4244) What bacteria is the leading cause of puncture wound infections?
   a) Staphylococcus aureus
4245) What bacteria is the most frequent cause of osteomyelitis from puncture wounds occurring through a rubber soled shoe?
   a) Pseudomonas
4246) Which antibiotics are recommended for prophylactic coverage of puncture wounds?
   a) Ciprofloxacin or Cephalexin
4247) What is the treatment of an Epinephrine autoinjector injury to a digit causing a painful pale digit?
   a) Subcutaneous injection of Phentolamine + Lidocaine solution to the site
4248) What type of injury typically causes a laceration over the metacarpophalangeal joints and increases the risk for infection?
   a) "Fight bite" injury
4249) Are prophylactic antibiotics recommended for "fight bites"
   a) Yes
4250) What types of bacteria are seen with "fight bite" wounds?
   a) Eikenella, Staphs, Strep, and Bacteroides
4251) Are you supposed to repair human and dog bites to the hand?
   a) No, due to the high risk of infection
4252) Can dog bite wounds on the scalp, face, torso, and proximal extremity be repaired?
   a) Yes
4253) Name the bacteria associated with cat and dog bites.
   a) Pasteurella
4254) What is the treatment for most cat and dog bites?

a) Amoxicillin/Clavulanate, Clindamycin + (Ciprofloxacin or Trimethoprim-Sulfamethoxazole)

4255) What type of bacteria is believed to cause cat scratch fever?

a) Bartonella henselae

4256) What condition can develop from cat scratch fever that causes lymphadenitis, conjunctivitis, and a fever?

a) Oculoglandular fever

4257) Which antibiotic treats cat scratch fever?

a) Azithromycin

4258) What bacteria are associated with livestock and large animal bites?

a) Brucella, Leptospira, and Francisella tularensis

4259) What is the recommended antibiotic used to treat bites from livestock and large animals?

a) Amoxicillin-Clavulanic acid

4260) Which antibiotic is used to treat rats, mice, squirrel, and gerbil bites?

a) Amoxicillin-Clavulanic acid

4261) List the different indications/injuries/wounds that prophylactic antibiotics are recommended with repair.

a) Open fractures, Wounds with Exposed Joints and Tendons, Animal bites, Human bites, and Intraoral lacerations

Analgesia and Sedation

4262) List the indications for use of conscious sedation in the emergency department.
  a) Fracture manipulation, Joint reduction, Abscess drainage, Laceration repair, Tube thoracostomy, Digital disimpaction, Cardioversion, or To obtain imaging

4263) List non-opioid medications used for pain.
  a) NSAIDs, Tylenol, and Aspirin

4264) What side effects can occur with chronic NSAID use?
  a) GI bleeding, Peptic ulcers, Platelet dysfunction, and Impaired coagulation

4265) At what age are NSAIDs contraindicated for use in pediatrics?
  a) < 6 months old

4266) List the opioid medications used for pain control and sedation.
  a) Morphine, Fentanyl, and Hydromorphone

4267) Which opioid medication is discouraged for analgesic use due to CNS toxicity and significant histamine release?
  a) Meperidine

4268) Give the two classes of local anesthetics.
  a) Amides and Esters

4269) What preservative in local anesthetics leads to most reactions?
  a) Methylparaben

4270) List the Amide local anesthetic medications.
  a) Lidocaine, Bupivacaine, and Prilocaine---(all have two i's)

4271) List the Ester local anesthetic medications.
  a) Procaine, Tetracaine, and Chloroprocaine

4272) What medication can be added to local anesthetics to help with the burning pain during injection?
  a) Bicarbonate buffer

4273) What medication is added to local anesthetics to extend the duration and slow the systemic absorption?
  a) Epinephrine

4274) What are the side effects that can occur from Lidocaine toxicity?
  a) Seizures, Cardiovascular depression, and Arrhythmias

4275) What is the maximum dose of Lidocaine with and without Epinephrine?
 a) 7 mg/kg with Epinephrine
 b) 4.5 mg/kg without Epinephrine

4276) What is the maximum dose of Bupivacaine with and without Epinephrine.
 a) 3 mg/kg with Epinephrine
 b) 2 mg/kg without Epinephrine

4277) What topical anesthetic combinations can be used instead of using local infiltration?
 a) Lidocaine, epinephrine, and tetracaine (LET)
 b) Lidocaine prilocaine (EMLA)
 c) Liposome-encapsulated lidocaine (LMX)
 d) Tetracain, adrenaline, and cocaine (TAC)

4278) Which topical anesthetics are reserved for non-intact skin?
 a) LET and TAC

4279) What other option is available for pain control in an extremity instead of local, topical, oral, or IV medications?
 a) Regional nerve blocks

4280) What medication can be given to reverse conscious sedation from benzodiazepines in the presence of hypoxia?
 a) Flumazenil

4281) What medication can be given to reverse conscious sedation from opioids in the presence of hypoxia?
 a) Naloxone

4282) What side effect can occur with rapid infusion fentanyl administration?
 a) Rigid chest syndrome

4283) What is a relative contraindication to using Nitrous oxide for sedation?
 a) History of pulmonary hypertension

References

1. "ABEM." *ABEM Exam Content*, 2019, www.abem.org/.
2. "Acute Flaccid Myelitis." *Acute Flaccid Myelitis*, June 2019, www.cdc.gov.
3. *Advanced Cardiovascular Life Support: Provider Manual*. American Heart Association, 2016.
4. Aehlert, Barbara. *PALS: Pediatric Advanced Life Support Study Guide*. Jones & Bartlett Learning, 2018.
5. "African Tick-Bite Fever." *African Tick-Bite Fever*, 8, May 2013, www.cdc.gov
6. Alaeddini, Jamshid. "Angina Pectoris." *Practice Essentials, Background, Pathophysiology*, 10 Nov. 2019, emedicine.medscape.com/article/150215-overview.
7. Alberino, Amanda, et al. "Caustic Ingestion." *WikEM*, Sept. 2019, wikem.org/wiki/Caustic_ingestion.
8. Allely, Peter. "Life in the Fast Lane • LITFL • Emergency Medicine Blog." *What Is Brugada Syndrome*, July 2019, litfl.com/.
9. American college of surgeons committee on trauma. *Advanced Trauma Life Support: Student Course Manual*. American College of Surgeons, 2018.
10. "Anterior Wall ST Segment Elevation MI ECG Review - Criteria and Examples: LearntheHeart.com." *Anterior Wall ST Segment Elevation MI ECG Review - Criteria and Examples | LearntheHeart.com*, Aug. 2019, www.healio.com/cardiology/learn-the-heart/ecg-review/ecg-topic-reviews-and-criteria/anterior-wall-st-elevation-mi-review.
11. Bhardwaj, Neerja. "Pediatric Cuffed Endotracheal Tubes." *Journal of Anaesthesiology, Clinical Pharmacology*, Medknow Publications & Media Pvt Ltd, Jan. 2013, www.ncbi.nlm.nih.gov/pmc/articles/PMC3590525/.
12. "Biliary Ultrasound." *Clinical Emergency Radiology*, by J. Christian Fox, Cambridge University Press, 2017, p. 211.
13. Brusch, John. "Infective Endocarditis." *Practice Essentials, Background, Pathophysiology*, 3 Jan. 2019, emedicine.medscape.com/article/216650-overview.
14. Burger, MacKenzie, and Derek J Schaller. "Physiology, Acidosis, Metabolic." *StatPearls [Internet].*, U.S. National Library of Medicine, 4 June 2019, www.ncbi.nlm.nih.gov/books/NBK482146/.
15. Burns, Ed. "Left Bundle Branch Block (LBBB) • LITFL • ECG Library Diagnosis." *Life in the Fast Lane • LITFL • Medical Blog*, 27 Apr. 2019, litfl.com/left-bundle-branch-block-lbbb-ecg-library/.
16. Burns, Ed. "Myocarditis ECG Changes • LITFL • ECG Library Diagnosis." *Life in the Fast Lane • LITFL • Medical Blog*, 16 Mar. 2019, litfl.com/myocarditis-ecg-library/.

17. Burns, Ed. "Pericarditis ECG Changes • LITFL • ECG Library Diagnosis." *Life in the Fast Lane • LITFL • Medical Blog*, 16 Mar. 2019, litfl.com/pericarditis-ecg-library/.

18. Burns, Ed. "Hypertrophic Cardiomyopathy (HCM)." *Https://Litfl.com/Hypertrophic-Cardiomyopathy-Hcm-Ecg-Library/*, 16 Mar. 19AD, litfl.com.

19. Burns, Ed. "Pericarditis ECG Changes • LITFL • ECG Library Diagnosis." *Life in the Fast Lane • LITFL • Medical Blog*, 16 Mar. 2019, litfl.com/pericarditis-ecg-library/.

20. "Campylobacter Jejuni Information for Health Professionals." Edited by CDC, *Centers for Disease Control and Prevention*, Centers for Disease Control and Prevention, 2 Oct. 2017, www.cdc.gov/campylobacter/technical.html.

21. "Cancer Facts for Men." *American Cancer Society*, 1 Aug. 2019, www.cancer.org/healthy/find-cancer-early/mens-health/cancer-facts-for-men.html.

22. "Cancer Facts for Women: Most Common Cancers in Women." *American Cancer Society*, 1 Aug. 2019, www.cancer.org/healthy/find-cancer-early/womens-health/cancer-facts-for-women.html.

23. CDC. "Travelers' Diarrhea - Chapter 2 - 2020 Yellow Book." *Centers for Disease Control and Prevention*, Centers for Disease Control and Prevention, Nov. 2019, wwwnc.cdc.gov/travel/yellowbook/2020/preparing-international-travelers/travelers-diarrhea.

24. Charshafian, Stephanie, and Hawnwan Philip Moy. "CE Article: Prehospital Resuscitative Thoracotomy: The Next Step in Improving Trauma Outcomes?" *EMS World*, 5 Dec. 2016, www.emsworld.com/215299/ce-article-prehospital-resuscitative-thoracotomy-next-step-improving-trauma-outcomes.

25. "Chlamydia." *Chlamydia*, 23, January 2014, www.cdc.gov

26. Cline, David, and John O Ma. *Tintinalli's Emergency Medicine: Just the Facts.* 3rd ed., McGraw-Hill Education, 2012.

27. Consolini, Deborah M., et al. "Fever in Infants and Children - Pediatrics." *Merck Manuals Professional Edition*, July 2018, www.merckmanuals.com/professional/pediatrics/symptoms-in-infants-and-children/fever-in-infants-and-children.

28. "Cryptosporidiosis Adult and Adolescent Opportunistic Infection." *National Institutes of Health*, U.S. Department of Health and Human Services, 16 July 2019, aidsinfo.nih.gov/guidelines/html/4/adult-and-adolescent-opportunistic-infection/323/cryptosporidiosis.

29. Cunha, Burke A. "Hospital-Acquired Pneumonia (Nosocomial Pneumonia) and Ventilator-Associated Pneumonia." *Overview, Pathophysiology, Etiology*, 30 July 2018, emedicine.medscape.com/article/234753-overview.

30. "Diverticulitis." *Practice Essentials, Background, Pathophysiology*, 10 Nov. 2019, emedicine.medscape.com/article/173388-overview.

31. Douketis, James D. "Deep Vein Thrombosis (DVT) - Heart and Blood Vessel Disorders." *Merck Manuals Consumer Version*, Mar. 2018, www.merckmanuals.com/home/heart-and-blood-vessel-disorders/venous-disorders/deep-vein-thrombosis-dvt.

32. "Ectopic Pregnancy." *Clinical Obstetrics & Gynaecology*, by Brian Magowan et al., Saunders, 2014.

33. Evers, Mark B. *"Carcinoid Tumors and Carcinoid Syndrome –Hormonal and Metobolic Disorders."* Merck Manuals Consumer Version, Dec. 2018, www.merckmanuals.com/home/hormonal-and-metobolic-disorders/carcinoid-tumors/carcinoid tumors-and-carcinoid syndrome.

34. Faden, H. *The Dramatic Change in the Epidemiology of Pediatric Epiglottitis.* Pediatric Emergency Care. 2006; 22(6):443-4 , 2006, reference.medscape.com/medline/abstract/16801849.

35. Fulop, Tibor. "Hypomagnesemia." *Background, Pathophysiology, Etiology*, 23 Aug. 2018, emedicine.medscape.com/article/2038394-overview.

36. Graber, Evan G. "Physical Growth of Infants and Children - Children's Health Issues." *Physical Growth of Infants and Children*, Feb. 2019, www.merckmanuals.com/home/children-s-health-issues/growth-and-development/physical-growth-of-infants-and-children.

37. Hamdy, Osama. "Hypoglycemia." *Practice Essentials, Background, Pathophysiology*, 10 Sept. 2019, emedicine.medscape.com/article/122122-overview.

38. Harness, Neil, et al. "Metacarpal Fractures." *Orthobullets*, Nov. 2019, www.orthobullets.com/hand/6037/metacarpal-fractures.

39. Hasbun, Rodrigo. "Meningitis Treatment & Management: Approach Considerations, Treatment of Subacute Meningitis, Treatment of Bacterial Meningitis." *Meningitis Treatment & Management: Approach Considerations, Treatment of Subacute Meningitis, Treatment of Bacterial Meningitis*, 11 Nov. 2019, emedicine.medscape.com/article/232915-treatment. Hemingway, Thomas. "Hyperviscosity Syndrome." *Practice Essentials, Pathophysiology, Epidemiology*, 21 Feb. 2018, emedicine.medscape.com/article/780258-overview.

40. Henry, Sharon. "ATLS 10th Edition Offers New Insights into Managing Trauma Patients." *The Bulletin*, 1 June 2018, bulletin.facs.org/2018/06/atls-10th-edition-offers-new-insights-into-managing-trauma-patients/.

41. Hnaide, Hazem Alsalman. "African Trypanosomiasis (Sleeping Sickness)." *Practice Essentials, Background, Pathophysiology and Etiology*, 9 Nov. 2019, emedicine.medscape.com/article/228613-overview.

42. Kaasinen, Valtteri, et al. "Akinetic Crisis in Parkinson's Disease Is Associated with a Severe Loss of Striatal Dopamine Transporter Function: a Report of Two Cases." *Case Reports in Neurology*, S. Karger AG, 26 Nov. 2014, www.ncbi.nlm.nih.gov/pmc/articles/PMC4280458/.

43. Kao, Amanda. "Identification of Children at Very Low Risk of Clinically-Important Brain Injuries After Head Trauma: A Prospective Cohort

Study." *The Journal of Emergency Medicine*, vol. 38, no. 2, 2010, pp. 273–274. doi:10.1016/j.jemermed.2009.11.011.

44. Kesser, Bradley W. "External Otitis (Acute) - Ear, Nose, and Throat Disorders." *Merck Manuals Professional Edition*, Aug. 2019, www.merckmanuals.com/professional/ear,-nose,-and-throat-disorders/external-ear-disorders/external-otitis-acute.

45. "Leptospirosis." *Leptospirosis*, 15,March 2019, www.cdc.gov

46. Levi, Marcel. "Disseminated Intravascular Coagulation." *Background, Pathophysiology, Etiology*, 7 Oct. 2018, emedicine.medscape.com/article/199627-overview.

47. Liebeskind, David. "Epidural Hematoma." *Background, Pathophysiology, Epidemiology*, 9 Nov. 2019, emedicine.medscape.com/article/1137065-overview. Liesveld, Jane, and Patrick Reagan. "Polycythemia Vera - Hematology and Oncology." *Merck Manuals Professional Edition*, Feb. 2019, www.merckmanuals.com/professional/hematology-and-oncology/myeloproliferative-disorders/polycythemia-vera.

48. Lin, Brian, and George Y Wu, MD, PhD. "Toxic Megacolon." Edited by Burt Cagir, *Background, Pathophysiology, Etiology*, 1 Mar. 2018, emedicine.medscape.com/article/181054-overview#a4.

49. "Lymphogranuloma Venereum." *Lymphogrnuloma Venereum*, 4, June 2015, www.cdc.gov

50. "Lyme disease."*Lyme disease*, 8, November 2019, www.cdc.gov

51. Maiese, Kenneth. "Brain Herniation - Neurologic Disorders." *Merck Manuals Professional Edition*, June 2019, www.merckmanuals.com/professional/neurologic-disorders/coma-and-impaired-consciousness/brain-herniation.

52. "Malaria."*Malaria*, 5, November 2019, www.cdc.gov

53. Mangla, shvarya, et al. "Brain-Type Natriuretic Peptide (BNP): Reference Range, Interpretation, Collection and Panels." *Brain-Type Natriuretic Peptide (BNP): Reference Range, Interpretation, Collection and Panels*, 15 Nov. 2019, emedicine.medscape.com/article/2087425-overview#a4.

54. Marx, John, et al. *Rosen's Emergency Medicine Concepts and Clinical Practice Expert Consult*. 8th ed., Saunders, 2013.

55. McKee, Michael D., et al. "Clavicle Shaft Fractures." *Orthobullets*, 2019, www.orthobullets.com/trauma/1011/clavicle-shaft-fractures.

56. Micek, Scott T., et al. "Health Care-Associated Pneumonia and Community-Acquired Pneumonia: a Single-Center Experience." *Antimicrobial Agents and Chemotherapy*, American Society for Microbiology Journals, 1 Oct. 2007, aac.asm.org/content/51/10/3568.

57. Moon, Charles, et al. "Ankle Fractures." *Orthobullets*, Nov. 2019, www.orthobullets.com/trauma/1047/ankle-fractures.

58. Ostapchuk, Michael, et al. "Community-Acquired Pneumonia in Infants and Children." *American Family Physician*, 1 Sept. 2004, www.aafp.org/afp/2004/0901/p899.html.

59. Pillai, Anil Kumar, et al. "Ureteroarterial Fistula: Diagnosis and Management: American Journal of Roentgenology: Vol. 204, No. 5 (AJR)." *American Journal of Roentgenology*, 2015, www.ajronline.org/doi/full/10.2214/AJR.14.13405.

60. Pokhrel, Prabhat K., and Sanaz A. Loftus. "Ocular Emergencies." *American Family Physician*, 15 Sept. 2007, www.aafp.org/afp/2007/0915/p829.html.

61. R Minnaganti, Venkat R. "Plague." *Background, Pathophysiology, Epidemiology*, 9 Nov. 2019, emedicine.medscape.com/article/235627-overview.

62. Schneck, Michael. "Leptomeningeal Carcinomatosis." *Practice Essentials, Background, Pathophysiology*, 27 Nov. 2017, emedicine.medscape.com/article/1156338-overview.

63. Simon, Eric E. "Hyponatremia." *Practice Essentials, Pathophysiology, Epidemiology*, 17 June 2019, emedicine.medscape.com/article/242166-overview.

64. "Schistosomiasis."*Schistosomiasis*, 11, April 2018, www.cdc.gov

65. Smith, Edward R, and Amin-Hanjani, MD Sepideh. "Evaluation and Management of Elevated Intracranial Pressure in Adults." *UpToDate*, Apr. 2019, www.uptodate.com/contents/evaluation-and-management-of-elevated-intracranial-pressure-in-adults.

66. Sudulagunta, Sreenivasa Rao, et al. "Posterior Reversible Encephalopathy Syndrome (PRES)." *Oxford Medical Case Reports*, Oxford University Press, 3 Apr. 2017, www.ncbi.nlm.nih.gov/pmc/articles/PMC5410886/.

67. Suk, Michael, et al. "Knee Dislocation." *Orthobullets*, July 2019, www.orthobullets.com/trauma/1043/knee-dislocation.

68. Suneja, Suneja. "Hypocalcemia." *Practice Essentials, Pathophysiology, Etiology*, 8 Aug. 2019, emedicine.medscape.com/article/241893-overview.

69. Swaminathan, Anand. "Neutropenic Fever." *REBEL EM - Emergency Medicine Blog*, 7 Feb. 2019, rebelem.com/neutropenic-fever/.

70. Tan, Walter. "Unstable Angina." *Practice Essentials, Background, Pathophysiology*, 10 Nov. 2019, emedicine.medscape.com/article/159383-overview.

71. Team, Orthobullets, et al. "Distal Radius Fractures." *Orthobullets*, Nov. 2019, www.orthobullets.com/trauma/1027/distal-radius-fractures.

72. Tintinalli, Judith, et al. *Tintinalli's Emergency Medicine A Comprehensive Study Guide*. 8th ed., McGraw-Hill Education, 2015.

73. "Vestibular Schwannoma (Acoustic Neuroma) and Neurofibromatosis." *National Institute of Deafness and Other Communication Disorders*, U.S. Department of Health and Human Services, 15 June 2018, www.nidcd.nih.gov/health/vestibular-schwannoma-acoustic-neuroma-and-neurofibromatosis.

74. Waitzman, Ariel A. "Otitis Externa." *Practice Essentials, Background, Anatomy*, 13 Nov. 2019, emedicine.medscape.com/article/994550-overview.

75. Waseem, Muhammad. "Otitis Media." *Practice Essentials, Background, Pathophysiology*, 13 Nov. 2019, emedicine.medscape.com/article/994656-overview.

76. Weber, Toni, et al. "Cuffed vs Non-Cuffed Endotracheal Tubes for Pediatric Anesthesia." *Pediatric Anesthesia*, vol. 19, 2009, pp. 46–54., doi:10.1111/j.1460-9592.2009.02998.x.

77. Weiner, Gary M, and Jeanette Zaichkin. *American Academy of Pediatrics and American Heart Association;* 7th ed., American Academy of Pediatrics and American Heart Association, 2016.

78. Weingart, Scott. "The Procedure of ED Thoracotomy." *EMCrit Project*, 4 June 2017, emcrit.org/emcrit/procedure-of-thoracotomy/.

79. Wiersinga, Wilmar M. "Myxedema and Coma (Severe Hypothyroidism)." Endotext (Internet). U.S. National Library of Medicine, 25 Apr. 2018, www.ncbi.nlm.nih.gov/books/NBK279007/.

80. "Women's Health Care Physicians." *ACOG*, Aug. 2019, www.acog.org/Patients/FAQs/Pelvic-Inflammatory-Disease-PID.

81. "Yellow fever."*Yellow fever*, 15, January 2019, www.cdc.gov

Index

I

M

N

O

Q

S

T

U

CPSIA information can be obtained
at www.ICGtesting.com
Printed in the USA
FFHW011633220120
57981994-63140FF